Health and the Modern Home

Routledge Studies in the Social History of Medicine

EDITED BY JOSEPH MELLING, *University of Exeter*
ANNE BORSAY, *University of Wales, Swansea, UK*

15. Contagion
Historical and Cultural Studies
Edited by Alison Bashford and Claire Hooker

16. Medicine, Health and the Public Sphere in Britain, 1600–2000
Edited by Steve Sturdy

17. Medicine and Colonial Identity
Edited by Mary P. Sutphen and Bridie Andrews

18. New Directions in Nursing History
Edited by Barbara E. Mortimer and Susan McGann

19. Medicine, the Market and Mass Media
Producing Health in the Twentieth Century
Edited by Virginia Berridge and Kelly Loughlin

20. The Politics of Madness
The state, Insanity and Society in England, 1845–1914
Joseph Melling and Bill Forsythe

21. The Risks of Medical Innovation
Risk Perception and Assessment in Historical Context
Edited by Thomas Schlich and Ulrich Tröhler

22. Mental Illness and Learning Disability Since 1850
Finding a Place for Mental Disorder in the United Kingdom
Edited by Pamela Dale and Joseph Melling

23. Britain and the 1918–19 Influenza Pandemic
A Dark Epilogue
Niall Johnson

24. Financing Medicine
The British Experience since 1750
Edited by Martin Gorsky and Sally Sheard

25. Social Histories of Disability and Deformity
Edited by David M. Turner and Kevin Stagg

26. Histories of the Normal and the Abnormal
Social and Cultural Histories of Norms and Normativity
Edited by Waltraud Ernst

27. Madness, Architecture and the Built Environment
Psychiatric Spaces in Historical Context
Edited by Leslie Topp. James E. Moran and Jonathan Andrews

28. Lunatic Hospitals in Georgian England, 1750–1830
Leonard Smith

29. Women and Smoking since 1890
Rosemary Elliot

30. Community Nursing and Primary Healthcare in Twentieth-Century Britain
Helen M. Sweet and Rona Dougall

31. Health and the Modern Home
Edited by Mark Jackson

Also available in Routledge Studies in the Social History of Medicine series:

Reassessing Foucault
Power, Medicine and the Body
Edited by Colin Jones and Roy Porter

Health and the Modern Home

Edited By

Mark Jackson

Routledge
Taylor & Francis Group
New York London

First published 2007
by Routledge
270 Madison Ave, New York, NY 10016

Simultaneously published in the UK
by Routledge
2 Park Square, Milton Park, Abingdon, Oxon OX14 4RN

Routledge is an imprint of the Taylor & Francis Group, an informa business

Typeset in Sabon by IBT Global
Printed and bound in the United States of America on acid-free paper by IBT Global

Library of Congress Cataloging-in-Publication Data

Health and the modern home / edited by Mark Jackson.
p. ; cm. — (Routledge studies in the social history of medicine, 31)
Includes bibliographical references and index.
ISBN-13: 978-0-415-956-10-9 (hardback : alk. paper)
ISBN-10: 0-415-95610-2 (hardback : alk. paper) 1. Housing and health—Great Britain—History. 2. Housing and health—United States—History. 3. Family—Mental health—Great Britain—History. 4. Family—Mental health—United States—History. 5. Family—Health and hygiene—Great Britain—History. 6. Family—Health and hygiene—United States—History. I. Jackson, Mark, 1959– II. Series.

[DNLM: 1. Environmental Illness—etiology—Great Britain. 2. Environmental Illness—etiology—United States. 3. Environmental Illness—history—Great Britain. 4. Environmental Illness—history—United States. 5. Housing—history—Great Britain. 6. Housing—history—United States. 7. Family Relations—Great Britain. 8. Family Relations—United States. 9. History, 20th Century—Great Britain. 10. History, 20th Century—United States. 11. Psychophysiologic Disorders—etiology—Great Britain. 12. Psychophysiologic Disorders—etiology—United States. WA 11 FA1 H4337 2008]

RA770.H42 2008
362.1—dc22 2007030644

ISBN10: 0-415-95610-2 (hbk)
ISBN10: 0-203-93241-2 (ebk)

ISBN13: 978-0-415-95610-9 (hbk)
ISBN13: 978-0-203-93241-4 (ebk)

Contents

Acknowledgments

The contributions to this volume were first presented as papers at a conference entitled 'Health, Heredity and the Modern Home 1850–2000,' organised by the Centre for Medical History at the University of Exeter in March 2005. The conference was supported by a grant from the Wellcome Trust, and I am grateful to the Trust not only for that financial support but also for regular advice and encouragement in recent years. I am particularly grateful to Claire Keyte and Mary Carter for organising the conference with customary expertise and for facilitating the production of this volume. I would also like to thank the speakers and participants at the conference, all of whom contributed to the congenial atmosphere and the intellectual quality of the presentations and discussions. Production of the final version of the book has been greatly assisted by the attention and advice of the series editor, Anne Borsay, of Max Novick, Katherine Carpenter, and Erica Wetter at Routledge, and of Eleanor Chan at IBT Global.

The illustrations for Chapter 10 are reproduced by kind permission of the Senior Archivist, Museum of Science and Industry in Manchester (Figure 1) and the National Gas Archive and Centrica (Figure 2). Illustrations for Chapter 11 are reproduced by kind permission of Local Studies, Sheffield Libraries (Figure 1), and Coventry Libraries and Information Services (Figure 2). Chapter 12 has been adapted from Gregg Mitman, *Breathing Space: How Allergies Shape Our Lives and Landscapes,* pp. 130–166 (Yale University Press, 2007), and is reproduced here by permission of Yale University Press. Excerpts from *The Complete Poems* by Anne Sexton. Copyright © 1981 by Linda G. Sexton. Reprinted with permission of Houghton Mifflin Company and sll/sterling Lord Literistic, Inc. Unpublished material from the Sexton archive is used with the permission of Linda Gray Sexton and the Harry Ransom Humanities Research Center, University of Texas at Austin.

Finally, I would like to thank Siobhán, Ciara, Riordan, and Conall for generating a frenetically creative, and yet sufficiently emotionally stable, domestic environment in which to think and write.

1 'Home Sweet Home'
Historical Perspectives on Health and the Home

Mark Jackson

INTRODUCTION

In an article published in the *New York Times* in 1980, Ralph Blumenthal highlighted government reports of the multiple health hazards supposedly present in modern American homes. 'Home sweet home it may be,' he wrote evocatively, 'but the coziest nest can mask a household of hazards.'[1] According to Blumenthal and other commentators, the indoor environment now contained a range of allergens, poisonous liquids, and toxic fumes that were responsible for making modern populations ill. As many contemporary clinicians were aware, the dangers of the domestic environment were particularly evident in allergy sufferers; hot and humid, carpeted and well-insulated homes provided an ideal breeding ground for house dust mites, which were known to be potent triggers of attacks of asthma, eczema and allergic rhinitis. According to some physicians, greater exposure to domestic allergens was a major factor in the explosion of allergies in most developed countries after the Second World War.[2]

This formulation of the poisonous, allergenic home was clearly not new in the 1970s and 1980s. As allergy emerged as a clinical specialty during the early decades of the twentieth century, the home environment was often cited as a critical factor in the development of allergic sensitivity. At one level, clinicians routinely referred to the material constituents and inhabitants of the home that could precipitate attacks, citing the role of dust, pets, plants, medicines, perfumes and cosmetics, and various foodstuffs in generating or exacerbating the symptoms of allergy.[3] Building on Victorian preoccupations with eradicating domestic dirt, dust and germs,[4] early twentieth-century allergists on both sides of the Atlantic advised patients and their parents on the best means of preventing or removing house dust, and proposed treating patients with asthma and hay fever in specially prepared, hermetically-sealed allergen-free chambers.[5]

At another level, it is evident that early twentieth-century concerns about the impact of the domestic environment on health were not restricted to material elements of the home. Contemporary allergists also attributed asthma and eczema, in particular, to disturbances in the psychological or emotional environment at home. Shaped partly by long-standing beliefs that asthma could be triggered by emotions, but also partly by novel psychoanalytical and psychosomatic approaches to both mental and physical diseases, leading clinical allergists such as John Freeman (1876–1962), director of the world's largest allergy clinic at St. Mary's Hospital in London, regularly referred to the manner in which either the absence or the over-expression of mother love, for example, could encourage the development of asthma and other allergic conditions in young children.[6] Drawing on his observations of the 'extraordinary prevalence of the Only Child' in his allergy clinics, Freeman suggested that, in addition to the usual array of physical allergens, the perils of 'the modern home' included a 'greater degree of emotionalism and nervous tension' within the 'asthmogenic family.'[7]

Although the first generation of clinical allergists were generally more concerned with identifying, isolating and preparing vaccines against outdoor allergens such as pollen or with charting the role of outdoor air pollution, than with elucidating and reducing the allergenic impact of the domestic environment, a number of broad political and economic factors served to promote their clinical interest in the relationship between the home and health in the decades after the Second World War. In the mid-1970s, for example, the Organization of Petroleum Exporting Countries increased the price of oil in an attempt to exert pressure on the West following the outbreak of war in the Middle East. Faced by rising fuel costs and rampant inflation, householders in developed, temperate countries became more conscious of the need to conserve energy and reduce heating bills: home-owners installed insulation, replaced older windows with double-glazing, and endeavoured to prevent draughts around doors. The net effect of these energy-saving alterations was to decrease ventilation, increase humidity, and provide a convenient environment for house dust mites to thrive in carpets, bedding, and other soft furnishings. Prompted partly by financial constraints, the impact of these major changes in home design was to increase exposure to domestic allergens such as mites and animal dander, particularly amongst modern Western populations; in response, allergists encouraged wives and mothers in particular both to keep their houses dust-free and to ensure the psychological stability of the home.

Although Blumenthal's concept of a 'household of hazards,' expressed in the *New York Times* in 1980, clearly comprised a continuation and reformulation of earlier twentieth-century interests in the domestic environment and allergies, it is however evident that it also constituted a radical departure from Victorian notions of the home. During the nineteenth century, the home was characteristically regarded as a haven, rather than a hazard, for asthma and hay fever sufferers. In addition to advising their patients to take 'hay fever holidays' in mountainous or coastal resorts where the air was cleaner and less likely to contain troublesome pollen, allergists on both sides of the Atlantic recommended staying indoors or at home during the summer pollen season. Even after house dust had been identified more clearly as a major indoor allergen during the inter-war years, the home remained a place of sanctuary for some allergy sufferers: an article in *The Times* in 1960 advised people with hay fever and asthma to 'shut themselves away at the hour of danger,' and to 'stay indoors with the doors and windows closed' during the peak pollen season in June.[8]

Complex and shifting understandings of the role of the home in determining the epidemiology and shaping the treatment of allergies raise several broader issues and questions that link the contributions to this volume. In the first instance, it is apparent that homes have changed substantially across time, not only in terms of their architectural features and furnishings, but also in terms of family structures and expectations. Perhaps more critically, the ideological contours and political meanings of the home also shifted, as the domestic space came to be seen as a promising site for intervention by medical experts and the state: from the early twentieth century, both public health advice and educational literature, directed at families and particularly at mothers, were devised and delivered by health visitors or psychiatric social workers who visited, inspected, and attempted to improve the home. Any exploration of the historical relationship between home and health needs to be sensitive to these material and ideological shifts across time.

Secondly, as the history of allergy suggests, the home has often been an ambiguous social space, constituting at the same time both a haven and a hazard. Thus, while homes were often extolled for the ways in which they fostered mental and physical health and happiness, they were also indicted as sites of oppression, neurosis and decay, particularly by feminist writers who, from the 1950s at least, began to construe any drive for domestic harmony as a means of subjugating women.[9] This ambivalence, or tension, has frequently been mirrored by broader, and often paradoxical, constructions of health and illness in the domestic setting. As several contributions to this volume suggest, the families of children labelled as maladjusted, delinquent, or asthmatic were often portrayed, at the same time, not only as victims of social circumstances beyond their control but also as innate, biological threats to the stability of society: 'problem families' were both a product and a cause of poverty, disease, and social unrest.[10]

Equally clearly, as discussion of shifting approaches to the aetiology of asthma demonstrates, there have been persistent but fluctuating tensions between identifying the material and psychological elements of homes as primarily pathogenic. While psychosomatic approaches to asthma were prominent during the 1940s and 1950s, for example, such psychoanalytically informed understandings of disease tended to fall into disfavour during the 1960s and 1970s as allergists and respiratory physicians returned with renewed vigour to their original focus on dust, perfumes, and pets. In part, this retreat into the material spaces of the home was driven by the promise of new pharmacological treatments, such as the antihistamines, selective bronchodilators, and inhaled steroids.[11] However, as the impact of oil prices on home construction and asthma suggests, shifting interest in the hazards of home were also shaped by broader socio-political, cultural, and epidemiological factors: by novel approaches to children, childhood, and education; by shifting patterns of disease; and by new expectations of parent-child relationships, fashioned themselves by concerns about imperialism, motherhood, crime and social order, infant mortality rates, degeneration, poverty, town planning, consumerism, and so on. Historical analysis of the ways in which homes were seen to influence health therefore demands close attention to the diverse social, political, and cultural contexts in which both modern homes and health were constructed.

HISTORIES OF HEALTH AND THE MODERN HOME

The central aim of this volume is to explore how the complex and shifting relationship between health (and illness) and the home was recognised, investigated, and exploited from the late nineteenth to the late twentieth century, through a series of specific, but often inter-linked, case studies. With this in mind, it is important from the outset to clarify, as precisely as possible, what we mean here by 'health,' 'modern,' and 'the home,' and to reflect on how those categories, and the relationships between them, have been explored in previous historical studies.

Health is a notoriously difficult concept to define and it is perhaps not surprising that historians of medicine have rarely addressed health directly. Most historical studies have focused on the history of specific diseases, or on the professional and political contours of clinical practice and health service delivery, rather than on the historical meanings and maintenance of health or on the strategies adopted in the past to promote health as well as to prevent and treat disease. Perhaps the only studies routinely to consider health and health promotion are those that have focused on public health and associated environmental health reforms, particularly during the nineteenth century,[12] or those that have explored strategies adopted in the twentieth-century to promote psychological health (or mental hygiene) and to prevent mental illness.[13] More recently, historical studies of cancer services, and particularly screening techniques, promise to offer novel insights into the prevention of potentially fatal diseases and the promotion of health and longevity.[14] Although the contributions to this volume undoubtedly take particular, albeit contested, medical conditions (such as suburban neurosis, maladjustment, lead poisoning, food allergies, or asthma) as their starting point, the analyses centre not only on the ways in which these conditions were defined and managed, but also on the manner in which intervention in the home came to be seen as a means of preserving, as well as restoring, physical and psychological health, understood primarily in terms of the absence of disease.

It is equally clear that historians of medicine have traditionally been preoccupied with the history of infectious, rather than non-infectious, diseases.

Thus, although studies of the epidemiological transition have focused constructively on the decline of acute infectious diseases (including on occasions the impact of housing on the pattern of diseases such as tuberculosis),[15] they have far less frequently offered insights into the rise of chronic degenerative conditions in the modern period. Apart from early excursions into the history of cancer and arthritis,[16] recent studies in occupational health history that have explored the environmental determinants and regulatory politics of chronic diseases such as asbestosis, silicosis, and lead poisoning,[17] or on-going studies of some of the modern 'diseases of civilization,'[18] historians have so far shown only limited interest in the dramatic downside of modern demographic and health transitions. One aim of this volume is to encourage greater historical interest in the wide range of chronic diseases that have increasingly impaired the health of, although have not necessarily killed, modern populations.

In chronological terms, the contributions to this volume explore historical constructions of health and home from the dying decades of the nineteenth century through to the turn of the millennium. In this sense, the term 'modern' refers primarily to a particular historical period. However, the term encompasses more than mere chronology; it also captures the processes of industrial modernisation and the complex political patterns of modernity, as well as the cultural aspirations of modernism. As some contributions to this volume demonstrate, Western forms of industrialisation during the nineteenth century dramatically altered the landscape and environment of modern populations, exposing them, for example, to novel forms of air pollution which increased the risk of developing debilitating and sometimes fatal respiratory diseases.[19] As concerns about the impact of modern industrial processes spread during the early decades of the twentieth century, governments on both sides of the Atlantic introduced legislation aimed at lowering levels of pollution, reducing its economic impact, and promoting respiratory health. Such intervention was not only directed at limiting environmental pollution by modern industry, but was also aimed at reducing the impact of domestic fuel consumption on health: transformed by industrialisation, modern homes, as well as modern manufacturing processes, threatened to pollute and kill.[20]

Since the writings of the German economist and sociologist Max Weber (1864–1920) in the early twentieth century, modernity has also been understood in terms of a particular set of social and political processes, which operated to challenge and replace traditional (Victorian) forms of social organisation. Modern governments thus endeavoured to engineer the rational management of society through the expansion of bureaucracy, a growing reliance on professional expertise and the systematic application of science and technology to work, home life, and warfare, the national and international integration of markets, the creation of more democratic forms of political organization, and the spread of literacy and education. Significantly, as Roger Cooter and Steve Sturdy have pointed out in one of the few focused historical studies of the relationship between medicine and modernity, the emergence of a modern, rational society involved 'the extension of bureaucratic structures into ever more intimate areas of social life.'[21] As several contributors to this volume argue, these processes not only penetrated and transformed the home, but also facilitated the recognition and formulation of new forms of illness, which were thought to be linked directly to the domestic (material and psychological) environment and therefore amenable to domestic management.[22]

As a cultural movement, modernism was closely linked to, and shaped by, the social, political, and industrial forces of modernity. Emerging in late nineteenth-century Europe as a form of rebellion against traditional patterns of social organisation and creativity, modernism strove not only to sweep away older art forms and generate new aesthetic visions, but also to transform urban and architectural landscapes. Encompassing new forms of tonality in music and novel literary styles, as well as cubism and surrealism in the visual arts, modernism thus also operated to change the style and contents of modern homes. During the early twentieth century, for example, the Swiss architect Le Corbusier (1887–1965) incorporated into his town plans and his domestic architectural designs the clean, pure lines and the open, airy spaces demanded by modernist rejections of cluttered Victorian interiors. Significantly, the modernist urge to create a fresh and dust-free domestic environment was fashioned partly by concerns about health. As Nancy Tomes has argued in her rich study of germs in modern American life, from the last decades of the nineteenth century fears that germs and infectious diseases could be transmitted by dust led home economists to criticise 'the overstuffed furniture, thick carpets, patterned wallpaper, and extensive bric-a-brac so beloved in Victorian decorating schemes. Instead, they promoted surfaces that were smooth, washable and free of ornamentation that might harbor dust, vermin, and germs.'[23] As anxieties about germs gradually receded during the middle decades of the twentieth century (in the wake of evidence of an epidemiological transition and the production of antimicrobial drugs), these formulations of a clean and healthy home environment found alternative expression in the clinical advice given to families (and particularly to mothers) to maintain a dust- and allergy-free home in order to prevent triggering or exacerbating attacks of asthma and other allergies in susceptible children.[24]

Home is arguably the most complex and flexible of the three categories under discussion in this volume. Although there are historical and sociological studies of the cultural meanings of the home and of domestic architectural style and interior fashion,[25] the changing nature of the home and its relation to health have rarely been explored in any depth by medical historians. Similarly, while there are numerous historical studies of public and environmental health reforms, which have concentrated on campaigns to reduce outdoor pollution and improve urban sanitation,[26] and some studies of medicine in relation to schools,[27] few medical historians have investigated the manner in which the domestic environment was thought to shape patterns of health and disease. One of the aims of this collection of case studies is to encourage closer historical attention to the ways in which homes were implicated in the distribution and manifestations of disease.

Within this volume, the term 'home' is understood and mobilised in several ways. At one level, home is taken to denote simply a physical place where people lived. As such, it describes the material construction, as well as the technical appliances and interior furnishings, of houses, any or all of which could make inhabitants ill.[28] However, as most of the contributions to this book demonstrate, clinical understandings of, and interventions in, the home were not confined to material elements. In many twentieth-century debates, the home also denoted a psychological or emotional space, created by and mediated through family relations and vulnerable to expert manipulation. Although there have been historical studies of the family,[29] and more particularly of the impact of family life on the experiences and welfare of women and children,[30] few researchers have concentrated on the manner in which family dynamics and the domestic emotional environment were construed in relation to health and disease, or on how shifting family ideologies and expectations shaped exposure to domestic hazards and produced new patterns of ill-health. By analysing modern constructions of the home as a material and psychological determinant of health and illness, this volume aims to expand the boundaries of medical history and to engage more closely with insights from recent environmental histories, which have begun to scrutinise and problematise historical patterns of exposure to both indoor home and occupational environments more vigorously.[31]

Finally, the notion of 'home' has also constituted an ideological and political entity, shaped by social and cultural values, and often existing in tension with the physical and psychological reality of people's homes.[32] Thus, the home has frequently been imagined as a source of physical and emotional comfort and stability. Images of the home as a permanent and solid foundation for healthy and productive family life are evident not only in the proliferation of popular phrases such as 'feeling at home,' 'home from home,' and 'home is where the heart is,' but also in the elaboration in the early twentieth century of the notion of an 'ideal home,' exemplified by the establishment of the Daily Mail Ideal Home Exhibition in 1908.[33] Significantly, as is evident in the themes portrayed at that exhibition over subsequent years, representations of the 'ideal home' were closely linked to broader socio-political currents, including persistent concerns about motherhood and the Empire, emergent preoccupations with the technological transformation of homes, industrial efforts to promote a financially viable commodity culture, and political recognition of the need, particularly in the post-Second World War years, to resolve critical housing shortages in original, and healthy, ways. The home thus became a site for political, and often explicitly medical, intervention aimed not only at preventing or reducing disease but also at realising the dreams of modernity.

THEMES AND DIRECTIONS

The contributions to this volume explore shifting historical constructions of the relationship between health and the home in the modern period from a variety of original perspectives. The volume is not intended to be comprehensive; rather, through a series of detailed case studies, it aims, firstly, to expose and analyse the manner in which notions of both health and home intersected and, secondly, to stimulate further research. Although historical in its focus, the volume is deliberately inter-disciplinary: the methods employed encompass not only a traditional historiographical reliance on documentary sources, but also techniques and insights from oral history, literary criticism, and film studies. Most of the chapters focus on Britain, but several contributions either explore the manner in which similar debates about the role of the home in shaping patterns of health and disease were pursued in a North American context or demonstrate the ways in which British and American clinicians borrowed heavily from each other's vocabularies, theories, and practices.

The book is divided into two sections. The first section explores the home and emotional health, particularly (but not exclusively) from the perspective of women and children, who traditionally spent more time at home and were regarded as more vulnerable to domestic hazards. The second section concentrates more closely on the manner in which the material elements of houses and homes (such as smoke, lead, food, dust, and insect infestations, for example) were implicated in patterns of chronic disease. Although the structure of the book helps to draw out certain prevailing themes and interconnections, the divide between the material and the psychological dimensions of the modern home is, of course, largely artificial; as several chapters demonstrate, the boundary between the emotional and physical causes and manifestations of many chronic diseases was particularly porous and negotiable.

In Chapter 2, Michael Clark offers a compelling dissection of Clemence Dane's play *A Bill of Divorcement,* first produced on the London stage in 1921 but set in an imaginary 1930s. Shaped by post-war fears that the stability of marriage and the authority of the traditional male-dominated family were under threat, the play explores the fate of an upper-middle-class family ruined by shell-shock and the fear of hereditary mental weakness. As Clark argues, although its structure, location, and characterisation were conventional, the play was in many ways about modernity, not primarily in the Weberian sense of socio-economic transformation, but more clearly in terms of 'a state of mind, a subjective experience of rupture and discontinuity' within personal and family lives. In particular, although the play exemplified Victorian attitudes to insanity, the domestic setting of the play also illustrated the manner in which the modern family and home environment, as well as the freedom offered to modern women, created new forms of emotional instability and mental illness.

The impact of the home on women's emotional health is pursued more closely in the next three chapters. In Chapter 3, Rhodri Hayward explores the manner in which the home was construed, especially by doctors such as Stephen Taylor, as a site of psychological oppression. During the 1930s, Taylor suggested that many of the minor complaints that afflicted isolated housewives in newly built suburbs were manifestations of a novel form of psychiatric illness, which he termed 'suburban neurosis.' As Hayward argues, Taylor's formulation drew on two competing models of anxiety: firstly, on Freudian suggestions that neurosis was the product of instinctive desires that had been thwarted or frustrated by modern civilisation, most clearly by the toxic domestic environment of the suburbs; and secondly, on a theory propounded by Taylor's colleagues at the Maudsley, namely, that the source of a housewife's neurosis 'lay not in her unconscious desires but in the inadequacy of her conscious thoughts.' In manipulating and merging these theories, Taylor linked psychological ill-health to the 'emotional poverty' of suburban homes.

One of the striking features of inter-war medical formulations of the neurotic housewife was the absence of the voices of women themselves. Women's experiences of the suburbs is explored in Jo Gill's analysis of the American confessional poet Anne Sexton. As Gill suggests, Sexton's assumption of a causal correlation between domestic environment, gender, occupation, and mental health clearly echoed Taylor's image of the neurotic British suburban housewife. However, Sexton's formulation of the suburbs, designated by town planners as female spaces, was ambiguous and ambivalent. At a broad level, the suburban home operated not only as a prison, from which Sexton ached to escape, but also as a sanctuary or haven, into which she could safely retreat from the dangers of urban life. In more discrete ways, modern domestic architecture and the proliferation of modern domestic appliances also functioned both to connect and expose, to integrate and separate: from Sexton's perspective, during the middle decades of the twentieth century, the home thus became a site of imprisonment and surveillance as well as safety and liberation.

As the following chapter by Ali Haggett demonstrates, Sexton's poetics not only influenced a range of post-war writers who focused on the suburbs, but also echoed and legitimated feminist critiques (by Betty Friedan and others) of traditional domestic roles and the banality of housework. However, broad assertions of feminist disaffection with domesticity should be challenged. Interviews with British women who stayed at home to raise children and manage the household during the 1950s and 1960s suggest that the impact of domesticity on women's mental health was far more complex than contemporary feminist critiques suggested. Women who developed anxiety and depression during the post-war years identified a failing marital relationship or much earlier problems in childhood as the cause of their illness far more often than they blamed the domestic role itself. Indeed, most of the women interviewed regarded their responsibilities for domestic work and for raising children as positive and rewarding. Of course, this does not necessarily imply that suburban isolation did not on occasions generate mental illness in both women and men; however, it suggests that feminist critiques of domesticity need to be tempered by careful attention to the lives and experiences of a much broader range of modern women.

The recognition that childhood experiences and circumstances could impact on mental and physical health (either in childhood or indeed much later in adulthood) was evident elsewhere during the middle decades of the twentieth century. As the following two chapters demonstrate, child guidance practitioners regularly investigated the home lives of troubled and troublesome children. In Chapter 6, John Stewart explores the manner in which psychiatric social workers, employed by child guidance clinics, used home visits not only to identify what they regarded as 'problem parents' and dysfunctional emotional domestic environments, but also to impart preventative strategies aimed at facilitating resilience to environmental pressures and restoring health. Linked closely to broader international attempts to promote mental hygiene in the early twentieth century, psychiatrists and social workers thus contended not only that maladjustment and delinquency were caused by disruptive home environments, but also that they were to be treated at home by experts in psychiatry.

Mid-century preoccupations with the homes of delinquent children are explored further by Sarah Hayes in Chapter 7. According to early child psychiatrists and psychologists, such as William Healy in the United States and Cyril Burt in Britain, a harsh domestic and social environment during childhood could lead either to delinquent 'rebels' or to neurotic 'rabbits.' However, it is striking that these formulations of the origins of maladjustment did not just focus on the role of parents. Although Burt, for example, regarded 'every tragedy of crime' essentially as a 'drama of domestic life,' he and other commentators recognised that a variety of factors both inside and outside the home influenced the development of delinquent children. Thus, while delinquency and neurosis might have been caused by a broken home, the prolonged absence of one or both parents, or weak discipline, they might also have been triggered by difficulties at school, the influence of peers, the effects of unemployment, and the potentially harmful impact of the cinema on children's expectations and behaviour.

Although psychiatrists and psychologists recognised that the domestic environment was only one of a complex constellation of factors shaping children's health, they nevertheless often emphasised the importance of maternal love in promoting and preserving health. As my own contribution to this volume suggests, psychoanalytical and psychosomatic preoccupations with mother–child relationships influenced approaches not only to behavioural problems and mental illness but also to physical illnesses. During the middle decades of the twentieth century, the onset of asthma and other allergic conditions was often explained in terms of domestic childhood traumas leading to the creation of an 'allergic personality.' For allergists such as John Freeman, for example, the 'asthmogenic home' included not only the physical allergens that might trigger attacks of wheezing, sneezing, and itching, but also a disordered emotional environment that disrupted health and generated disease: either 'smother love' or maternal deprivation could cause asthma. Although psychosomatic explanations and psychoanalytical therapies gradually lost favour, partly as the result of the introduction of new pharmaceutical approaches to treatment during the 1970s, they were popular in the immediate post-war period not only because they reinforced conservative attempts to restore domestic stability through the promotion of motherhood, but also because they appealed to holistic critiques of biomedical reductionism and Western capitalism.

The first chapter in the second part of this volume continues to focus on contemporary preoccupations with the role of women as the guardians of family (and national) health. In Chapter 9, Nancy Tomes explores the manner in which new advertising strategies aimed at improving public health as well as promoting certain health-related products targeted American mothers in particular. Within the modern home, mothers were encouraged to monitor and control the family's consumption of potentially hazardous food, medication, and cosmetics, as well as being expected to maintain the emotional stability of the home. However, the adoption by public health educators of commercial strategies to persuade housewives to purchase particular products was criticised by many medical practitioners, who decried the use of 'medical authority to sell mouthwash and toilet paper.' The American Medical Association, in particular, attempted not only to impose advertising codes but also to establish itself as the most reliable guide to the safety and efficacy of household remedies. This position, however, was in turn often challenged by consumer groups that criticised the established medical profession for failing to protect patients.

Tomes's analysis of health advertising in early twentieth-century America highlights the manner in which the modern home, and particularly modern mothers, were exposed to commercial and political exploitation. The economic and political dimensions of debates about health and home are also evident in British approaches to domestic smoke production and health throughout the twentieth century. As Stephen Mosley demonstrates in Chapter 10, responsibility for battling against the aesthetic and medical affects of smoke pollution in inter-war Britain placed 'an unrelenting strain on women.' According to publicity campaigns run by electricity and gas companies, the adoption of modern energy sources in the home would not only result in cleaner, healthier, and happier populations (with a much lower incidence of respiratory diseases, for example), but also in the liberation of women from the 'soul-destroying drudgery' of housework. However, such campaigns were slow to take effect, as British homeowners remained bound to the open fire by both sentiment and economy, as well as by persistent perceptions of the hearth as more hygienic than its smokeless rivals.

In spite of pressure from the National Smoke Abatement Society and publicity drives from electricity and gas companies, it was not until the London smog of 1952, in which several thousand people died from cardiorespiratory diseases, that the British government made a concerted effort to curb both industrial and domestic smoke production. As Catherine Mills argues in Chapter 11, the passage of the Clean Air Act in 1956 established a system for monitoring air quality and pollution levels, creating smokeless zones, and punishing offenders who continued to blacken the atmosphere with smoke. As Mills suggests, local implementation of the Act varied considerably, but intervention in the home was central to government strategies to combat pollution in the post-war decades. In Sheffield, clean air campaigners visited homes, distributed information leaflets, and exploited the media, targeting women's organisations and youth clubs in particular: the healthy modern home should be clean. Although propaganda was less intense in Coventry, local public health officers similarly visited homes and attempted to educate women and children about the benefits of modernising the domestic space by adopting smokeless fuels.

Strikingly, the strategies adopted by local authorities to reduce smoke emissions focused in the first instance on 'new corporation housing and the prosperous residential suburbs,' rather than on the urban, industrial terraces where smoke pollution was inevitably more pronounced. In this way, the socially disadvantaged were denied early access to clean air. Class, and more particularly race, determined exposure to domestic hazards in other ways during the middle decades of the twentieth century. As Gregg Mitman illustrates in Chapter 12, although asthma and hay fever had traditionally been regarded as aristocratic diseases, in post-Second World War America a wave of asthma deaths afflicted ethnic minorities in poverty-stricken, inner-city areas, where over-crowded and decaying housing, high infant mortality, crime, and disease were commonplace. Drawing on prevalent psychosomatic accounts of asthma, initial explanations of the rising mortality from asthma in poor immigrant communities focused on racial tensions linked, in popular political formulations, not only to the emotional turmoil unleashed by civil rights demonstrations, but also to the 'the damaged black psyche.' However, as Mitman argues, such explanations ignored fundamental environmental inequalities that exposed poor families to higher levels of allergens and pollutants: during the 1960s, the wave of asthma deaths was attributed to cockroach infestation, promoted by the ecological conditions generated by inferior quality housing.

Parallel British debates about the transmission of deprivation and disease within certain communities and families also focused in part on housing and the home environment. In Chapter 13, John Welshman explores these debates by focusing closely not only on Keith Joseph's articulation in 1972 of the 'cycle of deprivation' (in which the problems of one generation were repeated in the next), but also on the subsequent creation of a research programme that attempted to determine whether behavioural or structural factors were primarily responsible for 'transmitted deprivation,' a concept that encompassed the lack of social rights and responsibilities as well as the scarcity of material resources and amenities available to certain 'problem families.' Within this research framework, the impact of housing (rather than the home) became a prime consideration. Significantly, however, researchers disagreed about whether deprivation (in the form of homelessness, for example) was the result of personal inadequacies or, as most studies suggested, of broader economic and social factors that created 'persistent inequalities in the distribution of goods, resources and life chances in capitalist countries.'

Tensions between behavioural and structural explanations of deprivation and disease transmission, and indeed between psychological and physical accounts of disease, were also evident in formulations of lead poisoning in children. In the penultimate chapter, John Burnham traces critical transformations in clinical understandings of the role of the home environment in causing childhood plumbism. During the 1920s and 1930s, it was commonplace to assume that children ingested lead randomly from painted toys and domestic furniture. In the 1950s, however, attention shifted not only to the use of lead paint on walls, ceilings and floors, but also to the psychosocial environment of the family and home that might encourage children to eat non-food materials, a condition referred to as 'pica.' These concerns led some physicians to advocate removing vulnerable children from the poisonous home environment in much the same way (and for much the same reasons) that asthmatic children were removed from dusty and dysfunctional homes.[34] Significantly, as notions of the 'environment' broadened during the 1960s, clinical understandings of lead poisoning shifted once again. Focusing initially on invisible pollution from radioactivity and chemicals, modern environmentalists began to emphasise the dangers of exposure to small amounts of lead in the general atmosphere. From this perspective, the home was only one possible source of poisonous lead, and the boundaries between indoor and outdoor environments became increasingly ambiguous.

Growing clinical interest in children's exposure to lead and other domestic toxins did not displace or preclude close medical attention to the impact of diet on children's health and behaviour. In the final chapter, Matthew Smith explores the elaboration and reception of a novel American diet introduced in the early 1970s by Ben Feingold and aimed at reducing hyperactivity in children. The Feingold diet, as it became known, involved the elimination of food additives, which were thought to precipitate allergic reactions resulting in hyperactivity and other behavioural problems. Although the diet attracted considerable public and media attention, with over 200,000 families subscribing to the diet by the mid-1980s, Feingold spectacularly failed to convince mainstream paediatricians and allergists of its value and the diet's popularity faded, especially after Feingold's death in 1982. As Smith persuasively argues, this had little to do with the nature of the scientific evidence against the efficacy of the diet, and much more to do with wider political tensions both inside and outside the medical profession. In particular, the diet relied heavily on families, and especially mothers, to adhere rigidly to clinical advice and to constantly monitor the food consumed by their children. For many families, this proved impossible, partly because of the onerous nature of ensuring compliance and partly because it was difficult to control food consumed outside the home. A combination of genetic explanations for hyperactivity and the use of prescription drugs ultimately proved more appealing to families that were already struggling to maintain a healthy and happy home.

Collectively the chapters in this volume underline just how central the home has been to understandings of health and disease in the modern period on both sides of the Atlantic. Although the diverse, but often interlinking, contributions presented here can only begin to scratch the surface of historical constructions of the complex and shifting relationship between health and the home, they are intended to raise new questions, expose the value of novel sources, and suggest constructive points of contact between medical and environmental histories, as well as between history and literary and film studies. Perhaps most importantly, we hope that this book will stimulate further discussion and research not only into the manner in which the physical, psychological, and ideological ingredients of the modern home shaped patterns and experiences of health and disease, but also, conversely, into how anxieties about disease served to fashion the architecture, furnishing, decoration, and management of modern homes.

NOTES

1. Ralph Blumenthal, 'Changing hazards in the home,' *New York Times* (30 October 1980), C1. This report and its implications are discussed more fully in Gregg Mitman, *Breathing Space: How Allergies Shape Our Lives and Landscapes* (New Haven, CT: Yale University Press, 2007).
2. Mark Jackson, *Allergy: The History of a Modern Malady* (London: Reaktion, 2006).
3. See, for example, Warren T. Vaughan, *Primer of Allergy* (St. Louis, MO: C. V. Mosby Company, 1939), 43–4.
4. Nancy Tomes, *The Gospel of Germs: Men, Women, and the Microbe in American Life* (Cambridge, MA: Harvard University Press, 1998).
5. W. Storm van Leeuwen, *Allergic Diseases: Diagnosis and Treatment of Bronchial Asthma, Hay-Fever and Other Allergic Diseases* (Philadelphia, 1925). See discussions in: Carla Keirns, 'Better than nature: The changing treatment of asthma and hay fever in the United States, 1910–1945,' *Studies in History and Philosophy of Biological and Biomedical Sciences,* 34 (2003): 511–31; Jackson, *Allergy.*
6. For further discussion of these theories, see Chapter 8 in this volume; see also Jackson, *Allergy,* Chapter 3.
7. John Freeman, *Hay-Fever: A Key to the Allergic Disorders* (London: Heinemann, 1950), 161–88.
8. Anon., 'Outdoors ban for victims of hay fever,' *The Times* (7 September 1960), 8g.

9. For a discussion of this, see Jane Darke, 'Women and the meaning of home,' in Rose Gilroy and Roberta Woods (eds.), *Housing Women* (London: Routledge, 1994), 11–30. See also the chapter in this volume by Ali Haggett.
10. See in particular the chapters by John Stewart, Sarah Hayes, and John Welshman.
11. Jackson, *Allergy*, 103–47; see also Chapter 8 in this volume.
12. Christopher Hamlin, *Public Health and Social Justice in the Age of Chadwick: Britain, 1800–1854* (Cambridge: Cambridge University Press, 1998). On approaches to the promotion of public health in the twentieth century, see V. Berridge and K. Loughlin (eds.), *Medicine, the Market and the Mass Media: Producing Health in the Twentieth Century* (London: Routledge, 2005).
13. Mathew Thomson, *Psychological Subjects: Identity, Culture and Health in Twentieth-Century Britain* (Oxford: Oxford University Press, 2006).
14. A large programme of research into the history of cancer and cancer services is currently being conducted by Professor John Pickstone and his colleagues in the Centre for the History of Science, Technology and Medicine at the University of Manchester. See, for example, Carsten Timmermann, 'As depressing as it was predictable? Lung cancer, clinical trials, and the Medical Research Council in postwar Britain,' *Bulletin of the History of Medicine*, 81 (2007): 312–34.
15. See, for example, Neil McFarlane, 'Hospitals, housing, and tuberculosis in Glasgow, 1911–51,' *Social History of Medicine*, 2 (1989): 59–85.
16. Joan Austoker, *A History of the Imperial Cancer Research Fund 1902–1986* (Oxford: Oxford University Press, 1988); James T. Patterson, *The Dread Disease: Cancer and Modern American Culture* (Cambridge, MA: Harvard University Press, 1987); Evelleen Richards, *Vitamin C and Cancer: Medicine or Politics?* (Basingstoke: Macmillan, 1991); David Cantor, 'Contracting cancer: The politics of commissioned histories,' *Social History of Medicine*, 5 (1992): 131–42; Patrice Pinell, *Naissance d'un fléau: Histoire de la lutte contre le cancer en France (1890–1940)*, (Paris, 1992); S. Robert Lichter and Stanley Rothman, *Environmental Cancer: A Political Disease?* (New Haven, CT: Yale University Press, 1999).
17. David Rosner and Gerald Markowitz, *Deadly Dust: Silicosis and the Politics of Occupational Disease in Twentieth-Century America* (Princeton, NJ: Princeton University Press, 1991); Alan Derickson, *Black Lung: Anatomy of a Public Health Disaster* (Ithaca, NY: Cornell University Press, 1998); Christopher C. Sellers, *Hazards of the Job: From Industrial Disease to Environmental Health Science* (Chapel Hill: University of North Carolina Press, 1997); Geoffrey Tweedale, *Magic Mineral to Killer Dust: Turner & Newall and the Asbestos Hazard* (Oxford: Oxford University Press, 2000); Christian Warren, *Brush with Death: A Social History of Lead Poisoning* (Baltimore, MD: Johns Hopkins University Press, 2000).
18. Jackson, *Allergy;* Mitman, *Breathing Space;* Carsten Timmermann, 'Americans and Pavlovians: The Central Institute for Cardiovascular Research at the East German Academy of Sciences and its precursor institutions as a case study of biomedical research in a country of the Soviet Bloc (c. 1950–1980),' in Berridge and Loughlin (eds.), *Medicine, the Market and the Mass Media* (London: Routledge, 2005), 244–65; idem, 'A matter of degree: the normalisation of hypertension, c. 1940–2000,' in W. Ernst (ed.), *Histories of the Normal and the Abnormal: Social and Cultural Histories of Norms and Normativity* (London: Routledge, 2006).
19. See the chapters by Stephen Mosley and Catherine Mills.
20. Ibid. See also: Peter Brimblecombe, *The Big Smoke: A History of Air Pollution in London since Medieval Times* (London, 1987); Stephen Mosley, *The*

Chimney of the World: A History of Smoke Pollution in Victorian and Edwardian Manchester (Cambridge: The White Horse Press, 2001); Mark Jackson, 'Cleansing the air and promoting health: The politics of pollution in post-war Britain,' in Berridge and Loughlin (eds.), *Medicine, the Market and the Mass Media*, 219–41.

21. Roger Cooter and Steve Sturdy, 'Of war, medicine and modernity: Introduction,' in Roger Cooter, Mark Harrison, and Steve Sturdy (eds), *War, Medicine and Modernity* (Stroud: Sutton Publishing Limited, 1998), 1–21, at p. 1. For further discussion of modernity, see: Anthony Giddens, *The Consequences of Modernity* (Cambridge: Polity Press, 1990); Alan O'Shea's commentary on Marshall Berman's *All That is Solid Melts Into Air: The Experience of Modernity* (London: Verso, 1983), in Mica Nava and Alan O'Shea (eds.), *Modern Times: Reflections on a Century of English Modernity* (London and New York: Routledge, 1996), 8–13; Mark S. Micale (ed.), *The Mind of Modernism: Medicine, Psychology and the Cultural Arts in Europe and America, 1880–1940* (Stanford: Stanford University Press, 2004). I am grateful to Michael Clark for these references.
22. See, in particular, the chapters by Michael Clark, Rhodri Hayward, John Stewart, and Sarah Hayes.
23. Tomes, *The Gospel of Germs,* 144.
24. Jackson, *Allergy;* Carla Keirns, 'Short of breath: A social and intellectual history of asthma in the United States' (PhD thesis, University of Pennsylvania, 2004), 158–68.
25. For examples of pertinent historical and sociological studies of home, see: Witold Rybczynski, *Home* (London: Heinemann, 1988); Gwendolyn Wright, *Moralism and the Modern Home: Domestic Architecture and Cultural Conflict in Chicago 1873–1913* (Chicago: University of Chicago Press, 1980); Helena Barrett and John Phillips, *Suburban Style: The British Home, 1840–1960* (Boston: Little, Brown and Company, 1993); Annmarie Adams, *Architecture in the Family Way: Doctor, Houses, and Women, 1870–1900* (Montreal: McGill-Queens University Press, 1996).
26. See, for example, Hamlin, *Public Health and Social Justice;* Brimblecombe, *The Big Smoke;* Mosley, *The Chimney of the World.*
27. Bernard Harris, *The Health of the Schoolchild: A History of the School Medical Services in England and Wales* (Buckingham: Open University Press, 1995).
28. See, for example, Paul Blanc, *How Everyday Products Make People Sick: Toxins at Home and in the Workplace* (Berkeley: University of California Press, 2007).
29. Michael Peplar, *Family Matters: A History of Ideas about Family since 1945* (London: Longman, 2002); Mary Abbott, *Family Affairs: A History of the Family in 20th Century England* (London: Routledge, 2002); Eleanor Gordon and Gwyneth Nair, *Public Lives: Women, Family and Society in Victorian Britain* (New Haven, CT: Yale University Press, 2003).
30. Jane Lewis, *The Politics of Motherhood: Child and Maternal Welfare in England, 1900–39* (London: Croom Helm, 1980); Jane Lewis (ed.), *Labour and Love: Women's Experience of Home and Family, 1850–1940* (Oxford: Basil Blackwell, 1985); Angela Holdsworth, *Out of the Doll's House: The Story of Women in the Twentieth Century* (London: BBC Books, 1988); Sue Bruley, *Women in Britain since 1900* (Basingstoke: Macmillan, 1999); Roger Cooter (ed.), *In the Name of the Child: Health and Welfare, 1880–1940* (London: Routledge, 1992); Harry Hendrick, *Child Welfare: England 1872–1989* (London: Routledge, 1994); Marijke Gijswijt-Hofstra and Hilary Marland (eds.), *Cultures of Child Health in Britain and the Netherlands in the Twentieth Century* (Amsterdam: Rodopi,

2003); Harry Hendrick (ed.), *Child Welfare and Social Policy: An Essential Reader* (Bristol: The Policy Press, 2005).

31. See, for example, Michelle Murphy's challenging studies of the history of sick building syndrome: Michelle Murphy, 'The "elsewhere within here" and environmental illness; or, how to build yourself a body in a safe space,' *Configurations* 8 (2000): 87–120; Michelle Murphy, *Sick Building Syndrome and the Problem of Uncertainty: Environmental Politics, Technoscience, and Women Workers* (Durham, NC: Duke University Press, 2006).
32. In this context, it is worth noting that a forthcoming special issue of *Gender and History,* edited by Karen Adler and due to be published in 2010, will focus on 'homes and homecomings.'
33. Deborah S. Ryan, *Daily Mail Ideal Home Exhibition: The Ideal Home Through the 20th Century* (London: Hazar Publishing, 1997). See also Barry Curtis's review in *Journal of Design History,* 11 (1998): 266–8.
34. See the discussion in the chapter by Jackson in this volume.

Part One

Emotional Health and the Home

2 *A Bill of Divorcement*
Theatrical and Cinematic Portrayals of Mental and Marital Breakdown in a Dysfunctional Upper-Middle-Class Family, 1921–1932

Michael J. Clark

INTRODUCTION

During the years immediately following the end of the First World War, there was widespread public concern in Britain that the War had unleashed or accelerated certain irreversible processes of political, social, and cultural decline, and that the psychological effects of the conflict were undermining the mental and moral health of British society.[1] A series of apparently casual or motiveless killings involving shell-shocked ex-soldiers who had been unable to readjust to peacetime conditions were given widespread sensational coverage in the press, and for a time there existed a climate of fear verging on moral panic that the violence of the Western Front, so long kept at bay, was at last coming home to Britain.[2] At the same time, there was an equally widespread, though less vocal, apprehension that the stability of marriage and the traditional male-dominated family unit were in danger, not just from the traumatic experiences of the First World War but from far-reaching changes in the rights and roles of women that wartime conditions had either set in motion or accelerated.[3]

Against this background of cultural pessimism and moral alarmism, Clemence Dane's play *A Bill of Divorcement,* with its melodramatic tale of an upper-middle-class marriage ruined by shell-shock and hereditary mental taint, its attacks on the unfairness of English divorce law, and its apparent support for the medical regulation of marriage and procreation, caused a sensation when first produced by Basil Dean and the Reandean Company at St. Martin's Theatre, London in March 1921.[4] With its conventional three-act structure, country house location, and upper-middle-class characters, *A Bill of Divorcement* was far from being a 'modernist' play in either of the commonly understood senses of being socially realistic or formally innovative. However, its contemporary subject matter, near-future setting, and above all, the attitudes and beliefs expressed by the principal characters left audiences in no doubt that it was intended to be a drama of, and in some sense about, 'modernity.'[5]

Amid the gloom and uncertainties of the immediate post-1918 period, Clemence Dane deliberately sought to place *A Bill of Divorcement* in the vanguard of post-war British theatre, as a drama of contemporary social and medical issues and attitudes. Though sometimes mistaken for a propaganda tract, *A Bill of Divorcement* was not intended as a sociological text, and insofar as she had one, its author's conception of modernity was more a state of mind, a subjective experience of rupture and discontinuity, than one of far-reaching socio-economic transformation of the kind envisaged by Marx, Durkheim, or Weber. But by making the clash between the secular ideals and liberal moral outlook associated with the new century and the narrow religious beliefs and moral hypocrisy that she ascribed to the Victorian age central to the drama, Clemence Dane clearly sought to identify herself and her work with what she understood to be the spirit of the modern age. Yet even while apparently embracing the modernist challenge to Victorian social attitudes and moral values, the play also revealed a deep ambivalence and misgivings about the ultimate effects of modernity on the mental and moral health of British society in general and young British women in particular. In its hesitant and at times fearful response to modernity, *A Bill of Divorcement* seems to have struck a chord with the British theatre-going public,[6] making a powerful, if somewhat confused, contribution to ongoing public debates linking political and domestic violence, street crime and declining moral standards, the rise of radical secular ideologies and the decline of traditional religious belief, the unsettling effects of modernity and modern warfare on the national psyche, the rights and wrongs of women, and the future of marriage and the family. Like the First World War, the play seemed to symbolize the new age's sudden, catastrophic break with tradition, and in doing so, it both drew upon and powerfully contributed to the brittle, feverish mood of much British art and literature of the period.

The original stage production of *A Bill of Divorcement* ran for 401 performances before being adapted for the cinema as a silent film the following year, with some of the original cast also appearing in the film.[7] In 1932, a much more high-profile Hollywood sound film version was released by RKO Radio Pictures, a David O. Selznick production directed by George Cukor and starring John Barrymore, Billie Burke, and the young Katherine Hepburn.[8] A third and final screen version, directed by John Farrow and starring Maureen O'Hara, Adolphe Menjou, and Fay Bainter, was to follow in 1940.[9] Both the original stage play and the 1932 film version especially are of great interest to historians for the light that they shed on contemporary social attitudes toward mental illness, psychiatry, and eugenics, and for the doubts and anxieties that they reveal about the mental and moral state of the English middle-class family during the 1920s and '30s.[10] However, in order better to understand the interest and importance of the play and its cinematic versions for the medico-psychological and social history of the inter-war British family, let us first examine the life, work, and personality of its author more closely.

CLEMENCE DANE AND *A BILL OF DIVORCEMENT*

Winifred Ashton (1888–1965), a previously little-known novelist, artist, and former actress who adopted the pseudonym Clemence Dane in honour of her favourite London church, was a highly complex character.[11] Born into a respectable lower-middle-class family in Greenwich, south-east London, Ashton soon rebelled against her conventional Victorian upbringing and spent much of her youth as an art student and teacher in Germany, Switzerland, and Ireland before returning to England in 1913 to work as an actress on the London stage, under the name Diane Portis.[12] She began writing seriously after a breakdown in health in 1916–17, and first came to prominence in 1917 with her novel *Regiment of Women,* an uncomfortably frank portrayal of bullying and lesbian romance in a girls' boarding school.[13] In 1920, she began writing for the stage, and although she continued to work as an artist and to publish novels, short stories, essays, and poems, for the next 40 years she was to be known chiefly as a writer for the theatre, cinema, and radio, eventually publishing some 30 stage plays, 11 novels, 20 screenplays, and a dozen radio plays.[14]

From the mid-1920s onwards, Dane lived and worked mainly in London's Covent Garden, Midhurst, Sussex, and Brighton, where she became a familiar figure and a notable chronicler of the local artistic, literary, and theatrical scenes.[15] In 1947 she won an Oscar for 'Best Original Motion Picture Story' for the screenplay of Alexander Korda's *Perfect Strangers* (1945), and in 1953 she was awarded a C.B.E.[16] Though never rivalling Colette's imaginative genius, psychological sophistication or supreme literary artistry, Clemence Dane's life and work bear many surprising points of comparison with that of her French near-contemporary, and, matters of sexual orientation apart, Colette's semi-autobiographical novel *La Vagabonde* (1910, 1923) could in many respects have been a portrait of the young Clemence Dane.[17] Today, Clemence Dane is chiefly remembered, if at all, as the supposed model for her friend Noël Coward's dotty medium Madame Arcati in *Blithe Spirit* (1942),[18] but in the 1920s, she was probably a better known and more widely read author than Virginia Woolf. For the next 30 years, although increasingly burdened with the label 'English eccentric,' she remained a well-known and highly regarded artist and writer, whose work for stage and screen enjoyed considerable critical and commercial success, and whose contributions to contemporary debates around feminism, sexual politics, and national character were widely respected.[19]

Like its author, *A Bill of Divorcement* embodies and reflects a variety of complex and often confused reactions both to modernity in general and to the immediate post-war situation in particular. The plots of both the 1921 stage play and the 1932 Hollywood film adaptation are very similar, the screen version being merely a somewhat simplified version of the original stage play.[20] Both are set in an upper-middle-class English family and country house at Christmas time in the early 1930s—a near-future scenario at the time the play was first staged, but a kind of 'alternative present' by the time the 1932 film version was made.[21] All the action of the play, though not of the film, takes place indoors, which heightens the strong sense of psychological oppression and imprisonment by the past which pervades both stage and screen versions. On the fateful day in question, Hilary Fairfield (played by John Barrymore in the 1932 film), a former Army officer and, at least in the film, a gifted musician and composer, arrives home after escaping from a private asylum—'That place,' as he calls it—where he has been confined as a lunatic for the previous 17 years.[22] Hilary has a history of emotional instability and violent mood swings, but believes himself fully to have recovered from his illness, 'brought on', as we are told, by 'shell-shock' in the First World War, and is determined to pick up the threads of his former life with his beloved wife Margaret (Billie Burke).[23] However, unbeknown to Hilary, Margaret has obtained a divorce from him on the grounds of his prolonged mental unfitness, and is all set to remarry and begin a new life with her lover Gray Meredith (Paul Cavanagh).[24] Chaos ensues, as the wavering Margaret is torn between the demands of her old and new loves, and her teenage daughter Sydney (played by the 24-year-old Katherine Hepburn, in her screen debut) is forced to reappraise her own engagement to Kit (David Manners), the rector's son, in the light of her sudden introduction to the father whom she never knew, but allegedly so much resembles.[25] The impasse is only resolved when Sydney, who is altogether more clear-minded and decisive than her mother, enlists the help of the outwardly benevolent but authoritarian family doctor, Dr. Alliot (Henry Stephenson), and makes her mother's mind up for her, allowing Margaret to leave with her lover, while she herself chooses to dismiss her own fiancé and stay with her half-crazed father, renouncing her own prospects of marriage and motherhood when she learns from Dr. Alliot that insanity is hereditary in the Fairfield bloodline.[26] Both play and film end on a deeply unhappy, even tragic, note, with father and daughter locked into a kind of *folie à deux* of Hilary's making but Sydney's own choosing, all the more effectively conveyed in the 1932 film version by the crashing piano discords (instead of the usual swelling violins) that accompany the final frames.

A FAMILY AT WAR: VICTORIAN ATTITUDES, RESPECTABLE RELIGION, AND THE CHALLENGE OF MODERNITY

Much of the interest of *A Bill of Divorcement* for the history of the inter-war British family lies not so much in its artistic merits, but rather in the sheer profusion of contemporary social, legal, medical, and ethical issues that it seeks to address. Clemence Dane seems to have been determined to refer to as many controversial issues as possible, even at the expense of narrative fluency and artistic unity, and this makes both the play and, to a lesser extent, its screen versions particularly rich and fascinating sources for social and medical history.

Both play and film revolve around a number of contemporary social issues and cultural antagonisms, which set up powerful psychological tensions within and between all the principal characters, with far-reaching implications for their individual destinies and ultimately tragic consequences for the integrity and emotional well-being of the Fairfield family. The first and most obvious tension in both play and film is that between the long shadow of Victorian moral beliefs and social attitudes and the supposedly more open, honest, less conventional and more 'natural' mental outlook characteristic of the new century. In both play and film, the young Sydney Fairfield, the character who, it may be inferred, most nearly represents the author's own idealised self-projection,[27] aspires to be the complete modern woman. Independent-minded and determinedly unconventional in her attitudes and behaviour, she freely contradicts her elders and repeatedly insists that she is 'not nineteenth century,' unlike her mother, her Aunt Hester, and her fiancé Kit's clerical father and family.[28] Though affectionate, patient, and caring towards her mother, Sydney makes no secret of her impatience and even scorn for the antediluvian attitudes of her Aunt Hester, whom she describes as 'stand[-ing] for Noah and the flood,' and takes pleasure in shocking and embarrassing her by buying her a cigarette case as a Christmas present, confident that Aunt Hester will be only too glad to exchange it for Sydney's own unwanted present.[29] Gray Meredith, Margaret Fairfield's intended second husband, is another thrusting, dynamic representative of modern attitudes and values. He tells his beloved to her face that she is 'pure nineteenth century,'[30] while Dr. Alliot, yet another spokesman for modernity, primarily in its medical and scientific aspects, tells the womenfolk of the Fairfield family that social institutions, laws, morality, and even religious beliefs must either adapt to the conditions of modern life or face extinction: 'Grow or perish—it's the law of life.'[31]

In this vaguely organicist and social-Darwinistic perspective, the dynamic of modernity is facilely identified with the laws of 'Life' or 'Nature,' seen in both their scientific and moral aspects. The outlines of this brave new world remain largely unclear, but two important aspects become increasingly apparent in the course of the play: first, that in this new society, the treatment of the mentally ill and other 'unfit' and vulnerable groups is likely to be no less harsh and coercive than in previous, supposedly less 'enlightened,' eras; and second, that everyone—especially every woman—will be subject to far-reaching medical control in the interests of eugenics. This puts the female members of the Fairfield family in a difficult position. On the one hand, Sydney, the youngest and outwardly most 'modern' member of the family, would clearly like to be part of the new century, with its apparently greater individual freedom and intoxicating promises of emancipation and independence, especially for women. However, the new order, speaking through the voice of Dr. Alliot, in effect rejects her as 'unfit' because she is assumed to carry her father's legacy of hereditary mental taint, whereas even her mother Margaret can belatedly contribute to the eugenic improvement of society by bearing children to Gray Meredith.[32] Sydney thus unexpectedly finds herself outcast from society like her father Hilary, the only one of the principal characters not clearly identified as 'belonging' either to the nineteenth or to the twentieth century. So in a sense it is inevitable that Sydney and Hilary will be left to share each other's company, 'out of time,' as it were. They are, in effect, both victims or rejects of modernity, which thus appears in a deeply ambivalent light.

Together with the repudiation of Victorian attitudes and values, one of the strongest themes in the play, though significantly not of the 1932 film, is rejection of conventional religious belief. This is signalled at the beginning of the play, when Sydney, reproached by Aunt Hester for getting up late on Christmas day, gleefully retorts: 'I'm seventeen, I've left school, and I'm not going to church to-day, or any day any more ever,' except, she hastily adds, to accompany her mother and her intended to their wedding the following week.[33] Clemence Dane's deep-rooted hostility to institutional religion is most clearly expressed in the character of the rector, the Rev. Christopher Pumphrey, described in a stage direction as 'an insignificant man, with an important manner and a plum in his mouth.'[34] The Rev. Mr. Pumphrey epitomises the narrow-mindedness and hypocrisy of safe, respectable Anglicanism. At first, he attempts to use Hilary's presumed insanity as a smokescreen in order to deflect attention from his determination not to remarry a divorced woman (Margaret Fairfield) in church, and then further tries to force Margaret into abandoning her plans to marry Gray Meredith by threatening to block his own son Kit's intended marriage to Margaret's daughter Sydney.[35] The sheer odiousness of this attempt at moral blackmail, which Margaret interprets as a betrayal by the Church to which she belongs, momentarily stiffens her resolve to go ahead and marry Gray, if necessary in defiance of the Church to which she still feels attached and whose precepts she would like to obey. Margaret denounces the Rev. Pumphrey and her sister-in-law Hester as 'wicked' for trying to bully her with their hypocritical talk of a wife's 'duty,'[36] but her moral courage soon fails her and she too confuses the issue by invoking her dread of Hilary's violence, pathetically imploring them 'not [to] judge [me].'[37]

There is precious little of the spirit of Christianity in the Rev. Pumphrey's idea of pastoral care, but just as in the case of Victorianism, the legacy and habits of thought inculcated by the Christian religion, in particular the notions of sin, guilt, and Man's need for God's grace, are not so easily discarded. Hilary, for example, uses religious rather than scientific language to describe his state of mind when confined as a lunatic. Insisting that 'I was never like the rest of them. I was sane, always—but the face [of God] was turned away from me,' he describes himself as 'a lost soul' and the asylum itself as 'Hell! Hell!'[38] Again, when Margaret tells Gray that she cannot simply leave with him and abandon Hilary to his fate, Gray angrily accuses her of committing 'the sin without forgiveness. You're denying—not me—but . . . the spirit of life.'[39] When Dr. Alliot returns to the house, and manages to get rid of the Rev. Pumphrey, it becomes apparent that, in a confused sort of way, the author hopes that in a more rational, scientific age, medicine will come to exercise as strong and decisive an authority on the side of 'Life' as the Church once did on the side of God's laws for man, but in direct opposition to the outmoded and outworn dogmas of revealed religion. As Dr. Alliot tells Margaret: 'If your church forbids you, you must change your church; and if your God forbids you, why then, you must change your God.'[40] But even he says 'God be with you, child' to Margaret, when she goes to tell Hilary that she cannot go back to him, while to complete the confusion, Margaret then cries 'God help me' when forced to yield to Hilary's emotional entreaties.[41] No sooner, it seems, is God—or one god—driven out by the front door than he, or another god, returns in a new guise. And, as will soon become apparent, the modern age's new god of science will be invested with just as much arbitrary power over individual destinies as the God of the Christian Church ever was.

SOCIAL DARWINISM, MODERN ETHICS, AND THE INDIVIDUAL

The ethical messages in *A Bill of Divorcement* are equally ambivalent and confusing. Aunt Hester and the Rev. Pumphrey, the two self-confessed mouthpieces of conventional religion and anti-modernism, are represented as having no real moral principles, only prejudices coupled with an instinctive fear of change and a desperate concern for conventional ideas of respectability. However, Gray Meredith and Dr. Alliot, the two self-appointed spokesmen for modernity and a more naturalistic approach to morality, appear even less attractive with their callous, self-serving, social-Darwinist clichés and their complete lack of sympathy for the weaker members of society, in particular the mentally ill.[42] Thus Gray, on learning of Hilary's escape from the asylum and return home, at once asks: 'Is he dangerous?'[43] Stating that 'There's only one way to deal with an escaped lunatic,' Gray wants to call the police immediately, and later, when Margaret says 'I must be good to Hilary,' asks: 'What good is 'good' to him, poor devil?'[44]

Dr. Alliot's immediate reaction to the news of Hilary's escape is not quite so extreme, but if anything he is even harsher in his ruthless disregard for Hilary's feelings. 'Why, face it, man!' he bellows at Hilary. 'One of you must suffer. Which is it to be? The useful or the useless? The whole or the maimed? The healthy woman with her life before her, or the man whose children ought never to have been born?'[45] When Margaret attempts to remonstrate with him for 'go[ing] too far,' Dr. Alliot insists:

'Mrs. Fairfield, in this matter I cannot go too far.'[46] Later, the wavering Margaret tells a bewildered and furious Gray that she must stay with Hilary 'because he's weak [and] you're strong.'[47] She even claims that leaving Hilary for Gray would be tantamount to 'vivisection—like cutting a dumb beast [in order] to make me well. I can't do it. I'd rather die,' at which point Gray loses his patience and replies: 'Die then—you fool!'[48] By now, the audience must be wondering whether Margaret will not find Gray's passionate cruelty still harder to bear than Hilary's violent mood swings, and even after Sydney intervenes on her mother's behalf, Margaret has to work hard to persuade the disenchanted Gray to take her away with him after all.[49]

In effect, the play presents a spectrum of what might be called practical moral standpoints, ranging from the wavering sentimentality and excessive tender-heartedness of Margaret at one extreme to the cruelty and heartlessness of Gray and Dr. Alliot at the other. Sydney is caught somewhere between these two extremes, struggling to reconcile her own conflicting emotions and values while trying to remain, if not the master, at least the author of her own destiny. On the one hand, quite early in the play she says 'I . . . think it's morbid to have a conscience,' and cheerfully ignores her fiancé Kit's shocked reaction to her apparent hard-heartedness towards her insane father.[50] On the other hand, she is kind-hearted and caring towards her mother, and when she comes face to face with her father, behaves towards him in a deeply compassionate way. Though convinced of her own strength and ostensibly sharing the same 'modern' values as Gray and Dr. Alliot, Sydney refuses to follow them in riding roughshod over Hilary's rights and feelings. Knowing that she is 'free to be free,' Sydney chooses instead to stay with and protect her father, thereby sacrificing her own happiness for that of her mother.[51] On the face of it, this would seem a rather 'Victorian' conclusion to a supposedly modernist drama, yet Sydney's choice is clearly motivated as much by a profound sense of her own superiority and a kind of 'tough love' (for Kit) as by any apparent excess of filial duty. Throughout all these moral twists and turns, the author's own attitude remains deeply unclear. No sooner is one position taken up or apparently highlighted than it is subverted, undermined, or shown in an unflattering light, a pattern that is repeated frequently at many different levels throughout *A Bill of Divorcement*.[52]

ECCLESIASTICAL MARRIAGE, INSANITY, AND DIVORCE LAW REFORM

The title of *A Bill of Divorcement* is clearly intended to draw attention to the question of divorce, and when the play was first performed, some contemporaries took it to be a fervent plea for the reform of English divorce law.[53] In her prefatory note, Clemence Dane asks the audience 'to imagine that [in 1933, when the action is supposed to take place] the recommendations of the Majority Report of the Royal Commission on Divorce and Matrimonial Causes have become the law of the land,'[54] and the question of English divorce law reform is certainly an important element in the play, though not of the 1932 Hollywood film version. Indeed, through the medium of Dr. Alliot, the author even provides the audience with a brief history of English divorce law during the previous half-century.[55] However, once again, the messages are decidedly mixed.

Under the Divorce and Matrimonial Causes Act of 1857, which was still in force when *A Bill of Divorcement* was written, the only legal grounds for divorce in English law were a wife's adultery or a husband's adultery aggravated by persistent cruelty, incest, bigamy, bestiality, rape, sodomy, or desertion.[56] A Royal Commission on Divorce and Matrimonial Causes, otherwise known as the Gorell Commission, after its chairman, Lord Gorell (1848–1913), was appointed in 1909 'To inquire into the present state of the law and the administration thereof in divorce and matrimonial causes,' in response to widespread public concern that English divorce law was not only archaic, unenlightened, and manifestly unfair to women, but also tended to undermine the institutions of marriage and the family, by making it more economical for separated working-class spouses to live in sin or commit bigamy than to obtain a divorce.[57] The Majority Report of the Royal Commission, published in December 1912, recommended that the grounds for divorce should be equalized between men and women, that the law should be amended to allow divorce on grounds of incurable insanity after five years' confinement in an asylum, and that, under certain conditions, concealed madness, recurrent insanity, or incipient unsoundness of mind becoming apparent within six months of marriage should constitute legitimate grounds for annulment.[58] However, due to the strength of religious opposition to the proposals, the weakness of Asquith's Liberal government after the 1911 General Elections, and the interruption of the First World War, these recommendations were not enacted, and at the time *A Bill of Divorcement* was written in 1920, adultery still remained the only legally valid ground for divorce.

The main reasons for the appointment of the Royal Commission had in fact been public concern about the exorbitant costs of divorce proceedings and the difficulties of access to the courts, at a time when all divorce cases still had to be heard in London.[59] Characteristically, though, Clemence Dane chose to ignore these more mundane concerns and focus instead on the issue of whether incurable insanity should be a legitimate ground for divorce, an issue of potentially greater concern to metropolitan upper-middle-class audiences than the costs of divorce or access to the courts. However, in the process, not only the class aspect of the divorce issue but the whole question of the unequal treatment of men and women by the courts in divorce actions were in effect written out of the debate, making

A Bill of Divorcement an altogether less powerful statement of the case for divorce law reform than might otherwise have been the case.[60]

This weakening of the reformist impetus of the play is aggravated by what precedes the action. In both play and film, Margaret Fairfield has already obtained a divorce from Hilary, presumably on the grounds of his prolonged confinement as a lunatic, before the action begins.[61] Nothing is said about the cost of her divorce or indeed any other difficulties that she may have encountered in obtaining it, still less about the unequal treatment of men and women by the courts. All these problems are simply passed over in the initial assumption which the audience is asked to make. Rather, the focus is on the *psychological* aspect of divorce, and at this level, the effect of reform appears to be slight. In the play, Margaret has been divorced from Hilary for more than a year when he suddenly returns home, but she is still reluctant to marry Gray because, as Sydney explains to Kit, 'if mother isn't married in her own parish church, she'll think she's living in sin.'[62] As quickly becomes clear, though, Margaret stands no chance of being married by the Rev. Pumphrey in her—or rather, *his*—own parish church, and the Church's determined opposition to the remarriage of divorcees is thus set on a collision course with liberal demands for a more humane and compassionate approach to the reality of marital breakdown.[63] However, because the author has Hilary suddenly return home, and Margaret is briefly made to yield to his emotional entreaties to go back to him, this clash never fully materializes, and when Margaret finally does leave with Gray, it is not at all clear whether she is reconciled or resigned to 'living in sin' with her new husband. The message seems to be that so long as official religion remains resolutely opposed to any liberalization of divorce law and committed to maintaining the rules forbidding the remarriage of divorcees in church, a powerful stigma will continue to attach to divorce, and that some divorcees will experience strong feelings of guilt and anguish, whatever legal reforms may be enacted.[64] Far from inviting her audiences to see how much better society could be if, as is postulated in the prefatory note, the recommendations of the Majority Report of the Royal Commission were enacted, Clemence Dane seems to be warning them that legal reforms will make very little difference unless accompanied by a sea-change in social mores and religious practice. But this is more a counsel of despair than a strong plea for reform of English divorce law, and to this extent *A Bill of Divorcement* can hardly be said to have advanced the cause of divorce law reform, much less the legal or social emancipation of women.

SHELL-SHOCK, MADNESS, AND THE FAIRFIELD FAMILY

At the root of the many psychological and social problems confronting the Fairfield family is the chronic insanity of Hilary Fairfield, which, it is implied, took the form of violent, unpredictable mood swings together with emotional, if not actual physical, violence towards his young wife Margaret. This mental abnormality had, it seems, been apparent almost from the first days of their marriage, and has resulted in Hilary's confinement in an asylum for the past 17 years, during much of which time Margaret, acting on medical advice, has ceased to visit him.[65] Sydney, who has never even seen her father before the fateful Christmas Eve on which the action of the play takes place, has been led to believe that he is suffering from shell-shock sustained while serving as an officer during the First World War, before she was born.[66] But when she begins to question her Aunt Hester more closely about her father's illness, she learns that he had always been prone to violent mood swings even before his military service, that his sister Grace had 'not been herself' for many years before, and that all the members of the Fairfield family are more or less 'nervy.'[67] It is this family history of mental illness, rather than Hilary's own madness, that is the Fairfield family's real secret—'a shadow . . . a trouble . . . a ghost in the house,' as Sydney describes it,[68] which, as becomes clear from her conversation with Aunt Hester, now looms directly over her.

Hilary's madness, we are given to understand, has destroyed his marriage to Margaret, left his daughter Sydney fatherless, and left his sister Hester in a constant state of anxiety lest Sydney should start to show signs of her father's tendency to over-react to emotional upsets. In contrast to the earlier nineteenth-century view of the family as a therapeutic and emotionally protective environment,[69] *A Bill of Divorcement* reflects the very widespread tendency in late nineteenth- and early twentieth-century psychiatry to regard the family as a pathogenic milieu for the generation and transmission of all manner of nervous and mental disorders.[70] Yet while Hilary's madness is the ostensible cause of the barely suppressed tensions within the Fairfield family, there are many hints in the play that the real cause of this malaise is not hereditary mental illness brought on by shell-shock, but the more fundamental disturbance brought about by modernity. As Sydney remarks: 'Whenever your generation wants an excuse for anything they blame it on the war.'[71]

In both play and film, we are told very little about the specific characteristics of Hilary's madness, and next to nothing about shell-shock as such. Its status as a psychiatric disorder is simply taken for granted, and no mention is made of any of the medico-psychological controversies surrounding its diagnosis, nomenclature, treatment, and management.[72] Rather, shell-shock is made to function primarily as a metaphor for the fractured and fearful state of British society in the early 1920s, still reeling from the nightmare of the First World War and desperately trying to absorb the full impact of socio-economic, political, and cultural modernization.[73] In 1919, the Prime Minister David Lloyd George is reported to have said that 'The whole world is suffering from shell-shock,'[74] and *A Bill of Divorcement* is a neat expression of this mentality. For its author, shell-shock was a metaphor for the mental state of a society suffering not only from the horrors of war but from a pervasive sense of historical discontinuity, of cultural anxiety and disorientation, and of moral bewilderment in the face of apparently overwhelming and uncontrollable forces of change. As we have already seen, Clemence Dane's concept of modernity was more a state of mind than a broad general process of socio-economic or cultural change, and the narrative of shell-shock and hereditary mental taint in *A Bill of Divorcement* should similarly be interpreted more as a psychological allegory of the tortured relations between past and present and of the traumatic birth of the modern age than as a serious attempt to convey either the medical and social realities or the sufferer's experience of mental illness.

Ironically, though, despite its apparently central role in the play, one thing that seems to have been comparatively unaffected by modernity is madness itself and society's attitude to the care and treatment of the insane. *A Bill of Divorcement* presents a vivid picture of the stigma attached to mental illness, especially in well-off middle- or upper-class households, and of the sense of shame and desire for concealment felt by many relatives of insane people in early twentieth-century England.[75] However, while Hilary Fairfield is portrayed rather sympathetically, especially in the film version, in which he is a talented musician and composer, Clemence Dane appears to have had little sympathy or concern for the mentally ill as a social group. The First World War had to some extent broken down the formerly rigid separation between psychiatry and general medicine and made British psychological medicine more receptive to new ideas and initiatives.[76] But although the early 1920s saw increased public concern for the plight of the insane and widespread agitation for lunacy law reform, *A Bill of Divorcement* contains no echo either of contemporary critiques of asylum practice such as those of Montagu Lomax and Maurice Craig, or of the growing influence of more psychoanalytically inspired understandings of mental disorder and its treatment.[77] It is noticeable that what little we are told about mental illness in the play comes from Dr. Alliot, the Fairfields' family doctor, and that the views of psychiatry as a specialty thus go by default. Even in 1926, by which time she had clearly become more sensitized to the issue of lunacy reform, Clemence Dane could still write that 'Mental death has always had a peculiar horror for the young,'[78] and it is tempting to infer that the odd mixture of fear and pity for the insane apparent in *A Bill of Divorcement* may have sprung at least in part from some as yet unidentified personal experience of lunacy. Be that as it may, even while clearly drawing on the idea of shell-shock as a metaphor for the morbid state of post-war British society and culture, *A Bill of Divorcement* shows no sign of the influence either of any modern medico-psychological approach to the interpretation and treatment of mental illness, or of more liberal attitudes towards the legal restraint and institutional care of the insane. The play makes no concessions to psychiatric modernism, and remains strangely 'Victorian' in its apparently unquestioning belief in the hereditary transmission and incurability of insanity and the need for close confinement of the mentally ill.

PSYCHIATRY, HEREDITY, AND EUGENICS

Although the idea of heredity as an inescapable destiny and more specific notions of hereditary mental taint and the desirability of medical regulation of marriage and procreation on eugenic lines feature prominently in both stage and screen versions of *A Bill of Divorcement,* neither version goes into any detail with regard to genetics. 'It's in our blood, isn't it? . . . Latent insanity brought on by shell-shock?,' asks Sydney when she learns from her Aunt Hester that her father had always been emotionally unstable and that her late Aunt Grace was 'not herself' for many years,[79] but this is the most explicit statement about the presumed hereditary transmission of mental illness made anywhere in either the play or the film. The play refers explicitly to eugenics, when Sydney remarks in an aside that her fiancé Kit, the vicar's son, is 'as keen as I am on eugenics,' and refers briefly to a talk which he is preparing on the subject, but these passages were omitted from the film version.[80] However, Dr. Alliot's stern warnings about the danger of transmitting insanity to future generations survived in their entirety from play to film,[81] and the British and American theatre- and film-going publics can hardly have been left in any doubt as to their clear eugenic message. Indeed, the adaptation of the original stage play for the cinema had the effect of strengthening this particular message. For whereas much of the emphasis in Clemence Dane's play had been on the hypocrisy of conventional religious attitudes towards both madness and divorce and the unfairness of English divorce law, in the Hollywood version these more specifically English legal concerns and the attack on conventional religion were quietly dropped and the more universally interesting themes of the heredity of madness and the eugenic regulation of marriage and procreation were foregrounded instead.[82]

In fact, there is something peculiarly insubstantial and unconvincing about the medical and scientific references in both the play and its screen adaptations. While the supposed hereditary transmission of insanity is absolutely crucial to the plot, no details are provided as to the means of transmission, and no medical or scientific authorities are mentioned in support of this belief, which is simply taken as a given. Clemence Dane's own intellectual and cultural milieu was predominantly artistic, literary, and theatrical, and nothing is known of any medical or scientific associations that might particularly have influenced her or provided the rationale for the play's apparent advocacy of eugenic ideas.[83] Indeed, the more closely one examines *A Bill of Divorcement,* the more one suspects that the author was deliberately setting out to make a name for herself as a serious writer, and that she chose to write about shell-shock, the heredity of madness, and the need for eugenic regulation of marriage and procreation not out of any real interest in or knowledge of these matters, but because of their assumed resonance for contemporary theatre-going audiences. Clemence Dane had already published a novel, *Legend* (1919), about a young woman who renounces marriage in order to care for her celebrated but mentally unstable father in his declining years,[84] and *A Bill of Divorcement* looks rather like a reworking of *Legend* with a little psychiatry and eugenics thrown in for good measure. The medical references in both play and film are the bare minimum required to enable the audience to understand the development and accept the final resolution of the drama, and it is hard to avoid the conclusion that Clemence Dane was referencing psychiatry and eugenics, without really knowing what she was talking about.

For historians of science and medicine, perhaps the most striking thing about the medical and scientific ideas referred to in the play is not their detailed content, but rather the authority which the author chooses to ascribe to them. Particularly significant in this regard is Sydney Fairfield's reaction on learning that her family's hereditary tendency towards mental illness threatens her plans to marry Kit and have children. Although apparently so independent and free-thinking in her attitudes and behaviour, especially towards religion, Sydney only momentarily queries Dr. Alliot's statement of what she takes to be the medical facts about insanity in her family, and when he reaffirms his view, she immediately abandons her plans to marry and have children in order to accommodate this new knowledge.[85] In *A Bill of Divorcement,* Clemence Dane devotes much energy to attacking the outmoded and discredited claims to authority of conventional Christianity, yet she appears uncritically to advocate its replacement by a new scientific authority every bit as absolute and unchallengeable as its predecessor. In this respect, as in so many others in the play, the emancipation promised by modernity turns out to be more apparent than real and decidedly ambivalent in its implications for women especially.

CONCLUSION

A Bill of Divorcement was Clemence Dane's first major work to enjoy commercial success as well as critical notice, and represented a radical new departure from the light West End musical comedy sketches and neo-Elizabethan pageants with which she had previously been associated as an actress. The 1921 stage play ran in the West End for nearly 15 months,[86] and thereafter the name of Clemence Dane was to remain closely associated in the public mind with *A Bill of Divorcement,* not least because of the three film versions made in 1922, 1932, and 1940.

However, *A Bill of Divorcement* has not stood the test of time well, as Clemence Dane herself seems to have realised.[87] Though set in the near future and despite its highly controversial subject matter, *A Bill of Divorcement* was completely conventional in its dramatic form, while in its preoccupation with social and moral questions and its view of marriage and the family as ideal breeding-grounds for neurosis, it seemed to hark back to the social problem dramas of the pre-1914 period.[88] In fact, the stage play was written for a particular time and place and addresses a specific set of issues of concern mainly to upper-middle-class English audiences. Even just a few years later, the play had already lost much of its immediate relevance and had become almost impossible to stage. The 1932 screen adaptation gave it a somewhat extended lease of life by removing the most local and ephemeral concerns from the plot, but even this version now appears old-fashioned and outmoded both in its cinematic style and social attitudes. However, the 1932 Hollywood film version was a prestige production that enjoyed both critical acclaim and popular success at the time, and is still strangely moving even today for its compelling portrait of emotional instability, its tragic sense of human destiny, and for Katherine Hepburn's powerful, if uneven, performance in the role of Sydney Fairfield, a character who embodies much of Clemence Dane's own personality and shares many of her ambivalent attitudes towards feminism and modernity.

But for the medical and social historian, as distinct from the drama critic, classic cinema buff or film historian, the peculiarly ephemeral character of *A Bill of Divorcement,* together with its highly congested social, medical, and political agenda, make both play and film especially valuable as source-materials for the psychological and social history of the inter-war British family. Seen in this light, *A Bill of Divorcement* is of interest and importance precisely because it is so much a product of its time, and because many of its social attitudes so quickly came to seem inappropriate and outmoded. *A Bill of Divorcement* provides a series of vivid insights into middle-class beliefs about the role of heredity in shaping individual character and destiny, the emotionally traumatic effects of shell-shock and modern warfare, the incurability of mental illness, and the moral and scientific authority of medicine, in the early decades of the last century. While the domestic setting of both play and film often seems quite artificial and unconvincing, it does provide a powerful illustration of a family and home environment haunted by the spectre of mental illness, and which itself constitutes a fertile seed-bed for emotional instability. Although most contemporary expressions of hereditarian and eugenic concern about the hereditary transmission of insanity and mental defect concentrated on the threat posed by the 'underclass,'[89] *A Bill of Divorcement* focuses entirely on the effects of hereditary mental taint on an upper-middle-class family. For all its lack of any serious medical or scientific background, *A Bill of Divorcement* serves to remind us just how influential hereditarian and eugenic ideas were, even in supposedly progressive circles, in an era that knew nothing of DNA and clinical genetics nor yet of the horrors soon to be perpetrated by the Nazis in the name of eugenics. And for all its apparently clear-cut rejection of Victorian attitudes and uncritical embrace of the spirit of the new century, its pessimism and poignant conclusion signal deep underlying apprehensions about the impact of modernity on the emotional foundations of British family life.

Indeed, *A Bill of Divorcement* constitutes a prophetic warning of the psychological dangers of modernity and of the destructive effects, not just of modern warfare, but of the whole scientific and sceptical tendency of the modern age, on the ready-made moral answers, reassuring half-truths and false sense of security provided by traditional religion and the institutions of marriage and the family. While its author was deeply committed to the modernist values of openness, freedom of expression, and intellectual and moral honesty, she was under no illusion that greater individual freedom would necessarily bring with it greater happiness, especially for women. Modern women, Clemence Dane seems to suggest, can choose the freedoms offered by modernity, but only at a heavy price in emotional well-being and a sense of security and belonging. The implications of this choice for women's mental and physical health are left unstated, but it is difficult not to infer that modern woman will be freer but probably less healthy and less happy than her forebears. Although its central character appears to represent a modern feminist ideal of strong-minded, independent womanhood, *A Bill of Divorcement* affords few grounds for optimism about the effects of modernity on the health and happiness of young middle-class British women and their homes and families.

NOTES

1. On the psychological impact of World War I on British society and culture in the immediate post-war period, see: Ben Shephard, *A War of Nerves* (London: Jonathan Cape, 2000), Chapter 11; Daniel Pick, *Faces of Degeneration; A European Disorder, c. 1848–c. 1918* (Cambridge: Cambridge University Press, 1989), 231–33. The classic expression of post-war cultural pessimism was Oswald Spengler's *Decline of the West* (1918), which had already been widely discussed before the appearance of Charles Francis Atkinson's two-volume English translation (London: George Allen & Unwin, 1922).
2. See, for example, Douglas G. Browne and E.V. Tullett, *Bernard Spilsbury: His Life and Cases* (London: George Harrap & Co., 1951), 110, 113–114.
3. For wartime changes in women's employment and their political consequences, see Peter Clarke, *Hope and Glory: Britain 1900–1990* (London: Penguin Books, 1997), 90–95, 97–98. For the psychological impact of these changes on men, marriage and family life, see Joanna Bourke, *Dismembering the Male: Men's Bodies, Britain and the Great War* (London: Reaktion Books, 1996), 17–18, 166, 193–95, 200–01.
4. Clemence Dane, *A Bill of Divorcement. A Play in Three Acts* (London: William Heinemann, 1921). The play was written in May–June 1920. See also Samantha Ellis, 'A Bill of Divorcement, London, March 1921,' *Guardian Unlimited* (21/01/2004), 'Curtain Up,' No. 34, at http://www.guardian.co.uk/arts/curtainup/story/0,12830,1127731,00.html. For contemporary critical reactions, see: St. John Greer Ervine, '[Review of] *A Bill of Divorcement*,' *Observer* (20/03/1921), reprinted in A.C. Ward (ed.), *Specimens of English Dramatic Criticism. XVIIIth.–XXth. Centuries* (London and New York: Oxford University

Press, 1945), 282–89; Sydney W. Carroll, '[Review of] *A Bill of Divorcement,*' *Sunday Times* (20/03/1921); Stuart Petre Brodie Mais, *Some Modern Authors* (London: Grant Richards, 1923), 264–69; and Graham Sutton, *Some Contemporary Dramatists* (London: Leonard Parsons, 1924), 46–50.

5. The literature on modernization, modernity and modernism is too vast to be summarized here. But useful discussions are in: Anthony Giddens, *The Consequences of Modernity* (Cambridge: Polity Press, 1990), pp. 4–9, 36–40, 55–63, 137–39, 148; Alan O'Shea's commentary on Marshall Berman's *All That Is Solid Melts Into Air: The Experience of Modernity* (London: Verso, 1983), in Mica Nava and Alan O'Shea (eds.), *Modern Times: Reflections on a Century of English Modernity* (London and New York: Routledge, 1996), 8–13; Roger Cooter and Steve Sturdy, 'Of War, Medicine and Modernity: Introduction,' in Roger Cooter, Mark Harrison and Steve Sturdy (eds.), *War, Medicine and Modernity* (Stroud: Sutton Publishing, 1999), 1–21; Mark S. Micale, (ed.), *The Mind of Modernism: Medicine, Psychology and the Cultural Arts in Europe and America, 1880–1940* (Stanford: Stanford University Press, 2004).
6. This interpretation is indebted to Alan O'Shea, 'English Subjects of Modernity,' in Nava and O'Shea (eds.), *Modern Times* (1996), 7–37.
7. For the 1922 film version, directed by Denison Clift, see the entry in the Internet Movie Database (IMDb), at http://uk.imdb.com/title/n0315291. Malcolm Keen (1887–1970), who had played the part of Hilary Fairfield in the 1921 London stage production, appeared in the 1922 film version in the same role.
8. See the entry for *A Bill of Divorcement* (1932) in the Internet Movie Database, at http://uk.imdb.com/title/tt0022685; the article on David O. Selznick, Katherine Hepburn and *A Bill of Divorcement* on the Turner Classic Movies Website, at http://tcmdb.com/TCMDB/title/title.jsp?stid=68758&tid=6628 &category=overview, and follow the link 'Articles.' The 1932 film version is currently (September 2006) available on home video in VHS (NTSC) and VHS (PAL) format respectively in the U.S. and the U.K. from Video Collection International Ltd. and via Amazon, but not yet on DVD.
9. For the 1940 film version, see the entry in the Internet Movie Database at http://uk.imdb.com/title/tt0032252. Charles Aubrey Smith (1863–1948), who had appeared in the original stage production in the role of Gray Meredith, appeared in the 1940 film version as Dr. Alliot.
10. Both stage and screen versions of *A Bill of Divorcement* naturally lend themselves to a variety of critical approaches and theoretical interpretations. However, in this essay I shall concentrate on those aspects of the drama and the 1932 film version which are of particular interest to social and medical historians of the inter-war British family.
11. Clemence Dane left no autobiography as such, and no full-length biography has yet been published. However, useful sketches may be found in: Leonard R.N. Ashley, 'Ashton, Winifred [*pseud.* Clemence Dane] (1888–1965),' *Oxford Dictionary of National Biography* Vol. 2 (Oxford: Oxford University Press, 2004), 690–92; David Waldron Smithers, '*Therefore, Imagine': The Works of Clemence Dane* (Tunbridge Wells: Dragonfly, 1988); and Janice Oliver, 'Clemence Dane (Winifred Ashton),' in William M. Demastes and Katherine E. Kelly (eds.), *British Playwrights 1880–1956: A Research and Production Sourcebook* (Westport, CT, & London: Greenwood Press, 1996), 97–104. A more entertaining, though not entirely accurate, portrait of Clemence Dane is given in Cole Lesley, *The Life of Noël Coward* (London: Jonathan Cape, 1976), 226–28, 232, 371–73, 446. The National Portrait Gallery holds nine portrait images of Winifred Ashton/Clemence Dane, some of which may be viewed online at http://www.npg.org.uk/live/search/person.aspa?LinkID=mp01182.
12. Ashley, 'Ashton (Winifred),' 690.

13. Clemence Dane, *Regiment of Women* (London: William Heinemann, 1917), reprinted with an Introduction by Alison Hennegan (London: Virago, 1995).
14. See the useful select bibliographies of Dane's writings in: Smithers, '*Therefore, Imagine*' (1988), Appendix, 'The Works of Clemence Dane'; Oliver, 'Clemence Dane' (1996), 103–04; and at http://www.fantasticfiction.co.uk/d/clemence-dane. Clemence Dane's plays were collected and republished as *The Collected Plays of Clemence Dane* (2 vols.) (London: Heinemann, 1961). For Dane's work as a screen writer, see especially her entry in the Internet Movie Database (IMDb), at http://uk.imdb.com/name/nm0199304.
15. For Covent Garden, see Clemence Dane, *London Has a Garden* (London: Michael Joseph, 1964), and for Brighton, *The Moon Is Feminine* (London: Heinemann, 1938). See also Brighton Ourstory Newsletters 11 (Spring 2002), at http://www.brightonourstory.co.uk/newsletters/spring02/presents.htm, for an interesting appreciation of Dane's portrayal of Brighton's artistic and gay/lesbian worlds in the 1930s.
16. For Dane's 1947 Motion Picture Academy Award for 'Best Writing, Original Motion Picture Story,' see the entry for *Perfect Strangers* in the Internet Movie Database and follow the link 'Awards and Nominations,' http://uk.imdb.com/title/tt0037980/awards.
17. Colette (Willy), *La Vagabonde* (Paris: Fayard, 1910). In 1923, this novel was republished and adapted for the stage.
18. Noël Coward, *Blithe Spirit: An Improbable Farce in Three Acts* (London: Heinemann, 1942). This assumption is almost universally made in articles on Dane, although Coward himself does not suggest this anywhere in his autobiography, *Future Indefinite* (London: Heinemann, 1954). See, however, Lesley, *Life of Noel Coward* (1976), 228.
19. See Clemence Dane, *The Women's Side* (London: Herbert Jenkins, 1926).
20. The screenplay writer for the 1932 film version was Howard Estabrook. The action of the film closely follows the order of the original, and much dialogue is taken directly from the play. Unless stated, it should be assumed that all aspects of the plot or incidents of the action referred to in the text may be found in both stage and screen versions.
21. See Dane's prefatory note 'The People of the Play . . . Scene,' *Divorcement*, 1921 edition, which states that 'The action passes on Christmas Day, 1933.'
22. *Divorcement,* Act I, 36. All names in parentheses following the names of characters in *A Bill of Divorcement* should be understood as referring to the actors and actresses who played these roles in the 1932 film version.
23. *Divorcement,* Act I, 27–28, 35–36.
24. *Divorcement,* Act I, 7, 19–21; Act II, 47–48.
25. *Divorcement,* Act I, 27–28; Act II, 60–61; Act III, 74–80. Sydney is not actually engaged to Kit, but they have a mutual understanding and clearly expect to become engaged to be married in the near future.
26. *Divorcement,* Acts II & III.
27. See Clemence Dane's notes on Sydney's character, *Divorcement,* Act I, 4, and Sydney's final speech, *Divorcement,* Act III, 91–92, in which she describes herself and her artistic abilities in terms which might equally well have applied to the young Clemence Dane.
28. *Divorcement,* Act I, 17, 20.
29. *Divorcement,* Act I, 10.
30. *Divorcement,* Act I, 17.
31. *Divorcement,* Act II, 55.
32. *Divorcement,* Act II, 57; Act III, 85.

33. *Divorcement,* Act I, 5. Clemence Dane later described how she herself lost her religious faith in childhood, in *London Has a Garden* (1964), 58–59.
34. *Divorcement,* Act II, 58. In the 1932 film version, the character of the Rev. Christopher Pumphrey was entirely written out and Kit's surname was changed from Pumphrey to Humphreys.
35. *Divorcement,* Act II, 62.
36. *Divorcement,* Act II, 63.
37. *Divorcement,* Act II, 64.
38. *Divorcement,* Act I, 35, 36.
39. *Divorcement,* Act III, 87.
40. *Divorcement,* Act II, 55.
41. *Divorcement,* Act II, 65, 68.
42. This did not escape some critics at the time. See, for example: St. John Ervine, '[Review of] A Bill of Divorcement' in Ward, *English Dramatic Criticism* (1945), 288–89; and Mais, 'Clemence Dane,' *Some Modern Authors* (1923), 265–67.
43. *Divorcement,* Act II, 40.
44. *Divorcement,* Act II, 40–41, 43.
45. *Divorcement,* Act II, 57.
46. *Divorcement,* Act II, 57–58.
47. *Divorcement,* Act III, 85, 86.
48. *Divorcement,* Act III, 86.
49. *Divorcement,* Act III, 87–9.
50. *Divorcement,* Act I, 9, 22.
51. *Divorcement,* Act I, 7; Act III, 87–92.
52. This tendency has also been remarked in other works by Clemence Dane. See, for example, Alison Hennegan's Introduction to the Virago reprint edition of *Regiment of Women* (1995), x–xi. In this respect, though otherwise completely conventional in its dramatic form and staging, *A Bill of Divorcement* reads more like a post-modernist than a modernist work.
53. See, for example, Herbert Farjeon, 'A Divorce Problem,' *Daily Herald* (15/03/1921). In a wide-ranging survey of contemporary debates around the issue of divorce law reform in early-twentieth-century England, Janice Hubbard Harris discusses the Edwardian 'divorce novel' and stage plays at length, but does not mention *A Bill of Divorcement.* See Janice Hubbard Harris, *Edwardian Stories of Divorce* (New Brunswick, N.J.: Rutgers University Press, 1996), 104–49, 191–93.
54. *Divorcement,* prefatory note.
55. *Divorcement,* Act II, 54–55.
56. *An Act to Amend the Law Relating to Divorce and Matrimonial Causes in England,* 20 & 21 Vict., c. 85, s. 27. For historical commentary, see: Allen Horstman, *Victorian Divorce* (London & Sydney: Croom Helm, 1985), 78–79; Gail Savage, 'Divorce and the Law in England and France Prior to the First World War,' *Journal of Social History* 2 (1988): 499–513; and Lawrence Stone, *Road to Divorce: England 1530–1987* (Oxford: Clarendon Press, 1990), 368–382.
57. See: Harris, *Edwardian Stories,* 68–73; and the article on the Commission and its Report on the British Official Publications Collaborative Reader Information Service (BOPCRIS) Web site, at http://www.bopcris.ac.uk/bopall/ref7661.html
58. *Report of the Royal Commission on Divorce and Matrimonial Causes* (Cds. 6478–82) (London: His Majesty's Stationery Office, 1912–13). Both the Majority and Minority Reports agreed that unsoundness of mind or recurrent insanity should constitute grounds for annulment of marriage, though not for

divorce. 'Prolonged and incurable insanity' did not in fact become a ground for divorce for men or women in England until 1937. See Harris, *Edwardian Stories of Divorce,* 157.

59. See the BOPCRIS Web site article.
60. A more complete statement of Clemence Dane's views on divorce law reform is contained in her essay 'Canute and the Marriage Laws,' in *The Women's Side* (1926), 98–116, in which her concern for the equalization of the grounds for divorce between men and women is apparent. In 1922, shortly after *A Bill of Divorcement* was first produced, the Matrimonial Causes Amendment Act did in fact allow women equal rights to divorce on the grounds of adultery. See Harris, *Edwardian Stories of Divorce* (1996), 156.
61. This point was not lost on some contemporary critics: Mais, 'Clemence Dane' (1923), 264; Sutton, 'Clemence Dane' (1924), 47–48.
62. *Divorcement,* Act I, 20.
63. *Divorcement,* Act II, 62–63. In the play, the Rev. Pumphrey has only just discovered that Margaret Fairfield is a divorcée and not a widow, as he had previously supposed, leading to the sudden reversal of his previous willingness to marry Margaret and Gray in church.
64. Dane, 'Canute and the Marriage Laws' (1926), 109.
65. *Divorcement,* Act I, 21.
66. Ibid.
67. *Divorcement,* Act I, 27–28.
68. *Divorcement,* Act I, 29.
69. For the family as a therapeutic environment in early-nineteenth-century psychiatry, see: Akihito Suzuki, *Madness at Home: The Psychiatrist, the Patient and the Family in England, 1820–1860* (Berkeley: University of California Press, 2006); Andrew Scull, 'The Domestication of Madness,' *Medical History* 27 (1983): 233–248.
70. For the family as a pathogenic milieu or 'unit of degeneracy' in this period, see Janet Oppenheim, *'Shattered Nerves': Doctors, Patients and Depression in Victorian England* (New York and Oxford: Oxford University Press, 1991), 277.
71. *Divorcement,* Act I, 11.
72. For debates surrounding 'shell-shock' in World War I, see: Martin Stone, 'Shellshock and the Psychologists,' in W.F. Bynum, Roy Porter & Michael Shepherd, (eds.), *The Anatomy of Madness: Essays on the History of Psychiatry,* Vol. II (London: Tavistock Publications, 1985), 242–271; Elaine Showalter, *The Female Malady: Women, Madness and English Culture, 1830–1980* (London: Virago, 1987), 167–194; Harold Merskey, 'Shell-Shock,' in German E. Berrios and Hugh Freeman, (eds.), *150 Years of British Psychiatry, 1841–1991* (Ashford, Kent: Gaskell, 1991), 245–267; Shephard, *War of Nerves;* Peter Leese, *Shell Shock: Traumatic Neurosis and the British Soldiers of the First World War* (Basingstoke and New York: Palgrave Macmillan, 2002); and Edgar Jones and Simon Wessely, *Shell Shock to PTSD: Military Psychiatry from 1900 to the Gulf War* (Hove and New York: Psychology Press, 2005).
73. See Jay Winter's argument that, in post-1918 Britain, 'shell-shock . . . turned from a diagnosis into a metaphor,' and that 'in a host of ways, Britain has never recovered from the shock of the 1914–18 war': Jay Winter, 'Shell-Shock and the Cultural History of the Great War,' *Journal of Contemporary History* 35, No. 1 (Jan. 2000): 7–11.
74. Philip Gibbs, *The Realities of War* (London: William Heinemann, 1920), 452.
75. The classic source on stigma and mental illness is still Erving Goffman, *Stigma: Notes on the Management of Spoiled Identity* (Harmondsworth: Penguin Books, [1963] 1990). Akinobu Takabayashi (Wellcome Trust Centre for the

History of Medicine at UCL) is completing a Ph.D. on certification, psychiatric commitment, and stigmatization in British psychiatry around the time of the First World War.

76. For contrasting views of the impact of the First World War on British psychiatry, see Stone, 'Shellshock' (1985), 242–48, and Eric T. Dean, Jr., 'War and Psychiatry: Examining the Diffusion Theory in Light of the Insanity Defence in post-World War Britain,' *History of Psychiatry* 4 (1993): 61–82.
77. Montagu Lomax, *The Experiences of an Asylum Doctor: With Suggestions for Asylum and Lunacy Law Reform* (London: George Allen and Unwin, 1921). See also: Clive Unsworth, *The Politics of Mental Health Legislation* (Oxford: Clarendon Press, 1987), 118–31, 172–78: and Kathleen Jones, *Asylums and After: A Revised History of the Mental Health Services* (London: Athlone Press, 1993), 128–134.
78. Dane, *The Women's Side* (1926), 30.
79. *Divorcement,* Act I, 27.
80. *Divorcement,* Act I, 11. On eugenics in this period, see: Geoffrey Russell Searle, *Eugenics and Politics in Britain, 1900–1914* (Leyden: Noordhoff International, 1976); Greta Jones, *Social Hygiene in Twentieth Century Britain* (London: Croom Helm, 1986); and Mathew Thomson, *The Problem of Mental Deficiency: Eugenics, Democracy and Social Policy in Britain, c. 1870–1959* (Oxford: Clarendon Press, 1998).
81. *Divorcement,* Act II, 57–58.
82. For historical commentary on eugenic messages in inter-war English language films, see especially Martin Pernick, *The Black Stork: Eugenics and the Death of 'Defective' Babies in American Medicine and Motion Pictures since 1915* (Oxford & New York: Oxford University Press, 1996).
83. However, some contemporary eugenists and feminists did see the issue of divorce law reform, including the admission of insanity as a ground for divorce, as closely bound up with the achievement of social-hygienic reforms to help improve the quality of the race, and Clemence Dane may well have absorbed this view. See: Montague Crackanthorpe, 'Marriage, Divorce and Eugenics,' *The Nineteenth Century* 68 (1910): 686–702; and Havelock Ellis, *The Task of Social Hygiene* (London: Constable, 1912), 42.
84. Clemence Dane, *Legend* (London: William Heinemann, 1919).
85. *Divorcement,* Act II, 57; Act III, 73–74. Not all contemporary critics found this very convincing: St. John Ervine, 'A Bill of Divorcement' (1921) in Ward, *English Dramatic Criticism* (1945), 287; and Mais, 'Clemence Dane' (1923), 264.
86. Ellis, 'A Bill of Divorcement.'
87. See Dane, *Collected Plays* (1961), Vol. 1, 'Preface,' vii, where she says that she had included *A Bill of Divorcement* (pp. 131–198 in this volume) '[simply] because it was my first attempt at theatre.'
88. Allardyce Nicoll, *English Drama 1900–1930: The Beginnings of the Modern Period* (Cambridge: Cambridge University Press, 1973), 433–34.
89. David Garland, *Punishment and Welfare: A History of Penal Strategies* (Aldershot: Gower, 1985), 142–52; Pick, *Faces of Degeneration,* 176–221.

3 Desperate Housewives and Model Amoebae

The Invention of Suburban Neurosis in Inter-War Britain

Rhodri Hayward

INTRODUCTION

In March 1938, Stephen Taylor (1910–88), assistant editor of the *Lancet* and a rising medical politician, claimed to have identified a new class of neurotic patient.[1] He believed that the familiar figure of the working-class invalid chasing his consoling 'bottle of medicine' had been superseded in the outpatient clinics of London's great teaching hospitals by a new class of well-heeled young women presenting a variety of anxiety states. These women, Taylor argued, 'presented a definite clinical picture with a uniform background': they were in their late twenties or early thirties, cleanly dressed but lacking any sense of zest or glamour. Their permanent waves had been abandoned and their clothes, Taylor noted, adopting the patient's voice, were 'never as smart as the young hussies who work in the biscuit factory.'[2] Their breasts were flabby, their reflexes brisk, and they regaled young housemen with a succession of spurious complaints that included trembling hands, nagging headaches, swollen stomachs, jumpiness, buzzing ears, and insomnia.

Taylor believed that these collected complaints were manifestations of a newly emergent form of psychiatric illness, a 'suburban neurosis' that afflicted isolated young wives in the dormitory estates which had been built across England after the First World War.[3] Almost four million new houses were built between 1919 and 1938 and Taylor claimed that this sudden expansion had created new patterns of living that were fraught with psychological dangers.[4] He believed that the massive growth of owner occupation had combined with collapse of domestic service and the rise of commercialised leisure to create a peculiar new mental climate: a psychopathological atmosphere that was gradually poisoning the newly enfranchised women of inter-war Britain.[5]

Taylor illustrated this toxic process through a mixture of clinical history and character assassination. In his article, he described the life of an archetypal 'Mrs Everyman,' whose journey from schoolroom to suburb was a litany of disappointment and limitation. The brief financial and emotional independence she enjoyed as a shorthand clerk in a Brixton business house was compromised upon her entry into the marital home. The couple's joint savings were spent on 'Mr Jerry-builder's mortgage' and hire purchase furniture, and the sexual promise of the honeymoon squandered by the shocking and disappointing efforts of her inexperienced husband. A year after the birth of her first child she found herself condemned to a life of mind-numbing banality. As Taylor described it: 'She had developed a routine for doing the housework quickly. She had to think a little about the shopping but the cooking she did almost blindly. The *Peepshow* didn't take long to read, the wireless was always the same old stuff.'[6] Faced with a grumbling husband and a fretful child, the smallest provocation was enough to precipitate psychological collapse. In his narrative, Taylor conjectured that the arrival of a public health notice on the dangers of cancer would be enough to crystallise all her worries and fears. Imagined scenes of illness, bankruptcy, and the orphaning of her child eventually developed into a series of real physical complaints. The suburban neurotic was a victim of economic insecurity, cultural limitation, and social isolation.

The pitiful picture Taylor developed in his imaginary case history is now all too familiar to us. The idea of the suburbs as a kind of pathological force was a staple of inter-war literature and remains a standard trope among social historians today.[7] Commentators from J. B. Priestley to Clough Williams-Ellis won a wide audience with their dismal descriptions of the 'dull and monotonous' rows of 'nauseous little buildings' that characterised suburban growth.[8] There was a widespread feeling, as Guy Chapman put it, that Lloyd George's vision of a 'land fit for heroes' had turned out to be an 'Eldorado Banal.'[9] The suburbanite lived out a 'pseudo-human existence' organised around a 'religion of beggar my neighbour' and a 'science of faking and overcharging.'[10] It was a world of 'subtle swindles,' as Orwell's character George Bowling noted in *Coming Up for Air* (1939), a world of 'stockbroker tudor' and ersatz pixie glens, in which desperate men struggled to escape the infectious mediocrity of their suburban homes and wives.[11]

This image of the suburbs as a place of psychic opression remains a persistent feature of modern social histories.[12] Writing in *New Socialist* in 1983, Raphael Samuel claimed that the housewife of the 1930s was:

> less the mistress of her household than its drudge. There was no cook to supervise in the kitchen, no maid to answer the door; in a castle-like social system, she would find it difficult to exchange confidences with the 'daily' even if the family had money enough to employ one . . . On a newly settled estate there would be no relatives within hailing distance, to help out in a crisis or cushion an attack of 'nerves,' no callers to leave their visiting cards . . . in a life so self-enclosed, a visit to the local shops could count as a major expedition, and the visit of the tradesman's boy the principal day time event.[13]

In a similar vein, Ross McKibbin has speculated that the suburban woman of the 1930s was 'confined to the house, frantically raising an ever-diminishing number of children, dependent not upon an easygoing neighbourliness or nearby family network, but upon aspirins to see them through the day.'[14] Significantly, Taylor's report is now reprinted in undergraduate teaching materials and his pastiche praised for its insightful portrayal of suburban conditions.[15] Although uncomfortable with the sarcastic tone of Taylor's analysis, feminist historians such as Judy Giles have celebrated its 'potentially progressive nature,' claiming that its recognition that 'suburban domesticity is the cause of Mrs Everyman's illness contains the protofeminist analysis made so trenchantly by Betty Friedan and Hannah Gavron in the 1960s.'[16]

The power and persistence of Taylor's argument is perhaps unsurprising. His assumption of the atomised housewife's psychological anomie was fostered by critiques of suburban living which emerged on both sides of the Atlantic at the end of the Second World War.[17] In these accounts the modern housewife was depicted as a figure oppressed by a mixture of crass materialism and shoddy urban planning. In the United States, left-wing critics including David Riesman and Betty Friedan developed portraits of suburban domesticity as a kind of mental torture, in which the isolated housewife struggled with her existential emptiness among the wipe-clean surfaces and labour saving technologies of the modern home. In the United Kingdom, sociologists such as Michael Young argued that the migration of working-class families from the bombed out terraces of the East End to the new suburbs and out-of-town estates could be seen as an act of psychological destruction in which networks of friendship and family support were rent asunder by the utopian dreams of the urban planners.[18]

Post-war planning, as Lewis Mumford (1895–1990) noted in 1961, had created a new race of families trapped in space. In these suburban Swiss Family Robinsons, the mother lived out her life, 'surrounded with electrical or electronic devices that take the place of flesh and blood companions . . . her friends, her mentors, her lovers, her fillers-up of unlived life, are shadows on the television screen, or even less embodied voices.'[19] The suburban wife, Mumford noted, might answer these voices but she could never make herself heard. It was left to the sympathetic or psychologically aware historian to recover her voice. As Trevor Blackwell and Jeremy Seabrook insisted in their nostalgic exploration of post-war working class life: 'Those who listened hard might have detected the inner emptiness of the young woman in the new house on the estate in the middle of the morning, reflecting on the desertion of the streets and the bottles of milk on the doorsteps, felt absence of Mam, and burst into tears for no reason.'[20] Although few audiences could have failed to notice the housewife's desperate condition, within popular culture this inner oppression was sometimes conflated with sexual opportunity. The isolation and sadness noted by sociologists of post-war suburbia were re-scripted into a glamorous new persona: in media ranging from television romances to soft pornography and biblical tracts, the suburban housewife was feted as a coquettish neurotic whose alienation and repression only served to heighten her sexual and dramatic promise.[21]

The career of the suburban neurotic—from medical category via social critique to cultural icon—is remarkable and at the same time deeply deceptive. For the ubiquity of the desperate housewife disguises the contingency of her identity and the medical labour that underlay her construction. In the sections that follow I shall argue against the familiar model that portrays suburban neurosis as an emergent phenomenon generated solely through a particular conjunction of urban development, consumer opportunity, and individual psychology and shall suggest instead that its appearance was dependent upon new ways of imagining human nature, pathological anxiety, and epidemic infection that appeared in Britain after the end of the First World War. In particular, I will argue that the peculiar character of the suburban neurotic—her odd mixture of existential emptiness and sexual frustration—arose from the coincidence of two competing models of anxiety championed by rival groups of psychiatrists. Both theories understood anxiety as a form of hysteria. The first model drew upon the psychosexual assumptions of Freudian analysis, portraying anxiety as a biological reaction to the frustration of an animal instinct. The second model rejected this idea of biological frustration and instead depicted hysteria as a failure to achieve an emotional life. From this perspective hysterical anxiety appeared as a form of theatrical display put on to obscure a poverty of feeling. Taylor worked closely with proponents of both theories. As a student at St. Thomas's he trained with Henry Yellowlees (an enthusiastic champion of the new Freudian psychology), while his postgraduate work was carried out as an assistant medical officer at the Maudsley Hospital, whose senior staff worked hard to promote the theatrical model of hysteria.[22] It was Taylor's encounter with these two models and his effective combination of their salient characteristics that gave the suburban neurotic her unique and enduring character.

FREUDIAN PSYCHOLOGY AND THE FRUSTRATED DESIRES OF THE SUBURBAN NEUROTIC

In his description of the pathology of the suburban neurosis, Taylor provided an implicit model of psychological health. Indeed, he argued that the very shape and form of his patients' illnesses could be read as a sketch-map of normal but frustrated desires. As he noted, the patient's 'miserable little story' revealed a complex and 'deep seated aetiology': 'The stomach which swells represents perhaps an unconscious urge to further motherhood, the sleepless nights a longing for a full sex life.' These frustrated animal urges had been made manifest since '[e]xistence in the suburbs is such that the self-preserving, race-preserving herd instincts can be neither adequately satisfied or sublimated.'[23] The normal and healthy woman implicit in these aetiological models was not the prim and subservient figure imagined by Victorian commentators but an altogether more vibrant and primitive creature. Her implied psychology was a Neanderthal confusion of sexual and herd instincts that had been thwarted by contemporary architecture and design.[24]

The story that Taylor constructed would have seemed familiar to inter-war audiences. Doctors, therapists, playwrights, and novelists were keen to remind each other of the unconscious agendas that lay behind the manifestation of women's psychosomatic complaints.[25] Craft teachers and marriage counsellors urged their charges to practice positive sublimation, using pickle making and embroidery to channel the potentially disruptive effects of animal drives.[26] New forms of literary narration and self-experiment encouraged the introspective apprehension of a rich instinctual life, allowing readers to connect their everyday upsets to deeper biological longings.[27] Naomi Mitchison (1897–1999), a prominent feminist novelist and close friend of Taylor, described her own sense of the sexual and herd instincts, complaining that these vital impulses were obscured by the housewife's role. She argued that modern woman is 'several kinds of being.'

> One is the social being, part of the community, with social relationships, and, as this, one is not really an 'I' at all—one is not *whole,* any more than a single bee taken from his hive is, biologically speaking, a true bee at all. The community goes on and is, if not really eternal, sufficiently so for one's needs for immortality: that is the biological side of things. And then one is a personal being, and that includes one's mortal body, tossed about by hormones or emotions or whatever—and all one's apeish longing for closer contact.[28]

This idea of an instinctive self and the conviction that it was the hidden source of individual anxieties rested upon a debateable set of assumptions. It partly originated in Freud's early claim that anxiety should be understood as the physical expression of blocked toxic sexual energy rather than a straightforward reaction to some environmental threat.[29] This claim had been amplified during the First World War. Many British military doctors who were sympathetic to psychoanalysis argued that anxiety should be seen as a form of hysteria in which manifest fears of battle acted as covers for deeper unconscious conflicts. Through this approach cases of shellshock were traced back to unconscious homosexual fantasies and episodes of wartime anxiety were seen as simple rehearsals of older confrontations with violent fathers.[30] The new mechanisms posited in these accounts encouraged a hermeneutic approach to worry, representing it not as a reaction to present difficulties but as an historical sign of thwarted desires and forgotten fears.[31]

The Freudian account represented worry and psychogenic illness in terms of a 'familial romance'; they were seen as reactions to childhood incidents and conflicts with parental authority.[32] Taylor's account of the suburban neurosis, however, went beyond this reductive aetiology. It presented the disorder as a species of environmental illness created and sustained by new forms of domestic and commercial organisation. As Taylor noted, 'It is only when the environment fails so hopelessly that the neurosis becomes manifest,' and he blamed the advent of contraception, the companionate marriage and low maintenance suburban home for generating the mental squalor of the modern woman. As he noted, 'the small labour saving house, the small family and the small friends have left the women of the suburbs relatively idle, they have nothing to look forward to, nothing to look up to and nothing to live for.'[33]

This conception of the suburbs as a toxic environment was a literary commonplace yet it also received intellectual support from the new holistic philosophy of Neo-Hippocratism that was championed by leading physicians after the First World War.[34] These doctors rejected simplistic models of bacterial infection and argued instead that illness was generated through the complex interrelationship between the physical and psychical constitution of individuals and their surroundings. This intellectual position was underwritten by the development of new statistical and experimental techniques that allowed psychological morbidity to be connected to patterns of social organisation.[35]

Statistical evidence for the Neo-Hippocratic model was provided in part by new data on the distribution of illness generated in the administration of Lloyd George's National Health Insurance scheme.[36] In the hands of intellectual sympathisers such as Major Greenwood (1880–1949) of the London School of Hygiene and Tropical Medicine and James Halliday (1898–1983) of the Scottish Department of Health, records on the changing rates of insurance claims were deployed to show how recent social and economic changes shaped the psychopathology of the British population.[37] Halliday argued that manifestation of psychological distress had been transformed in Britain after the end of the First World War. Although old-fashioned hysteria with its intendant aphonias, aphasias, and paralyses had declined, there was a massive increase in psychosomatic disorder and anxiety states.[38] This rising incidence of psychosomatic illness could be attributed to increasing economic insecurity and the 'neglect of innate biological rhythms' as Britain succumbed to the twin forces of urbanism and industrialisation. The psychological effects of these changes, as Mark Jackson has described, could be seen in the rise of affections such as asthma, migraine, colitis, and rheumatism.[39] Moreover, the falling birth rate demonstrated the particular sickness of women when faced with 'the increasing noxious pressure being exerted by the communal environment.'[40] Once a psychological mechanism was assumed, the inefficient operation of just about any biological function could be taken as a sign of wider environmental failings.

Halliday's interpretation of the birth rate transformed individual decisions or problems of particular couples into an index of the nation's psychological health. His position was widely supported.[41] In 1938, the nerve specialist A. J.

Brock (1879–1947) wrote to the *British Medical Journal* complaining that the declining birth rate was a manifestation of the national drift towards race suicide. It could be attributed to the irresponsibility of modern women, who, like the work-shy psychoneurotic, wished to avoid the pains of true labour.[42] With pathogenic infection ruled out as a causative agent, character, culture, and environment emerged as the new sources of illness. This change of perspective, facilitated by the growth of the new statistics, was reinforced by new forms of social investigation. These medical inquiries received their most famous articulation in the 'Peckham Experiment,' which throughout the inter-war period epitomised the new social approach to health.

The Peckham Experiment had started in 1926 as a form of medical club offering 'periodic health overhauls' to some 100 families in south-east London.[43] It was run by George Scott Williamson (1884–1953), an eccentric pathologist, and Innes Pearse (1889–1979), an endocrinologist working at the Royal Free Hospital. Although the initial club collapsed in 1929, their ambition remained undaunted. In 1935, they built the Pioneer Health Centre and over the next five years almost 1,500 Peckham families subscribed as members. This establishment marked a unique departure. Although rival medical centres worked towards the reduction or prevention of disease, Peckham aimed at the achievement of positive health.[44] Although medical treatment of patients was eschewed, the centre provided a mixture of antenatal and infant welfare classes, social activities, and recreational opportunities including swimming, ping pong and roller skating. Although the work and guiding philosophy of the centre have been comprehensively analysed by Jane Lewis and Barbara Brookes, it is worth pausing to recover certain aspects of the Peckham project insofar as it contributed to the conceptual development of the suburban neuroses.[45]

The work of the Pioneer Centre was informed by the same model of human nature that Taylor deployed in his analysis of the suburban neuroses. Indeed, Taylor referred warmly to Pearse and Williamson's efforts.[46] They assumed the existence of a primitive potential in each human being, explaining: 'the Pioneer Health Centre is an experiment in the field of human biology. It is an attempt to study the power or "urge" behind human living, as any physical scientist might set out to study any form of energy in the physical world. The experiment presumes the existence of such an energy or "urge"'.[47] Pearse and Williamson, however, did not base their arguments on contemporary psychopathology.[48] Their approach was holistic and idiosyncratic. They insisted that the basic organism was the family, since the single individual was incapable of reproduction, and only the family could manifest instinctive urge for life.[49] It was a model rooted in the emergent discipline of cell biology, and Pearse and Williamson looked to the amoeba to provide a model of healthy existence.[50] The life of the modern suburban neurotic was characterised by a state of fearful withdrawal, whereas the amoeba demonstated a vigorous engagement with its environment. As Pearse explained:

> When the amoeba encounters food in the immediate environment, the *whole* entity flows towards the attractive morsel; it stretches out its body in the form of embracing limbs—pseudopodia, surrounds the food particle, and, dragging its whole body forward in the direction of its embrace, engulfs the prize. Whatever attracts it, the appearances, to all intents and purposes are identical—an all or nothing type of enveloping action for each and every new experience embraced.[51]

Pearse and Williamson believed that the operation of this amoeboid lust for life and the adverse effects of civilization would be revealed through careful observation of families who joined the centre. After initial consultations and health checks, family members would be granted access to the centre's various social activities, but their use of these facilities was carefully monitored.[52] Ongoing surveillance of the centre families revealed the deformatory effects of modern existence.[53] On first joining, members were shown to be shy and withdrawn and exhibited none of the social and sexual striving that characterised amoeboid life. In *Experiment in Living* (1943), Pearse and her educational assistant, Lucy Crocker, described a fat, flabby, constipated working-class couple, 'Mr and Mrs X,' who in their seven years of marriage had retreated into lives of suspicious disillusion. Their children—a 'furtive,' 'lisping,' 'bedwetting' four year old and a 'listless,' 'sweaty,' 'rubberoid' toddler—brought them little pleasure: 'Night by night,' as Pearse and Crocker noted, 'their long drawn out silences are cloaked in the blare of a thirty shilling loud speaker.'[54]

Pearse and Crocker compared the process to the decay and encystment of the senile amoeba, noting how the modern couple 'encyst themselves in their houses, using them as medieval keeps with the drawbridges up because of their foreboding of their relative incapacity to contact any change in their self-limited environment.'[55] This process occurred when the vital sources of the family's energy—companionship, lovemaking, and home-cooked food—were replaced with the dead world of commercial goods and leisure.[56] It was a natural reaction of any couple who failed to find sustaining social surroundings:

> Out of Nature's ample endowment, the young family builds through no fault of their own, not a rich protean body—a *home* that grows out from the nucleus of parenthood, but a poor hovel of sleeping and eating, breeding and clothing. For all too often the family holds no converse with the outside world; its functional scope is restricted to its own hearth and there is little to sustain and feed its members but what happens within the four walls of the house. Compelled thus by circumstance endogenously to consume its own products, the exploratory tentacles of the family are withdrawn, and, shrunken around its nucleus, there forms a hard resistant crust of suspicion and defence.[57]

The imposition of the metaphorical language of cell biology onto the routines of everyday suburban living turned the mundane events of family life into signs of protoplasmic decay. The Peckham Experiment, as many journalists noted, provided clear evidence as to the nature and extent of suburban neurosis.[58] The unconstrained activity of the instinctive amoeba had thrown the stagnant conditions of modern civilisation into sharp relief.

MAUDSLEY PSYCHIATRY AND THE MAKING OF A MENTAL SLUM

The literary techniques of Freudian novelists, the social epidemiology of the Neo-Hippocratics, and the social experiments of the Peckham Centre all rested upon the assumption of a primitive instinctual life that could provide a benchmark against which to judge the effects of modern civilisation. Yet Taylor remained ambivalent about the generality of the sex and herd instincts, and his description of the suburban neurosis oscillated between the psychodynamic model and a more radically constructivist understanding of desire that had been pioneered by his colleagues at the Maudsley Hospital.[59] Against those commentators who saw anxiety as resulting from the frustrations of desire by the wider culture, the Maudsley group argued that desire and emotion were simple artefacts of this wider culture itself. Increased anxiety, as Taylor noted, had been made possible by the growth of leisure time and the adoption of what he called 'a false set of values.'[60]

Connections between sexual drive and the growth of leisure were often made in the inter-war period. In 1928, Viscountess Rhondda (1883–1958), the feminist editor of *Time and Tide* magazine, complained that the modern woman, despite the advantages of her education, was becoming:

> after a year of two of idle uselessness in the home . . . much the same kind of creature that the leisured girl of 1870 became; she overestimates the sexual side of life since sex appears to be her sole *raison d'etre*—spends half her time thinking about her clothes, regards herself as an inferior kind of creature who is not of sufficient importance in the scale of things for it to matter how she spends her time amusing herself.[61]

A similar analysis was offered by the popular philosopher C. E. M. Joad (1891–1953) in 1932:

> The middle class woman has found her basis of task and function in the home cut away from under her feet. The intensive application of science to the home has reduced domestic work to the performance of a few routine duties . . . Thus she finds herself with time on her hands and boredom in her heart, a drug in the market of society, and gives to sport and sexual pleasure the energies for which the world has apparently no use. Bored, restless and discontented, driven to exploit her sexual attractiveness from

> sheer lack of satisfactory occupation, in the traditional partnership of man and wife the middle class woman is no longer a partner but a passenger—a passenger robbed by science of her functions.[62]

There was little basis for this fantasy image of the bored and leisured housewife and, as economic historians have shown, the actual uptake of labour saving domestic technology was extremely small.[63] As Geoffrey Gorer commented in 1938, the fact that society seemed to be moving from conspicuous consumption to conspicuous leisure only served to conceal the sheer amount of work that the apparently leisured lifestyle involved.[64] Yet Taylor was convinced that the modern housewife was burdened with a new level of physical inactivity and mental opportunity, 'a process,' according to Taylor, 'for which she is completely unadapted':[65]

> At school she was not taught to use her brain for her own amusement. Since then, all the stimuli reaching her not very adequate cerebrum have been designed to inhibit rather than stimulate thought. The papers she reads and the films she sees are all of the "flash in the pan" wish fulfilment variety. The wireless of necessity dare not be provoking. She has no knowledge of what books to read, nor how to set about getting them. The wisdom of the world, if she did but know it, is waiting for her on the station book stall, at six-pence a time.[66]

This concentration on 'false values' marked a new departure. It shifted the basis of Taylor's argument from the psychodynamic models of the new psychology onto the clinical descriptions of British neuropsychiatry. The source of the housewife's neurosis, in this analysis, lay not in her unconscious desires but in the inadequacy of her conscious thoughts. Her emptiness stemmed from the failure of her home life or mass culture to provide the materials capable of sustaining her identity. As Taylor noted, the 'suburban woman has made a fetish of the home,' aping the 'the kind of life successfully led by people to whom books, theatres and the things of the intellect matter'; yet this fetish brought no satisfaction since she failed to realise that these things only became meaningful through their place in a wider culture.[67] The sense of emptiness was exacerbated by her intellectual reliance on the '*Daily Peepshow*' and the weekly cinema: 'In both, she sees continuous, "tempests of emotion"—uncouth marriages of elderly clergymen to young parishioners, torsos daily discovered in trunks, romantic love triumphing over New York's press men, and plumbers made rich beyond dreams by Saturday's football pools.'[68]

From this perspective, the suburban neurosis emerged not so much from the housewife's respectable suppression of her own emotions, but from her vicarious observation of the emotional life of others. Against our modern ideas of suburban repression as the determinative factor in the creation of the desperate housewife, Taylor suggested a radically constructivist model in which the housewife's pathological interiority was itself a pure fabrication: just as her outer environment was, in Taylor's words, 'a tawdry jerry built box', so too was her inner life an artificial construction built out of the cheap and flimsy materials of popular entertainment. Certainly, Taylor did not employ a straightforward psychodynamic view of the emotions. The suburbanite was not struggling with her internal torrents and tempests; rather, the emotions themselves were simply a form of display. 'The objects of the emotions' as Taylor noted, 'are gradually seen through, and the emotions themselves begin to lack conviction . . . The same applies to the failure of conation [i.e. the feeling of will or intention]. The loss of urge to strive is combined with a very reasonable appreciation of the hopelessness of striving.'[69]

Taylor's model of the emotional life becomes clearer if we turn to a paper he wrote in 1940 on 'Mental illness as a clue to normality.'[70] The paper was written as a critique of the artificial categories of psychiatric classification and it reflected a nominalist approach pioneered by his colleagues at the Maudsley Hospital—Frederick Golla, Edward Mapother, and Aubrey Lewis—in the years leading up to the Second World War.[71] Yet within this argument, Taylor provided a sketch of the hysteric that condensed many of the main points developed in his earlier portrait of the suburban neurotic. He argued that it was impossible to know whether the emotions experienced by the hysteric were genuine: as when, to use Taylor's example, 'a wife switches on a torrent of emotion at her late homecoming husband.'[72] The absence of conation resulted in the conflation of her inner life with the superficial thrills of popular culture. As Taylor noted, the 'noble virtues seem to have no place in the hysteric's make up, and instead she adopts a cheap sentimental set of values, clearly reflected in her daily paper, the *Daily Peepshow.* She will weep over a "poor little doggie," yet a war leaves her unmoved. Though she revels in pseudo-distress yet she is completely without shame . . . Her real feelings are as shallow as her emotional expression is extravagant . . . She is a sad creature, knowing neither true happiness nor true sorrow.'[73]

Although the apparent persona of the suburban neurotic might have been shaped by the new Freudian ideas of sexual desire and repression, that new identity itself emerged, according to Taylor's Maudsley colleagues, as new ways of acting and pretending became available. As F. L. Golla (1877–1968), the director of the Maudsley's Pathological Laboratory, had explained in his 1921 Croonian Lectures:

> [the hysteric is] an egocentric individual without strong or durable emotions though anxious to impress the outer world with the gravity and intensity of his experiences . . . The total personality conveys an impression of flimsiness. He appears to be a very different person to the volcano of ill-suppressed sexual passions that some writers on psychotherapy have portrayed. The symptoms of hysteria convey to

the observer a certain general impression of what can be called theatricality—though possibly the stage ill deserves such a comparison.[74]

This disregard for the patient's professed feelings was made possible by the invention of new electro-physiological technologies in the late nineteenth century. Although these were relatively crude devices, measuring physiological processes such as blood pressure or the electrical resistance of the skin, they were understood to have a much larger import.[75] As Otniel Dror has shown, these machines were seen as making visible the emotional interior of the individual.[76] Indeed, machine and emotion were often conflated. Thus, the failure of the apparatus to generate an expected experimental result—a movement of the galvanometer light or a scratch on a smoked drum kymograph—became a demonstration of the emptiness of the patient's professed feelings.[77]

This technological demonstration of the hysterical woman's inner emptiness was endorsed by many of Taylor's colleagues. Aubrey Lewis and Edward Mapother complained that '[u]nsatisfied with their own capacities, [hysterics] seek to cut a better figure than their endowment warrants, and are constantly posing and pretending.'[78] C. P. Blacker concurred, claiming that the outpatients he treated lacked any 'pivotal values' beyond the '*Daily Thought*.'[79] Henry Devine (who taught on the DPM course at the Maudsley) claimed that hysterics, despite their superficial passions, were crippled by 'emotional poverty' and the absence of 'an adequate effective rapport with their surroundings.' Like the rustic gables and clapboard porticos of the jerry-built suburban house, the hysteric presented an image which far outstripped their situation.[80]

Yet if the mind and personality of the suburban neurotic were a slipshod construction from the cheap and flimsy materials of popular entertainment, so too was her theoretical definition. It emerged, as we can now see, at the nexus of two different psychiatric arguments: a neuropsychiatric approach that deployed electrophysiological technology to undermine the neurotic's claim to an emotional life, and a new psychodynamic psychology that insisted upon the disruptive potential of housewives' primitive amoeboid emotions. The tensions between the two approaches were concealed through a virtuoso display of patrician contempt creating a Leavisite, or culturally elitist, psychiatry, in which the failure of the suburban neurotic lay both in the management of her desires and in the achievement of a meaningful interior life.[81] Taylor argued that for such women 'a carefully graded reading list is perhaps more useful than a bottle of medicine,' but this itself was only a sticking plaster solution. The effective prevention of neurosis would require a complete re-engagement with the problems of urban life. Doctors would have to become the 'social architects of the future.'[82] As he concluded: 'We have, I fear, let matters go too far in the jerry-building, ribbon-development to institute an entirely satisfactory scheme of prophylaxis. We have allowed the slum which stunts the body to be replaced by a slum which stunts the mind.'[83]

CONCLUSION

This project of 'mental slum' clearance was to occupy Taylor for much of his subsequent career. During the war he served with Home Intelligence, monitoring and managing the tide of public opinion.[84] The work reinforced his belief that public anxiety could only be tackled through political intervention.[85] In July 1945 he won a seat in the new Labour government and worked as Parliamentary Private Secretary to Herbert Morrison, Lord President of the Council.[86] Yet despite his political involvement, it was not until his parliamentary career had ended in the election of 1950 that Taylor was given an opportunity to become directly involved with the creation of a new kind of urban environment that would be capable of satisfying the animal appetites and emotional emptiness of its inhabitants. This urban utopia was Harlow.

Harlow was one of the fifteen new towns created by the New Towns Act of 1946, although construction did not begin until 1949. Its master planning was under the control of the modernist architect Sir Frederick Gibberd, whilst Taylor acted as one of his commissioners on the board of the Harlow Development Corporation.[87] The design embodied the new social hygiene necessary to combat the possibility of suburban neurosis. The 'emotional poverty' of residents was countered through the formation of an Arts Trust that brought in a resident string quartet and sculptures by Henry Moore and Barbara Hepworth (a corporate raffle prize from the Festival of Britain).[88] Social isolation was offset by the creation of 'neighbourhood units' of between 3000 and 5000 people, which encouraged community interaction and the satisfaction of the population's latent herd instinct.[89] And although many believed that the openness of the new houses' interior and exterior design stifled sexual opportunity (especially the bedroom picture windows), the high birth rate in the young population gave the lie to this complaint.[90] The concept of the suburban neurosis was central to the design of Harlow, yet the new town would ultimately prove to be the concept's undoing.

In 1959, with the support of the Mental Health Research Fund, Taylor began a series of surveys into the psychiatric condition of Harlow's population.[91] He worked with Sidney Chave (1914–85), a post-graduate student who had taken part in the large-scale London School of Hygience and Tropical Medicine (LSHTM) investigation into rates of illness on an LCC estate in Hertfordshire.[92] The Harlow study was set up as a comparator to these earlier investigations. Its aim, as Chave noted, was to see whether 'the social planning embodied in the new town could lessen the prevalence of neurosis when compared with a typical housing estate where such planning is largely absent.'[93] The approach was comprehensive: surveys were made of the rates of admission to local mental hospitals, referrals to psychiatric out-patient clinics, and psychological consultations with general practitioners; market research was undertaken into the inhabitants' satisfaction with the urban environment, and a field investigation was made into self-reported psychiatric symptoms.[94]

The results, as Taylor and Chave admitted, were surprising.[95] Although there was a lower rate of major psychiatric referrals, the rates of primary-care consultation for minor neuroses were roughly equivalent to the rates found in the LSHTM survey, and these again were almost 30% higher than the national averages established by the General Register Office in 1957.[96] Furthemore, psychiatric interviews testing for symptoms of nerves, depression, undue irritability, and sleeplessness revealed that the incidence of reported complaints was similar to the figures produced in Chave's earlier study of Tottenham—the borough from which most of Harlow's population had emigrated.[97] The distribution of these symptoms did not correlate with the image of the anxious young housewife produced in Taylor's original work and cultivated in Young and Willmott's surveys of East London.[98] It was the 45- to 54-year-old woman who was at greatest risk—and the children that had once been blamed for confining the mother to the house were now feted as 'social catalysts' bringing about community integration.[99]

As Chave and Taylor realised, their survey effectively undermined both the psychological claims of new town design and the idea of suburban neurosis from which it had been conceived. They concluded that 'sub-clinical neurosis is not a product of immediate environment' and instead claimed that it was a disease entity 'with its roots deep in the physical or emotional background of the individual.'[100] The problem, as Chave later noted, was not one of urban design but of individual recalcitrance:

> Our search for symptoms has thus enabled us to identify a group of people who displayed the signs of individual and social malaise more than the others. Was this due to the new town? Is this the "suburban neurosis"? The "new town blues" of which we have heard? We think not, we believe that these, the symptoms and the discontents, are all the marks of underlying emotional disturbance; that these are the people who carry their neurosis with them wherever they go and project their inner disharmony upon their environment. But our evidence suggests that such people are to be found everywhere and in about the same proportion if we look for them systematically.[101]

In their reassessment of the suburban neurosis and the psychological limitations of the planned environment, Taylor and Chave transformed the focus of their analysis. They recognised, as many of their peers were beginning to, that economic factors were pre-eminent in the generation of anxiety and that insecurity over access to resources could not simply be removed through education or architectural design.[102] At a deeper level, their identification of a problem group 'who project their inner disharmony onto the environment' restored a certain agency to neurotics. They were no longer the victim of psychological circumstance; rather, they were actively involved in shaping perceptions of their surroundings. This change of role is striking and it reminds us just how silent and quiescent the figure of the suburban neurotic had been. Constructed from conflicting positions in psychiatry and drawn from a patrician suspicion of mass culture, her ephemeral nature was only revealed when psychiatric investigators turned into oral historians and began to transcribe and collate the comments of actual patients.[103] As Ali Haggett has suggested in her contribution to this volume and elsewhere, when the 'suburban neurosis' re-emerged in the 1960s, it was an identity driven less by the problems of the environment than by the availability of new forms of anti-depressant medication.[104]

NOTES

1. On Taylor, see his autobiography, *A Natural History of Everyday Life* (London: The Memoir Club, 1988); 'Lord Taylor of Harlow, MD, FRCP, FRCGP, FFOM,' *British Medical Journal* 1 (1988): 578.
2. Stephen Taylor, 'The suburban neurosis,' *Lancet* (26 March 1938): 759–761.
3. See also [Stephen Taylor], 'Grains and scruples by a Voice in the Wilderness,' *Lancet* (1 and 29 October 1938), 801–03, 1021–22 repr. 'The biology of war and a word on the modern woman,' in Henry Bashford (ed.), *Doctors in Shirt Sleeves* (London: Kegan Paul, Trench, Trübner and Co., 1939), 241–48. On the flight to the suburbs see: J. Burnett, *A Social History of Housing* (London: Methuen, 1986), 254–7; D. Feldman, 'Migration,' in M. Daunton (ed.), *The Cambridge Urban History of Britain* (Cambridge: Cambridge University Press, 2000), 185–206, esp. 202–04.
4. Approximately 2,886,000 private homes were built between 1 January 1919 and 31 March 1939: Marian Bowley, *Housing and the State* (New York: Garland, [1954] 1985), 271, appendix II, table II. Roughly half of these (49.1%) were owner occupied: M. Swenarton and S. Taylor, 'The scale and nature of the growth of owner occupation in Britain between the Wars,' *Economic History Review* 2, 38 (1985): 373–92 (383).
5. On the growth of leisure, see Claire Langhamer, *Women's Leisure in England, 1920–1960* (Manchester; Manchester University Press, 2000).
6. Taylor, 'Suburban neuroses', 759.
7. D. Matless, *Landscape and Englishness* (London: Reaktion Books, 1998), 34–8; R. Colls, *Identity of England* (Oxford: Oxford University Press, 2002), 217–19; D. L. North, 'Middle Class Suburban Lifestyles and Culture in England' (D. Phil. diss, University of Oxford, 1989), 29–39; M. Swenarton, 'Tudor Walters and Tudorbethan: reassessing Britiain's inter-war suburbs,' *Planning Perspectives* 17 (2002): 267–76.
8. J. B. Priestley, *English Journey* (London: Heinemann, [1934] 1984), 92. Clough Williams Ellis, *England and the Octopus* (London: Geoffrey Bles, 1928), 40. For overviews of inter-war suburban contempt: D. L. North, 'Middle Class Suburban Lifestyles,' 41–54; Andrzej Olechnowicz, *Working Class Housing in England between the Wars: The Beacontree Estate* (Oxford: Clarendon Press, 1997), 145–48; Paul Oliver, Ian Davis and Ian Bentley, *Dunroamin: The Suburban Semi and*

its Enemies (London: Barrie and Jenkins, 1981), 27–53, 86–90; V. Cunningham, *British Writers of the 1930s* (Oxford: Oxford University Press, 1988), 256–60.

9. Guy Chapman, *Culture and Survival* (London: Edward Arnold, 1940).
10. Charles Duff, *Anthropological Report on a London Suburb by Professor Vladimir Chernichowski* (London: Grayson and Grayson, 1935), 60.
11. G. Orwell, *Coming up for Air* [1939], (London: Penguin Books, 1998). On 'stockbroker tudor' and suburban architectural taste, see: Osbert Lancaster, *Pillar to Post* (London: John Murray, [1938] 1956). On the dangers of men being infected by their wives' suburban aspirations, see James Hammerton, 'Pooterism or partnership? Marriage and masculine identity in the lower middle class, 1870–1920,' *Journal of British Studies* 38 (1999): 291–321.
12. D. Beddoe, *Back to Home and Duty: Women between the Wars, 1918–1939,* (London: Pandora, 1989); Adrian Bingham, '"An era of domesticity": histories of women and gender in interwar Britain,' *Cultural and Social History* 1 (2004): 225–33.
13. R. Samuel, 'Suburbs under siege,' *New Socialist* (May/June 1983): 29.
14. R. McKibbin, *Classes and Cultures: England, 1918–1951* (Oxford: Oxford University Press, 1998), 82–3.
15. J. Giles and T. Middleton (eds.), *Writing Englishness 1900–1950* (Basingstoke: Macmillan, 2005), 230–9.
16. J. Giles, *Women, Identity and Private Life in Britain, 1900–50* (New York: St. Martin's Press, 1995), 80.
17. Mark Clapson, *Invincible Green Suburbs, Brave New Towns: Social Change and Urban Dispersal in Post War England* (Manchester: Manchester University Press, 1998), 5–16.
18. M. Young and P. Willmott, *Family and Kinship in East London* (London: Pelican, 1957).
19. L. Mumford, *The City in History* (Harmondsworth: Penguin Books, [1961] 1975), 512.
20. T. Blackwell and J. Seabrook, *A World Still to Win* (London, 1985) quoted in Mark Clapson, *Suburban Century: Social Change and Urban Growth in England and the USA* (Oxford: Berg, 2003), 127.
21. Beth Jones, *Satisfied Lives for Desperate Housewives: God's Word on Proverbs 31* (Portage, MI: Valley Press, 2005); Robert Strand, *Desperate Housewives of the Bible* (Mobile, AL: Evergreen Press, 2005).
22. On training with Yellowlees, see: Taylor, *Natural History,* 189. For Yellowlees' promotion of psychodynamic approaches, see his, 'Psychology and medicine,' *Lancet* 217 (1929): 1129–1135 repr. in *Clinical Lectures on Mental Diseases* (London: Heninemann, 1932), ch. 15.
23. Taylor, 'Suburban neurosis,' 760.
24. For discussions of the sexual instinct in British social psychology, see: W. MacDougall, 'The definition of the sexual instinct,' *Proceedings of the Royal Society of Medicine* 7–3 (1913–14): 65–78. On the herd instinct, see: W. McDougall, *An Introduction to Social Psychology,* 23rd ed. (London: Methuen, [1908] 1936); idem, *The Group Mind* (Cambridge: Cambridge University Press, 1920); Wilfred Trotter, 'The herd instinct and its bearing on the psychology of civilised man,' *Sociological Review* 1 (1908): 227–48; idem, *Instincts of the Herd in Peace and War* (London: T. Fisher Unwin, 9th ed. [1916] 1924); R. N. Soffer, 'New elitism: social psychology in pre-war England,' *Journal of British Studies* 8.2 (1969): 111–40; Mathew Thomson, '"Savage civilisation": Race, culture and mind in Britain, 1898–1939,' in W. Ernst and B. Harris (eds.), *Race, Science and Medicine: Racial Categories and the Production of Medical Knowledge, 1700–1960* (Routledge, 1999).
25. F. G. Crookshank, 'Organ States and Emotional Correlatives,' *Psyche* 10 (1930): 65–79; Karin Stephen, *Psycho-analysis and Medicine: A Study of the*

Wish to Fall Ill (Cambridge: Cambridge University Press, 1933), 19–28; A. Blanco-White, *Worries in Women* (London: Gollanz, 1941), 46–47; A. Goodwin, 'The health of a married woman,' *Journal of State Medicine* 44 (1936): 253. For literary examples, see, May Sinclair's characters Anne Magendie in *The Helpmate* (London: Archibald Constable, 1907) and Priscilla Lethbridge in *Life and Death of Harriett Frean* (New York: Modern Library, [1922] 2003). For further discussion, see Rhodri Hayward, 'From Clever Hans to Michael Balint: Emotion, influence and the unconscious in British medical practice,' in Fay Bound (ed.), *Medicine, Emotion and Disease* (Basingstoke: Palgrave, 2006), 144–68.

26. Edward F. Griffith, 'Marriage and family life,' in Noel G. Harris (ed.), *Modern Trends in Psychological Medicine* (London: Butterworth Medical, 1948), 155–56. For interwar notions of positive sublimation, see: Katherine Holden, '"Nature takes no notice of morality": Singleness and *Married Love* in Interwar Britain,' *Women's History Review* 11.3 (2002): 481–504; Alison Oram, 'Repressed and thwarted, or the bearer of the new world? The spinster in inter-war feminist discourses,' *Women's History Review* 1.3 (1992): 413–33; Fiona Hackney, '"Use your hands for happiness': Home craft and make-do-and-mend in British women's magazines in the 1920s and 1930s,' *Journal of Design History* 19 (2006): 23–38.
27. See for example Marion Milner's widely read self analysis in Joanna Field (pseud.), *A Life of One's Own* (Harmondsworth: Pelican, [1934] 1952), esp. Ch. 10.
28. N. Mitchison, *Home and the Changing Civilisation* (London: Bodley Head, 1934), 150. On Taylor's friendship with Mitchison, see his *Natural History of Everyday Life*, 237.
29. S. Freud, 'The justification for detaching from neurasthenia a particular syndrome: the anxiety neurosis,' in *The Standard Edition of the Complete Psychological Works of Sigmund Freud vol. III*, eds. J. Strachey and A. Freud (London: Hogarth Press, 1962), 87–115.
30. Hugh Crichton-Miller, 'Anxiety states: The mother complex,' in Hugh Crichton-Miller (ed.), *Functional Nerve Disease: An Epitome of Wartime Experience for the Practitioner* (London: Hodder and Stoughton, 1920), 120.
31. See: E. Jones, 'The psychopathology of anxiety,' *British Journal of Medical Psychology* 9 (1929): 17–25; W. R. D. Fairbairn, 'Some points of importance in the psychology of anxiety,' *British Journal of Medical Psychology* 9 (1929): 303–31.
32. G. Deleuze and F. Guattari, *Anti-Oedipus: Capitalism and Schizophrenia* (Minneapolis: University of Minnesota Press, 1996), 48–9.
33. Taylor, 'Suburban neurosis,' 761; Taylor, 'Grains and scruples,' 1021.
34. C. Lawrence, 'Still Incommunicable: Clinical Holists and Medical Knowledge in Inter-war Britain,' in Christopher Lawrence and George Weisz (eds.), *Greater than the Parts: Holism in Biomedicine, 1920–50* (Cambridge: Cambridge University Press, 1998), 94–111; David Cantor, 'The Name and the Word: Neo-Hippocratism and Language in Interwar Britain,' in David Cantor (ed.), *Reinventing Hippocrates* (Aldershot: Ashgate, 2002), 280–301.
35. Olga Amsterdamska, 'Demarcating epidemiology,' *Science, Technology and Human Values* 30.1 (2005): 17–51; A. J. Mendelsohn, 'Medicine and the making of bodily inequality in twentieth-century Europe' in Jean-Paul Gaudillière and Ilana Löwy (eds.), *Heredity and Infection: The History of Disease Transmission* (London and New York: Routledge, 2001), 21–79, esp. 33.
36. Edward Higgs, 'Medical Statistics, Patronage and the State: The Development of the MRC Statistical Unit, 1911–1948,' *Medical History* 44 (2000): 323–40; E. Magnello, 'The introduction of mathematical statistics into medical research,' in E. Magnello and A. Hardy (eds.), *The Road to Medical Statistics* (Amsterdam: Rodopi, 2002), 95–123.

37. Major Greenwood and May Smith, 'Some pioneers of medical psychology II,' *British Journal of Medical Psychology* 14 (1934): 158–191; J. Halliday, 'Principles of aetiology,' *British Journal of Medical Psychology* 19 (1943): 367–380.
38. J. L. Halliday, *Psychosocial Medicine: A Study of the Sick Society* (London: William Heinemann Medical Books, 1949), 111–26.
39. J. L. Halliday, 'The rising incidence of psycho-somatic illness,' *British Medical Journal* (2 July 1938): 11–14. M. Jackson, *Allergy: The History of a Modern Malady* (London: Reaktion, 2006), 185–86; see also Chapter 8 in this volume.
40. J. L. Halliday, 'Psycho-somatic medicine and the declining birth rate,' *Lancet* (12 May 1945): 605; Halliday, *Psychosocial Medicine* (London: William Heinemann, 1949), 138.
41. E. Charles, *The Menace of Under-Population* (London: Watts, 1936); essays by Charles and Glass in Hogben, *Political Arithmetic* (London: Allen and Unwin, 1938).
42. Brock, 'Social pathology,' *British Medical Journal* (8/10/1938): 762. On Brock, see: David Cantor, 'Between Galen, Geddes, and the Gael: Arthur Brock, Modernity, and Medical Humanism in Early Twentieth-Century Scotland,' *Journal of the History of Medicine and Allied Sciences* 60.1 (2005): 1–41.
43. I. H. Pearse and G. S. Williamson, *The Case for Action* (London: Faber and Faber, 1931).
44. Jane Lewis and B. Brookes, 'The Peckham Health Centre, "PEP" and the concept of general practice during the 1930s and 1940s' *Medical History* 2 (1983): 152–53; Abigail Beach, 'Potential for participation: health centres and the ideal of citizenship, c. 1920–1940,' in C. Lawrence and A-K. Mayer (eds), *Regenerating England: Science, Medicine and Culture between the Wars* (Amsterdam: Rodopi, 2000), 203–30.
45. Jane Lewis, 'The Peckham Health Centre: An inquiry into the nature of living,' *Bulletin of the Social History of Medicine* 30–31 (1982): 39–43; idem, 'A reassessment of the work of the Peckham Health Centre, 1926–51,' *Milbank Memorial Fund Quarterly* 61.2 (1983): 307–51.
46. Taylor, 'Suburban neurosis': 761.
47. I. Pearse, 'Pioneering in London: the Peckham Experiment,' in [Community Service Society], *The Family in a Democratic Society* (New York: Columbia University Press, 1949), 170.
48. On their neglect of psychological models, see: I. H. Pearse and L H. Crocker, *The Peckham Experiment: A Study of the Living Structure of Society* (London; George Allen and Unwin, 1943), 272–73.
49. See Lewis and Brookes, 'Reassessment,' 313–14.
50. See the posthumous statement in G. S. Williamson and I. H. Pearse, *Science, Synthesis and Sanity: An Inquiry into the Nature of Living by the Founders of the Peckham Experiment* (London: Collins, 1965), 76–84.
51. I. H. Pearse and L H. Crocker, *Peckham Experiment,* 21–22.
52. On the surveillance mechanisms deployed at Peckham, see: David Armstrong, *The Political Anatomy of the Body* (Cambridge: Cambridge University Press, 1983), 36–38.
53. I. H. Pearse and G. Scott Williamson, *Biologists in Search of Material* (London: Faber and Faber, 1948), 47.
54. Pearse and Crocker, *Peckham Experiment,* 249–50; Pearse and Williamson, *The Case for Action,* 32–3.
55. Pearse and Crocker, *Peckham Experiment,* 259.
56. Wellcome Library for the History and Public Understaning of Medicine, Contemporary Medical Archives (CMAC), SA/PHC/D.3/22/1/10 G. Scott Williamson,, 'Homsesteads and Nutrition as the Basis for Industrial Planning' [1945], 2–3; Pearse and Williamson, *The Case for Action,* 52–6.

57. Pearse and Crocker, *Peckham Experiment,* 248; Pearse, 'Houses vs. Homes,' CMAC SA/PHC/e.9; Pearse, 'Pioneering', 182.
58. 'Did your ears burn?,' *Daily Herald* (9 February 1938); 'Science aids the Friendless,' *The People* (19 February 1939); and other cuttings held in CMAC SA/PHC/A.
59. Taylor, 'Grains and scruples,' 851.
60. Taylor, 'Grains and scruples,' 1022; Taylor, 'Suburban neurosis,' 760.
61. Viscountess Rhondda, *Leisured Women* (London: Hogarth Press, 1928), 28–9.
62. C. E. M. Joad, 'The plight of marriage in the jazz age,' in Samuel D. Schmalhausen (ed.), *Our Neurotic Age: A Consultation* (New York: Farrar and Reinhart, 1932), 286–308, 295–96. See also, B. Russell, *The Conquest of Happiness* (London: George Allen and Unwin, 1930), 188–89, 210–50.
63. Susan Bowden and Avner Offer, 'The technological revolution that never was: gender, class and the diffusion of household in interwar England,' in Victoria de Grazia and Ellen Furlough (eds.), *The Sex of Things: Gender and Consumption in Historical Perspective* (Berkeley: University of California Press, 1996), 244–75.
64. Geoffrey Gorer, *Hot Strip Tease and Other Notes on American Culture* (1937) quoted in G. Chapman, *Culure and Survival* (London: Jonathan Cape, 1940), 195.
65. Taylor, 'Suburban neurosis,' 759; Taylor, 'Grains and scruples,' 1021.
66. Ibid.
67. On the equivalence of the home and the interior life in inter-war culture, see: Alison Light, *Forever England: Feminity, Literature and Conservatism between the Wars* (London: Routledge, 1991), pp. 121–28; J. Giles, 'A home of one's own: Women and domesticity in England, 1918–1950,' *Women's Studies International Forum* 16.3 (1993): 239–55; idem, *Women, Identity and Private Life in Britain, 1900–50* (New York: St, Martins Press, 1995), 141–4; Claire Langhammer, 'The meanings of home in post-war Britain,' *Journal of Contemporary History* 40.2 (2005): 341–62.
68. Taylor, 'Suburban neurosis,' 760.
69. Ibid., 761.
70. S. Taylor, 'Mental illness as a clue to normality,' *Lancet* 238 (1940): 677–80, 730–4.
71. E. Mapother, 'Tough or tender? A plea for nominalism in psychiatry,' *Proceedings of the Royal Society of Medicine* 27 (1934): 1687–1712. For commentary: R. Hayward, 'Making psychiatry English: The Maudsley Hospital and the Munich model,' in Volker Roelcke and Paul Weindling (eds.), *Inspiration, Co-operation, Migration: British-American-German Relations in Psychiatry, 1870–1945* (Rochester: University of Rochester Press, forthcoming).
72. Taylor, 'Mental illness as a clue to normality,' 731.
73. Ibid., 731–32.
74. F. L. Golla, 'The objective study of neurosis,' *Lancet* (20 August 1921): 377.
75. Otniel E. Dror 'The affect of experiment: The turn to emotions on Anglo-American physiology, 1900–1940.' *Isis* 90 (1999): 205–237; Robert Frank, 'The telltale heart: Physiological instruments, graphic methods and clinical hopes, 1854–1914,' in William Coleman and Frederic Holmes (eds.), *The Investigative Enterprise: Experimental Physiology in Nineteenth-Century Medicine* (Los Angeles: University of California Press, 1988).
76. Otniel E. Dror 'Techniques of the brain and the paradox of emotions, 1880–1930,' *Science in Context* 14.4 (2001): 643–60; Otniel E. Dror, 'The scientific image of emotion: experience and technologies of inscription,' *Configurations* 7 (1999): 355–401; Rhodri Hayward, 'The tortoise and the love-machine: Grey Walter and the politics of electro-encephalography,' *Science in Context*

14.4 (2001): 615–641; Geoff Bunn 'The lie detector, Wonder Woman and liberty: the life and work of William Moulton Marston,' *History of the Human Sciences* 10 (1999): 91–119.
77. F. L. Golla, 'The organic basis of the hysterical syndrome,' *Proc. RSM (Section of Psychiatry)* 16 (1923): 1–13; A. D. Waller, 'The measurement of human emotion and of its voluntary control,' *Proceedings of the Royal Society of Medicine* 13 (1919–20): 41–56; Eric Wittkower, 'Studies on the influence of emotions on the functions of the organs,' *Journal of Mental Science* 81, (1935): 533–682.
78. A. Lewis and E. Mapother, 'Psychological medicine,' in F. W. Price (ed.), *A Textbook of the Practice of Medicine,* 5th ed. (London: Oxford University Press, 1937), 1870.
79. C. P. Blacker, *Human Values in Psychological Medicine* (Oxford: Oxford Medical Publications, 1932), 80, 84.
80. H. Devine, *Recent Advances in Psychiatry* (London: J. & A. Churchill, 1929), 86; D. K. Henderson and R. D. Gillespie, *A Textbook of Psychiatry* (Cambridge: Cambridge University Press, [1927] 1956), 154–55.
81. North, 'Middle-class suburban lifestyles,' 315–20.
82. Taylor, 'Grains and scruples,' 802.
83. Taylor, 'Suburban neurosis,' 761.
84. Ian McLaine, *Ministry of Morale: Home Front Morale and the Ministry of Information in World War II* (London: Allen and Unwin, 1979).
85. S. Taylor, *Battle for Health: A Primer of Social Medicine* (London: Nicholson and Watson, 1944), 123–24; S. Taylor, 'Socialism and public opinion,' in David Munro (ed.), *Socialism: The British Way* (London: Essential Books), 223–55. On links between the Labour party programme of social and psychological reconstruction, see: Stephen Fielding, 'To make men and women better than they are? Labour and the building of socialism in the 1940s,' in J. Fyrth (ed.), *Labour's Promised Land? Culture and Socieity in Labour Britain, 1945–51* (London: Lawrence and Wishart, 1995), 16–25; J. Nuttall, *Psychological Socialism: The Labour Party and the Qualities of Mind and Character* (Manchester: Manchester University Press, 2006).
86. Taylor, *Natural History,* 393–95.
87. Sir Frederick Gibberd, *Harlow New Town: A Plan Prepared for Harlow Development Corporation* (London: HMSO, 1947).
88. Taylor, *Natural History,* 397–98.
89. Mark Llewellyn, 'Producing and experiencing Harlow: Neighbourhood units and narratives of New Town life 1947–53,' *Planning Perspectives* 19 (2004): 155–74.
90. J. Attfield 'Inside pram town: A case study of Harlow house interiors, 1951–61,' in J. Attfield and P. Kirkham (eds.), *A View From the Interior: Feminism, Women and Design* (London: The Women's Press, 1989), 215–37; Taylor, *Natural History,* 397–98.
91. See Sidney Chave, 'Making the Plan' [Diary], CMAC: GC/178/A2/1.
92. M. Warren, 'Prologue: an appreciation of Sidney Chave,' in M. Warren and H. Francis (eds.), *Recalling the Medical Officer of Health: Writings by Sidney Chave* (London: King Edward's Hospital Fund, 1987), 15–18; F. M. Martin, J. H. F. Brotherston, and S. P. W. Chave. 'Incidence of neurosis on a new housing estate,' *British Journal of Preventative and Social Medicine* 11 (1957): 196–202.
93. S. Chave, 'Mental health in Harlow New Town,' *Journal of Psychosomatic Research* 10 (1966): 39.
94. S. Taylor and S. Chave, *Mental Health and Environment* (London: Longmans, 1964).

95. Sidney Chave 'Diary' (Wellcome CMAC: GC/178/A.2/10). Entry for 5 September.
96. W. P. D. Logan and A. Cushion, *Morbidity Statistics from General Practice 1* [General Studies on Medical and Population Subjects no. 14] (London: HMSO, 1958).
97. J. H. F. Brotherstone and S. P. W. Chave, 'General practice on a new housing estate,' *British Journal of Preventative and Social Medicine* 10 (1956): 200–07; F. M. Martin, J. H. F. Brotherstone, and S. P. W. Chave, 'Incidence of neurosis in a new housing estate,' *British Journal of Preventative and Social Medicine* 11 (1957): 196–202; [Anonymous], 'Suburban neurosis up to date,' *Lancet* (18 January 1958): 146–47.
98. Young and Willmott, *Family and Kinship*, pp. 147–64; H. V. Dicks, 'The Predicament of the Family in the Modern World,' *Lancet* (5 February 1955): 295–97.
99. Taylor and Chave, *Mental Health and Environment*, 125–26.
100. Ibid., pp. 169, 168.
101. Chave, 'Mental health in Harlow New Town,' 43.
102. As Harlow's doctors commented, anxiety states 'tend to be self-curing as hire purchase payments come to an end,' C. Taylor et. al, 'The health centres of Harlow: An essay in cooperation,' *Lancet* (22 October 1955): 863.
103. For examples of suburban contentment in comparison to other housing, see: [Mass Observation/Advertising Service Guild], *An Enquiry into People's Homes* (London: John Murray, 1943): 178, 191; Stella Instone, 'The Welfare of the Housewife,' *Lancet* (4 December 1948): 899–901; Dagmar Wilson, 'Surveying the Housewife,' *Public Health* 62 (1949): 139–42
104. See: Chapter 5 in this volume; Ali Haggett, 'Housewives, neuroses and the domestic environment, 1945–70,' PhD thesis, University of Exeter, 2007. See also: Christopher M. Callahan and German E. Berrios, *Reinventing Depression: A History of the Treatment of Depression in Primary Care* (New York: Oxford University Press, 2005); Nikolas Rose, 'Neurochemical Selves,' *Society* (November/December, 2003): 46–59.

4 Anne Sexton's Poetics of the Suburbs

Jo Gill

INTRODUCTION

> 'I am actually a "suburban housewife" only I write poems and am sometimes a little crazy.'[1]

In this characteristically nuanced and deceptive declaration, the American poet Anne Sexton (1928–74) first posits, then complicates, and finally demurs from a particular personal identity. The defiant main clause (beginning 'I am actually') aims for clarity, as though to explain once and for all who she is. But the scare quotes around 'suburban housewife' signal a degree of unease with the label and its perceived signification, and the conjunctions ('only') and diminutives ('sometimes a little') that herald the subordinate clauses further undermine the certainty of the original assertion. In this way, Sexton acknowledges—albeit tacitly—the complexity of the contradictory parts that she is required to play and the difficulty that she has in reconciling them. As she goes on to explain: 'I fear I am not myself here in my suburban housewife role.' Sexton's assertion assumes and thereby leaves implicit a causal connection between place, gender, occupation, and mental health. It is this assumption to which Sexton's work returns again and again, and which is the subject of this chapter.

Taking the ambivalence of Sexton's self-description as its starting point, this chapter explores the relationship between space, gender, history, and subjectivity in Anne Sexton's poetry, drawing particular attention to the construction and representation of suburban identity in her work.[2] Where confessional poetry has typically been read as focusing on the subject's inner life, or the landscape of the mind, I will suggest that Sexton's writing deviates from this model, valorising instead a distinct, unexpected, and poetically fertile locale. For Sexton, the American suburbs represent both a literal place and a figurative space, one whose meanings and parameters have to be constantly negotiated and repeatedly tested in order fully to accommodate the multiple identities (housewife, poet, and madwoman) that she proposes to install there.

Her poetry shows us a historically specific suburban world of open-plan lounges and modern kitchen appliances, of picture windows, backyards, and barbecues. Against this backdrop, Sexton presents a world of intense neighbourliness, high-pressure childrearing, carefully demarcated gender roles, and highly vulnerable marriages. The 1972 poem 'The Risk' presents us, in just twelve lines, with a picture of suburban domesticity in crisis where 'a daughter tries suicide,' 'the kitchen blows up its shiny kettle / and the vacuum cleaner swallows its bag.'[3] The mother in this poem—stereotypically the dominant figure in the feminised suburbs—collapses onto the 'marriage bed' in an abject state of self-destruction. The 1973 sequence 'The Divorce Papers,' written while Sexton was preparing to divorce her husband Kayo, paints a similar picture. The accoutrements of the average suburban life—of wedding rings and children, vacations and kitchens, of televisions, aprons, washers and driers—are juxtaposed in surreal and disturbing ways.[4] Marsha Bryant has noted the same strategy in the work of Sexton's contemporary, Sylvia Plath. In both cases, the effect is to illuminate the 'unstable boundaries of postwar domesticity.'[5]

The post-war American suburbs, whose growth was intended to meet the needs of a rising marriage and birth rate, were designated by planners and critics alike as female spaces. They were conceived and built according to—arguably distorted—expectations of what women wanted. Kenneth T. Jackson explained the design of houses in the prototype of post-war suburban architecture, Levittown: 'the floor plan was practical and well-designed, with the kitchen moved to the front of the house near the entrance so that mothers could watch their children from kitchen windows and do their washing and cooking with a minimum of movement. Similarly, the living room was placed in the rear and given a picture window overlooking the backyard.'[6] From these early days, though, there was concern among commentators about the effects of suburban development on the experiences and behaviours of its occupants. In 1967, President Johnson commissioned a task force to report on suburban problems—the most 'pervasive' and 'elusive' of contemporary concerns, according to Senator Edmund S. Muskie, one of the task force's participants.[7] According to Kenneth T. Jackson, by the 1960s critics such as Betty Friedan had 'challenged the notion that the dream home was emotionally fulfilling for women.' Jackson cites Gwendolyn Wright's observation that suburban housewives' 'isolation from work opportunities and from contact with employed adults led to stifled frustration and deep psychological problems.'[8]

This chapter begins by examining the rhetorical and metaphorical uses to which Sexton puts this profoundly ambivalent space, for example, in poems that depict the self in the modern suburban home as dislocated and fragmented or in poems that devise a complex rhetoric of voyeurism and display entirely appropriate to contemporary suburban experience. It goes on to consider Sexton's suburban poems in their particular historical moment. Deborah Nelson has convincingly argued that the ascendance of the confessional mode of poetry with which Sexton has habitually been associated coincided with two key factors: the emergence of the suburbs as the apotheosis of American living; and the pervasiveness in Cold War America of a culture of anxiety, hostility, and surveillance.[9] Nelson showed that Sexton's work was produced and read within an environment that was characterised by suspicion and that bestowed contradictory messages about privacy and community. These messages were, in turn, replicated, affirmed, and re-circulated in the new architecture of the period with its open-plan layouts and picture windows. Both of these seemed to invite association and deny privacy (or to assert the 'visibility principle,' as contemporary observer William M. Dobriner put it) while functioning to enforce strict geographical, gender, and familial boundaries.[10]

An important hypothesis pursued throughout this chapter is that there is a productive relationship between the profound self-reflexivity that I perceive to be characteristic of Sexton's work and its suburban origins.[11] My point is that the self-consciousness of her writing (its awareness, in particular, of its relationship with its audience, its concerns about truth and deception, its anxiety about personal revelation) replicates a wider self-consciousness about privacy and surveillance, about seeing and being seen, and about social and gender conformity that characterised suburban domestic life during her lifetime.

The historical facts of Sexton's suburban origins have been noted by others, primarily as an accusation, as a way of signalling the domestic nature of her art, or as a way of showing what the suburbs 'did' to women of the *Feminine Mystique* generation.[12] Such readings have situated Sexton in a passive relationship with these discourses. In contrast, I will argue that Sexton actively, persistently, and consciously—albeit often with considerable ambivalence—evoked the suburbs as the site of her poetry, as the source of her poetic voice, and as a badge of difference with which to counter dominant metropolitan and masculine literary models. Although in some of her poems contemporary ideologies of the suburbs were implicated in the growing psychological crisis of the female subject, in others the suburbs offered familiarity, security, and a vantage point that could be used to her benefit.

SUBURBAN FLIGHT

Anne Sexton was raised in some style on the outskirts of Boston and spent the summers at her grandparents' affluent home on the Massachusetts coast, a place that was immortalised in 'Funnel,' discussed later in this chapter. She moved to the new suburbs of Boston, as did so many others of her generation, as a young housewife and mother and took sporadic jobs outside the home (selling cosmetics door to door, for instance). However, with her husband away for long periods of time as a salesman, she remained in the suburbs as the main home maker.[13]

Throughout her adult life, Sexton experienced periods of profound psychological trauma that resisted firm diagnosis. Her illness was apparently precipitated by post-partum depression and was first labelled 'hysteria' and subsequently a form of manic depression. It was characterised at different times by a variety of symptoms including dissociation, fugue states, deep depressions, and suicidal impulses.[14] Her treatment included sustained psychotherapy, medication with Thorazine and lithium, and repeated periods of hospitalisation or visits to the 'summer hotel,' as Sexton put it, arguably parodying the middle-class ritual whereby mothers and children escaped from the suburban home for the long summer vacations while the fathers continued to commute into the city to work.[15] Sexton's psychiatric condition was complicated over the years by her growing dependence on alcohol and sleeping pills.[16] Lori Rotskoff has analysed changes in attitudes towards, and the consumption of, alcohol in post-Prohibition, post-World War Two America. In this period, which saw a change from alcoholism being regarded as a moral sin, to alcoholism being regarded as a form of sickness, the proper place for moderate 'healthy' drinking was in the 'domestic sphere, in the private homes of men and women.'[17] The culture of suburbia encouraged conformity in this respect. As Rotskoff put it, quoting a contemporary critic: 'suburbia was a place where everyone "buys the right car, keeps his lawn like his neighbour, eats crunchy breakfast cereal, and votes Republican." He might have added "and drinks the same drinks"'. During the 1950s and 1960s there was growing concern among a small group of alcoholism experts that 'domesticity itself could be a major source of discontent leading to alcoholism.' For some suburban women, it was becoming increasingly clear, 'domestic pressures and dissatisfactions could cause excessive or pathological drinking.'[18]

Sexton began to write poetry in 1957 after her first severe adult breakdown. This was in part at the suggestion of her therapist; Sexton's extreme circumstances notwithstanding, the turn to psychiatric therapy and other forms of expert guidance was a defining feature of the time and place.[19] However, her interest in poetry was also stimulated by seeing the literary critic I. A. Richards in a PBA television programme about the sonnet. The widespread introduction of television sets into the suburban home was also a characteristic of this period and, according to Deborah Nelson, implicated in unsettling the boundaries between private and public spheres. As Lewis Mumford explained in his 1961 book *The City in History*, the suburban housewife lived an isolated existence: 'surrounded with electrical or electronic devices that take the place of flesh and blood companions: her real companions, her friends, her mentors, her lovers, her fillers-up of unlived life, are shadows on the television screen, or even less embodied voices.'[20]

Sexton was an acquaintance of the poets Robert Lowell and Sylvia Plath. She commented in her brief memoir of Plath, 'We did grow up in the same suburban town . . . but she was about four years behind me and we never met.'[21] However, there were significant differences among the three poets, not least Lowell's association with the metropolis and with Brahmin Boston culture, and Plath's escape from the American suburbs via New York (immortalised in her novel *The Bell Jar*) and England.[22] Although Sexton has typically been compared with Lowell, I argue that one of the ways in which she resisted the association was by a conscious recognition and articulation of the different spaces that each inhabited, as for example in her poem 'Man and Wife,' her response to his 'To Speak of Woe that Was in Marriage,' discussed later.

Sexton's move to the suburbs in 1953 was entirely characteristic of her generation of young American newlyweds. As Gordon, Gordon, and Gunther noted in their 1961 book *The Split-Level Trap:* 'Between 1950 and 1959, nearly two-thirds of [America's] increase appeared in the suburbs; the central cities . . . increased in population by about 1½% during those years; the suburbs increased 44%.'[23] Like so many other 'babyboomers,' the Sextons settled first in one suburb, Newton Lower Falls, and then in another. In 1964 they moved to a new house—'a two-story modern colonial' in a 'better neighbourhood, with better schools nearby.'[24] William M. Dobriner cites the 'better-for-children' rationale as one of the key factors in contemporary flight from the cities to the suburbs. However, as his case studies show, 'better-for-children' sometimes masks the desire among those he questioned either to raise children away from urban Black populations or, in the case of Jewish and Catholic respondents, within the same 'ethnic and religious community.'[25]

Suburban flight was, then, almost exclusively a White phenomenon. According to Elaine Tyler May, although the suburban population more than doubled between 1950 and 1970, 'blacks were excluded from the suburbs by *de facto* segregation and the FHA's [Federal Housing Authority's] redlining policies.'[26] Many of the poems in Sexton's first collection, rather like those in Lowell's first avowedly 'confessional' work *Life Studies,* take as their ostensible subject a particular kind of privileged White American up-bringing or, more specifically, the threats to its stability and status as turn-of-the century standards gave way to Depression years, to the economic growth stimulated by America's role as supplier to the Second World War effort, and to the retrenchment and counter-cultural movements of the Cold War era.[27]

The unease evident in Lowell's and Sexton's work of this period mimicked the larger tensions generated in contemporary society by contradictory imperatives on the one side to modernise and prosper and on the other to retain the standards and mores of the past. During the late 1950s and 1960s this was experienced, as Joan Didion explained in her account of the birth of the hippy movement in the Haight-Ashbury area of San Francisco, as a new kind of 'generational rebellion'—one with a profoundly ideological basis. The hippy movement, for Didion, was 'not a traditional generational rebellion. At some point between 1945 and 1967 we had somehow neglected to tell these children the rules of the game we happened to be playing . . . Maybe there were just too few people around to do the telling. These were children who grew up cut loose from the web of cousins and great-aunts and family doctors and lifelong neighbors who had traditionally suggested and enforced the society's values.'[28] Gordon, Gordon, and Gunther observed that 'emotional breakdowns . . . occur vastly more often in the mobile suburbs than in integrated communities.'[29] It was to this historical, generational, ideological, gender, and, one might add, geographical upheaval that many of Sexton's poems addressed themselves.

Sexton's early poem 'Funnel,' probably written in 1958, registers the emotional and material disappointment attendant on the move from the city to the suburbs, from the extended to the nuclear family, from the traditions of the past to the uncertainties of the present.[30] 'Funnel' records the containment and mediocrity of modern suburban life, particularly when contrasted with the freedom and abundance of the past. It opens with an account—Biblical in its idiom and heroic in its proportions—of the scale and importance of the past:

> The family story tells, and it was told true,
> of my great-grandfather who begat eight
> genius children and bought twelve almost new
> grand pianos

But from this expansive opening (the mouth of the 'funnel'), the poem begins to retract and diminish. The hyperbolic adjectives of these opening lines are replaced with weaker, lesser ones: 'hushed, 'marginal,' 'musted.' The grandeur of the past (the family of 'eight children,' the extensive grounds planted with 'thirty-six pines,' the confidence with which the patriarch or 'bearded man' surveys his domain with 'giant steps') gives way to the mediocrity of present-day life in the suburbs:

> Back from that great-grandfather I have come
> to puzzle a bending gravestone for his sake,
> to question this diminishing and feed a minimum
> of children their careful slice of suburban cake.

Sexton referred to poetry as a life line, as a means of escape from the debilitating conditions of suburbia or 'disturbia' as *The Split-Level Trap* labels it.[31] To the poet Oscar Williams she wrote on her receipt of a generous travel award: 'I am off this August (out of the suburbs as you always told me, as you always told me I must go out of the suburbs).'[32] In a similar context, she wrote of her need to be 'unchained' from her everyday life.[33] To Fred Morgan, editor of *The Hudson Review,* who had accepted some of her early poems, she wrote: 'I would be here in the suburbs and going nowhere if it weren't for such as you.'[34] And to poet Carolyn Kizer she confided, 'I would be no one at all without my new tight little world of poet friends. I am kind of a secret beatnik hiding in the suburbs in my square house on a dull street.'[35] Her comments confirm Lewis Mumford's point: 'Beginning as a mechanism of escape, the suburb has turned into its very opposite.'[36]

Nevertheless, the suburbs were elsewhere—and this is a crucial contradiction both in Sexton's representation of the suburbs and in their very nature—depicted as a sanctuary, as a welcome relief from the frightening conditions of urban life. Sandy Robartes, one of Sexton's neighbours who was dragooned into accompanying her into Boston for her Robert Lowell poetry classes, explained that at first Sexton was too frightened to leave her own house. Sexton's biographer commented that 'Anne, who still panicked when she had to walk alone on a city sidewalk, liked being able to run across the lawns' to see her suburban neighbours.[37] The suburbs, then, were simultaneously a prison and a haven.

In her life and her work, Sexton manipulated readerly expectations of the role of suburban housewife and mother, provisionally identifying with that label and then utterly traducing its efficacy. She did this by the sardonic or despairing tones of the poems discussed later. Interestingly, too, she did it visually in her use of photographic portraits and public performances of her work. In both cases she exploited to great effect the transgressive value of the apparently passive suburban housewife turning and assertively speaking. Arthur Furst conceded as much in his introduction to *Anne Sexton: The Last Summer,* the book of still photographs that he took at Sexton's home in the summer of 1974 and published in 2000. Furst, like others before him, noted the discursive impact of the incongruity he perceived between Sexton's suburban setting and demeanour and the anger, sexuality, and explicitness of the poems:

> Anne was sitting at her kitchen table, amid the gingerbread men and women of her wallpaper and matching curtains, her back to the refrigerator, the message board and phone . . . Virginia Slims, lighter and ashtray were positioned in front of her. Her hair was carefully coiffed, and she was wearing a silk blouse and slacks. It was the dark side of the 1960s image of a homemaker, if you could imagine Betty Crocker composing "The Fury of Cocks" and "When Man Enters Woman."[38]

It is the body rather than the text that is subject to interpretation here, that is being read. This was also the case in response to Sexton's physical appearance in staged readings of her work. William Pritchard reported of a Sexton performance: 'she read with spellbinding intensity, to the extent that one wasn't quite sure just what one was responding to—the poems? Or something else—the life that was all tied up with them.'[39]

Sexton's flamboyant championing of the suburbs marked a defiant assertion of poetic identity, a self-conscious annexing of this implicitly gendered place and of the complex perspectives, relationships, experiences that it represented. Moreover, the modern home provided a rich source of metaphor, in particular giving Sexton the means to explore and critique some of the tensions and contradictions of contemporary women's experience. *The Feminine Mystique* had so recently shown that beneath the public face of the 'suburban housewife' lay a private narrative of violence, breakdown, failure and resentment, a secret life that Sexton's poetry explored.[40] As an example of Sexton's self-positioning or perhaps self-invention as suburban housewife and poet I want to examine one poem in particular, 'Man and Wife.' I will then turn to other poems that represent the female self in the modern suburban home as dislocated, fragmented and split ('Self in 1958') or as inauthentic ('Housewife'), and to poems that figure the female confessional subject as food, as offering herself up in and to a culture that overvalues consumption ('The Death Baby').

'MAN AND WIFE'

The title 'Man and Wife' alludes to the Christian marriage service and already signals the loss of identity for the woman who is here no longer 'woman' but 'wife,' defined by her relationship with the man.[41] Moreover, the title and epigraph, '*To speke of wo that is in marriage,*' look back both to Chaucer's 'Wife of Bath's Prologue' and to Robert Lowell's poems 'Man and Wife' and 'To Speak of the Woe that is in Marriage' (both from his 1959 volume *Life Studies*). Here Lowell's metropolitan milieu (Marlborough Street in Boston, and New York's Greenwich Village) is defiantly countered by the modern suburban landscape of Sexton's experience. Sexton's poem diagnoses the condition of married life in the suburbs as one of alienation, dislocation, and despair. Idealistic expectations of marriage as a union of love, or companionship, or, failing that, of bare familiarity, are emphatically exposed. We should note the disclaimers, negations, and denials ('not lovers,' 'not even,' 'nothing') in these opening lines:

> We are not lovers.
> We do not even know each other.
> We look alike
> but we have nothing to say
> We are like pigeons . . .

Sexton's speaker likens the couple not to the doves or love-birds of lyric convention but to a pair of lost pigeons; pigeons are well known for mating for life, a potential sign of commitment or, as in this poem, of claustrophobic restriction. The simile conveys the couple's dislocation and disorientation as they land, seemingly inadvertently, in the suburbs. It is ironic, given the separation between the couple conveyed here, that the only thing that does bind them is their shared misery in this suburban home. Their despair is experienced 'in unison'; the first-person plural 'we' is used throughout.

Just as idealised expectations of married life are undermined, so too are preconceptions of suburbia. While in stanza two, the city ('Boston') from which the couple have fled signifies squalor, deprivation, and danger—with 'blind walls' against which the subjects collide, 'traffic that kept stamping

/ and stamping,' and 'worn out' fruit stalls onto which the couple's own exhaustion is displaced—the suburbs prove little better. Indeed, the speaker describes herself and the husband as 'that pair who came to the suburbs / by mistake.' Lewis Mumford describes the move from city to suburbs as a quest for 'liberation from the sometimes dreary conventions and compulsions of an urban society,' and, ironically in Sexton's case given her personal history of mental illness and hospitalisation, as a search for 'asylum.'[42] 'Man and Wife' shows us the abject failure of such aspirations.

Sexton drafted this poem in 1958 and sent a copy to Robert Lowell as part of her application to join his Boston University poetry class. She then returned to and revised it in May 1963, almost certainly while she was reading, with great enthusiasm, Friedan's newly published *The Feminine Mystique*. On 6 June 1963, Sexton wrote to a friend 'Have you read The Feminine Mistique (spelling?) [sic]. If not, hurry and do so. Motherhood is beautiful but it sure ain't everything.'[43] Friedan's book famously analyses the 'problem that has no name,' the problem of profound dissatisfaction experienced by a generation of women in mid-century and specifically *suburban* America. As the opening lines of Friedan's book explain, 'the problem lay buried, unspoken, for many years in the minds of American women. It was a strange stirring, a sense of dissatisfaction, a yearning that women suffered in the middle of the twentieth century in the United States. Each suburban wife struggled with it alone.' Friedan's study found that women's lives in 'the suburbs, those ugly and endless sprawls which are becoming a national problem,' were characterised by frustration, *ennui* and ultimately an amorphous pathological condition diagnosed as 'housewife's fatigue.'[44] Sexton's poem dramatises such a context, and such a condition, the 'problem' that resists articulation and reveals itself only somatically in physical and emotional collapse: 'They are two asthmatics / Whose breath sobs in and out / Through a fuzzy pipe.' In stanza three, 'green rain' (signifying the clean country air which was one of the reputed advantages of the retreat from the city, or, conversely, the poisoned environment indicted in Rachel Carson's *Silent Spring,* published just months before this poem was written), instead of energising or rejuvenating the couple, serves only to clarify. It opens their eyes to the dreadful nature of their new plight: 'Now there is green rain for everyone / as common as eyewash.'

Elaine Tyler May opens her study of American Cold War culture with a vignette about *Life* magazine's 1959 feature on a newlywed couple who elected to spend their honeymoon in a fallout shelter. In a letter of September 1961 to Tony Hecht, Sexton notes 'everyone in the suburbs is building fallout shelters.'[45] 'Man and Wife,' written in May 1963, only months after the Cuban missile crisis of October 1962, imagines such a scene in its true horror. Saturated by the 'green rain' of nuclear fallout ('green rain for everyone'), her couple are forced into a squalid and finally antagonistic intimacy. The military metaphors are significant given this Cold War nuclear context:

Now they are together
like strangers in a two-seater outhouse,
eating and squatting together.
They have teeth and knees
but they do not speak.
A soldier is forced to stay with a soldier
because they share the same dirt
and the same blows.

Starved of companionship, starved of space and air, the couple's condition exemplifies the squalid intimacy of suburban marriage in all its alienation, violence and tension. Gordon, Gordon, and Gunther identify 'increased tension' and 'tremendous emotional stresses' as characteristic of suburban life in this period.[46] In unpublished lecture notes for this poem, Sexton comments on its evocation of 'forced intimacy, dumb instincts.'[47] The paradoxical situation of being 'together / like strangers' speaks both of the couple and of the wider suburban community of which they are a metonym. They seem paralysed by their situation, trapped in a suburban prison of their own choosing, symbolised here by the 'window pane' so redolent of contemporary suburban architecture and of an ideology that both invites and repels intimacy. Silent 'exiles' who 'neither talk nor clear our throats,' they cannot fully participate in the life of which they dream. Instead, they 'gasp in unison beside our window pane / drunk on the drunkard's dream.' The window here, as in a number of other poems, is a metaphor for isolation and belonging, for privacy and communication, for seeing and being seen.

SURVEILLANCE

Plate glass, picture windows, and glazed patio doors were a notable feature of post-war suburban architecture. To a generation who moved to the suburbs from over-crowded and ill-lit urban housing, one of the most attractive features of new suburban housing developments was the space, light, and perspective that such windows promised. However, these windows carried an ideological as well as a practical significance. Lynn Spigel notes that the introduction of plate and sliding glass doors 'mediated the twin goals of separation from and integration into the outside world.'[48] Sexton's work frequently uses images of plate glass and picture windows to represent contradictory processes of observing and being observed fundamental both to life in the suburbs and to confessional poetry. In a vital sense these images function as a metaphor for the way in which the speaker of the confessional poem (the 'I') is simultaneously subject and object of the narrative, both the person observing and the person being observed. Windows stand figuratively for the confessional text, which seeks also to integrate the inside and the outside, self and other, subject and reader, penitent and confessor.

In 'For John, Who Begs Me Not to Enquire Further,' for example, a sequence of metaphors—of glass bowls and mirrors, of transparent, translucent, reflective or refracting surfaces—privileges and ultimately confuses these processes of seeing and being seen, of self-scrutiny and self-display.[49] The glass bowl in that poem both isolates the speaker and, paradoxically, confirms her contiguity with the world around her; it suggests a form of self-identity and a means of identification with others who share the same conditions. The fractured condition of the 'cracked mirror' / 'awkward bowl' that dominates the poem operates both as a metaphor for the damaged, fissured identity of the subject, and as a signifier of the distorted perspective that life in the suburbs offers. The poem, widely regarded as Sexton's manifesto, speaks from and for the inevitably unstable position of suburban housewife and poet articulated by Sexton in the quotation with which I opened this chapter. It closes with a confirmation of that 'separation' and 'integration,' which Spigel defines as characteristic of suburban life. Here, the 'invisible veil' is both a barrier and the absence of a barrier, serving both to separate and to integrate:

> This is something I would never find
> in a lovelier place, my dear,
> although your fear is anyone's fear,
> like an invisible veil between us all . . .
> and sometimes in private,
> my kitchen, your kitchen,
> my face, your face.

Another poem, 'What's That,' written just a month later in March 1959, shows that the window, like the parameters of the suburban home and the boundaries of the female self, is permeable and thus potentially vulnerable.[50] There is a collapse in 'What's That' of the barriers between private and public, internal and external, self and other (hence the equivalence of 'calling me, calling you' at the end of the poem). In this curious poem, it is never clear whether the un-named presence that lurks outside the 'kitchen window' is to be feared or welcomed.

> Before it came inside
> I had watched it from my kitchen window,
> Watched it swell like a new balloon,
> Watched it slump and then divide,
> Like something I know I know—
> A broken pear or two halves of the moon

The object ('it') might signify some alien threat or a fear of recurrent depression. Yet the images might also signify some kind of inspiration, even a visitation from the muse (in classical mythology a female figure). The dilemma that the poem contemplates is all the more acute and astonishing because it takes place in such an unlikely, and specifically suburban, environment:

> It is as real
> as splinters stuck in your ear. The noise we steal
> is half a bell. And outside cars whisk by on the suburban street
> and are there and are true.[51]

Although, as I have suggested, glass windows were celebrated as a technological and aesthetic advance in modern suburban America, Sexton and other writers and commentators of the period voiced misgivings about the exposure that they invited. John Keats's tellingly entitled book *The Crack in the Picture Window* featured a caricature of a suburban couple, John and Mary Drone. Welcomed into their newly built suburban home, one of countless built as a consequence of the post-war G.I. Bill, John and Mary Drone found 'a nine-by-twelve rug spread across the largest room wall to wall, and there was a sheet of plate glass in the living-room wall. That, the builder said, was the picture window. The picture it framed was of the box across the treeless street.' What the Drones learned was that having the means to look out inevitably gives someone else the power to look in: 'through their picture window, a vast and empty eye with bits of paper stuck in its corners, they could see their view—a house like theirs across a muddy street, its vacant picture eye staring at theirs.'[52] There was a reciprocity here that betokened either communality or a stultifying anxiety about constantly being on view.

The suburban home then represented both a place of privacy and safety and one of vulnerability and public scrutiny. To quote Lynn Spigel, the modern home with its large picture windows and open-plan living areas was 'designed as a space for looking . . . the new tract homes of the mass-produced suburbs featured sliding glass doors, bay windows, and open plans that were designed to maximise the visual field.'[53] This led to a specific kind of exposure, and a particular threat to privacy and autonomy, one felt acutely by women, who were typically at home much more than husbands who were employed outside the suburbs. As Betty Friedan explained, the design of typical open-plan homes gave 'the illusion of more space for less money . . . there are no true walls or doors; the woman in the beautiful electronic kitchen is never separated from her children . . . A man, of course, leaves the house for most of the day. But the feminine mystique forbids the woman this.'[54] The point was confirmed by Nelson: 'the suburban home was supposed to offer the opportunity to live out the democratic dream of privacy in post-war America. And yet . . . suburban homes . . . were associated with a profound *deprivation* of privacy as well.'[55] In a letter to Hollis Summers on her return from a writers' conference, Sexton herself complained: 'my suds, I'm back in the suburbs, the children are having an acorn fight on the front lawn, it is 95 in the shade . . . a ham is cooking itself and me in the oven (my desk is situated in the dining room, but at the door leading into the kitchen . . .).'[56]

Gordon, Gordon, and Gunther's *The Split-Level Trap* indicted the home as a place of fear, anxiety and claustrophobia. In the prologue to their book, they visualised 'one of the split-level houses [where] a young mother is crying. She is crouched in a dark closet. Voices in the walls are telling her she is worthless.'[57] Similarly, John Keats described 'today's housing developments,' which 'actually drive mad myriads of housewives shut up in them.'[58] For Sexton it was not only the internal architecture of the home, but the larger social environment that proved so debilitating. For the speakers in her poems, the threat came not necessarily from within but from wider suburbia. In 'Leaves that Talk,' the danger is represented by the malicious green leaves that whisper to her through the windows of her home—windows that render her visible and thus vulnerable and that form an inadequate protection against the outside world: 'they call, though I sit here / sensibly behind my window screen.'[59]

What is interesting in many of these poems is that, the speaker's vantage point on the outside world notwithstanding, she is engaged primarily in a process of inner surveillance or *self*-policing characteristic both of suburban life in Cold War America *and* of confession. In 'Three Green Windows,' for example, the speaker is simultaneously seeing and being seen; she is subject and object of observation.[60] Trapped in a Benthamite panopticon, behind 'three green windows' looking west, south, and east, the speaker both occupies an excellent vantage point and feels herself to be open to everyone else's gaze. Most importantly, though, she is scrutinising, judging, correcting, her own behaviour. The poem proceeds in a mood of free-floating reverie, but the reverie is guarded. It is interrupted repeatedly by negated and therefore, according to Freud, real anxieties about family and friends and about personal and social responsibilities ('the sewers and the drainage / the urban renewal and the suburban centers').[61] It is her own perceptions and observations that the subject must keep under closest watch, must correct or deny:

> I have misplaced the Van Allen belt,
> the sewers and the drainage,
> the urban renewal and the suburban centers.
> I have forgotten the names of the literary critics.
> I know what I know.

There are some things that she cannot permit herself to have seen and known, although the presence of these issues and objects is ineradicably confirmed by the succession of denials and negations through which they are detailed: 'I do not think of the rusty wagon on the walk. / I pay no attention to the red squirrels.'

'Flight' similarly attempts to efface the real, investing instead in the desired, imagined or ideal.[62] The poem has two movements and two tones.

On the outward journey, the speaker is travelling toward the airport, joyfully anticipating flying away to join her absent lover: 'Thinking that I would find you,' the poem opens, 'thinking I would make the plane / that goes hourly out of Boston.' In this mood of exuberant optimism, the speaker can afford to risk a journey from the safe suburbs (the first draft of the poem was entitled 'Letter from the Suburbs') 'into the city.' She can afford to notice aspects of life that, particularly in her position as resident of the White suburbs, she would usually choose to ignore or deny, admitting into consciousness—and conceding shared desires with—thirsty men and Black women:

> I drove into the city.
> Thinking that on such a night
> every thirsty man would have his jug
> and that the Negro women would lie down
> on pale sheets

'Thinking that I would find you,' the speaker can tolerate finding the unlooked-for. On the return journey, though, when the airport is closed down by fog and all flights are 'grounded,' things look different. The repressed others return. Their difference and ugliness is newly visible to the perceiver as she drives home down the aptly named 'S[t]orrow Drive':

> Knowing I would never find you,
> I drove out of the city.
> At the airport one thousand cripples
> sat nursing a sore foot.

The image gestures, perhaps, towards Sophocles' Oedipus, so-named after the injury inflicted on his feet by his parents, Jocasta and Laius, as they abandoned him on the hillside in the hopes of circumventing the Oracle's prophecy that the child would kill his father and marry his mother. In the context of Sexton's poem, and of her work more generally, the story of Oedipus and Jocasta stands as a metaphor for the desperate tension between seeking to know and tell the truth, and avoiding such dreadful insight.

Later poems, 'Hurry Up Please, It's Time,' for example, demonstrate a growing impatience with the restrictive conventions of suburban life and, metaphorically, the taboo against speaking confessionally.[63] Here the speaker is not ashamed of her spectacular self-display, but is proud of her intimate revelations, happy to acknowledge and provoke her voyeuristic audience:

> Ms. Dog prefers to sunbathe nude.
> Let the indifferent sky look on.

So what!
Let Mrs. Sewal pull the curtain back,
from her second story.
So what!
Let United Parcel Service see my parcel.
La de dah.
Sun, you hammer of yellow,
you hat on fire,
you honeysuckle mama,
pour your blonde on me!
Let me laugh for an entire hour
at your supreme being, your Cadillac stuff,
because I've come a long way
from Brussel sprouts.
I've come a long way to peel off my clothes
and lay me down in the grass.

The laughter and the flamboyant self-display replicate comments that Sexton made in correspondence about her own circumstances. In an unpublished letter of 31 March 1966 to Fred Morgan, Sexton jokes, 'I am laughing, Fred, at the ridiculousness of my life here in suburbia; and if you don't think it amusing, you ought to try living with me,' and to Philip Legler in a letter of May of the same year, she affirmed with some pride, 'I am the shock of the proper Boston neighbourhood in my bikini suits.'[64] Elisabeth Bronfen has read the spectacular self-display reported in Sexton's psychotherapy sessions as symptomatic of the specific ideological context in which she lived. According to Bronfen, 'Anne Sexton's hysterical disorders can be read as symptoms for all that was wrong in her culture's relation to female subjectivity; in fact, they perform the daughter's discontent with these constraints. Her dissociations, her chameleon-like ability to take on any illness, and her role playing can be seen as a desperate somatic parody of what was expected of the suburban housewife and mother at the time . . . Her confessional poetry then came to repeat, by making completely public, this illness that for many women grew out of the restricted roles postwar, American culture offered them.'[65]

Other poems, too, are explicit about the spectacular and gendered nature of contemporary suburban existence. 'The Touch' and 'Housewife' figure the female body as an extension of, and indivisible from, the modern home. Le Corbusier's 'machine for living in' becomes, in Sexton's eyes, a mechanism of domination and despair. In 'The Touch,' the father 'comes with the house and even at night / he lives in a machine made by my mother.'[66] As 'Housewife' declares:

Some women marry houses.
It's another kind of skin; it has a heart,
A mouth, a liver and bowel movements.

The walls are permanent and pink.
See how she sits on her knees all day
Faithfully washing herself down.[67]

Women and the home are here linked in a perpetual cycle of consumption and waste. In another poem, 'The Sickness Unto Death,' the speaker likens herself to 'a house full of bowel movement.'[68] In 'Housewife,' the modern home demands abjection, sacrifice, and obeisance from the woman, who is implicated in an endless ritual of cleansing. For Lynn Spigel, describing contemporary suburban architecture, the 'antiseptic model of space was the reigning aesthetic at the heart of the postwar suburbs.'[69] In 'Hurry Up Please, It's Time,' too, the kitchen demands the life blood, the very breath, of the woman who becomes its primary caregiver: 'My kitchen is a heart. / I must feed it oxygen once in a while / and mother the mother.'[70]

In 'The Death Baby,' the modern kitchen is the altar for the immolation of the female subject.[71] A curious and disturbing poem, the speaker reports and then plays out her own sister's dream:

My sister at six
dreamt nightly of my death:
"The baby turned to ice.
Someone put her in the refrigerator
and she turned as hard as a popsicle"

Modern domestic appliances, which had seemed to promise liberation to housewives of the period, here signal their imprisonment and annihilation. Ruth Schwartz Cowan has shown that middle-class women setting up home on either side of the Second World War typically had a smaller home than their own mothers, fewer if any servants, and more domestic appliances, accompanied by the tacit expectation that these women would operate them.[72] These poems' concerns about scrutiny and annihilation, their desire to display their female speakers, and their anxiety about the repercussions of such display speak not only of the plight of the modern woman, but of the particular circumstances of the female confessional poet who both invites and resists attention, who both offers herself up for consumption by an audience and seeks to avoid such an exchange.

'Self in 1958,' originally 'The Lady Lives in a Doll House,' was drafted in 1958 and completed in 1965.[73] In her unpublished lecture notes Sexton comments: 'in the next poem we have me stopped as the perfect housewife, as the advertised woman in the perfect little ticky tacky suburb . . . It is a picture of me before madness became my friend.'[74] Her comment suggests both a critical distance on, and some kind of accommodation with, the conditions the poem describes. 'Stopped' is an interesting choice of word, connoting a state of frozen inanimation or arrested development. Sexton proceeds to interrogate the situation the poem describes: 'Why do I call myself a plaster doll? Why do I live in a doll's house? (because I feel unreal, because the furniture, the scenery is perfect but I am unreal' [punctuation in the original]. The suburbs transmit a sense of inauthenticity, incompleteness, self-alienation.

The poem opens with a huge question ('What is reality?'), which introduces the sequence of images of impermanence and superficiality that follow ('plaster,' 'shellack,' 'nylon,' 'advertised clothes'). Femininity is seen as a form of masquerade or performance ('I am a plaster doll; I pose'), although if we read 'poses' as meaning 'poses questions' the poem invites a different interpretation. If the 'I' poses questions, or im/poses her perspective ('I pose / with eyes that cut open without landfall or nightfall'), she becomes altogether more difficult and challenging, acquiring more agency than the surface image suggests.

Nevertheless, 'Self in 1958' depicts a profound inauthenticity—hence the strange syntax of line six, 'Am I approximately an I. Magnin transplant?'—which is tied up with rituals of consumption and display ('I. Magnin' is the name of a department-store). Femininity in this poem is medicalised or pathologised ('plaster,' 'cut,' 'transplant') and it is dangerous ('cut open,' 'steel'). As in 'Housewife,' femininity is remorseless, continuing 'without landfall or nightfall' and requiring endless reiteration. Again, we might read all of these elements as figuring both the modern woman and the confessional poet—relentlessly cutting herself open, displaying her inner demons for the edification of some anonymous audience.

Femininity is played out in front of the mirror (implicitly in stanza one, the speaker is looking at her own reflection although we cannot read this as a Lacanian moment of pleasurable self-realisation; there is blankness here, dislocation and disorientation), or it is played out in front of a camera ('life enlarges,' 'flash') that is also a gun ('life takes aim'). Crucially, femininity is played out in an 'all-electric kitchen.' Stanza three opens: 'Someone plays with me, / plants me in the all-electric kitchen.' Sexton gestures here towards the infamous 'kitchen debates' of 1959 between Soviet leader Khrushchev and U.S. Vice-President Nixon. These took place at the 1959 Moscow trade fair, at the height of the Cold War, when Russia and America were in competition for military and ideological dominance. For Nixon, superior domestic appliances stood for all that was best about modern America and, by extension, for an idealised femininity. Friedan confirmed the point: 'The American housewife—she was the dream image of the young American woman and the envy, it was said, of women all over the world.'[75] Sexton's speaker/doll demurs from this position and questions the ideal. She is placed in the kitchen against her own volition and uncertain how to perform once she is there, hence the repeated questions, exclamations, and parenthetical dashes. Although for Nixon the 'all-electric kitchen' liberates ('what we want is to make easier the life of our housewives'), for Sexton's speaker, it is a kind of prison.

She 'should,' and thus presumably cannot, 'spring open the doors'; she remains 'rooted' to the wall.

CONCLUSION

There is a deep ambivalence in Sexton's poetry not only about being a woman in Cold War America, but about being a woman and a confessional poet. Anne Sexton handles this ambivalence by confronting, manipulating, even exaggerating it. Profoundly equivocal about each and any of the contradictory roles available to her (madwoman, suburban housewife, poet), her poetry refuses to settle on any one, exchanging and interweaving elements of each in unsettling and transgressive ways.

Sexton was not the first or the only poet to explore the ramifications of suburban life. In the generation immediately preceding hers, Phyllis McGinley had earned the moniker 'housewife poet,' and even William Carlos Williams was identified as a poet whose ambiguous territory was the New Jersey suburbs.[76] Poets since, including Mona Van Duyn and James McMichael, have made the suburbs their locus. In prose fiction, John Updike, John Cheever, Joyce Carol Oates, and many others have written about suburban values, experiences, and crises. What is interesting and unique in Sexton's case is the way in which her own experience of psychological disturbance in a domestic framework is welded with an acute and informed reading of contemporary ideology and a sophisticated and self-conscious aesthetic to form a new poetics of the suburbs.

NOTES

1. Linda Gray Sexton and Lois Ames (eds), *Anne Sexton: A Self-Portrait in Letters* (Boston: Houghton Mifflin, 1979), 143.
2. My argument is informed in part by recent work in cultural geography. As Edward Soja notes, 'as we approach the *fin de siecle,* there is a growing awareness of the simultaneity and interwoven complexity of the social, the historical, and the spatial, their inseparability and interdependence': Edward Soja, *Third Space: Journeys to Los Angeles and Other Real-And-Imagined Places* (Oxford: Blackwell, 1996), 3.
3. Anne Sexton, *The Complete Poems* (Boston: Houghton Mifflin, 1981), 491.
4. Sexton, *Complete,* 509–35.
5. Marsha Bryant, 'Ariel's Kitchen: Plath, *Ladies Home Journal,* and the Domestic Surreal,' in Anita Plath Helle (ed.), *The Unravelling Archive: Essays on Sylvia Plath* (Ann Arbor: University of Michigan Press, forthcoming), 269–95 (287).
6. Kenneth T. Jackson, *Crabgrass Frontier: The Suburbanization of the United States* (New York: Oxford University Press, 1985), 235–6.
7. Charles M. Haar, *The End of Innocence: A Suburban Reader* (Glenview, IL: Scott, Foresman and Company, 1972), Foreword. President Johnson's taskforce was asked to consider the 'economic, social and physical problems of suburbs and the people who live there' (13–15). No specific mention was made of issues relating either to psychological problems or gender.

8. Jackson, *Crabgrass,* 243–4.
9. Deborah Nelson, *Pursuing Privacy in Cold War America* (New York: Columbia University Press, 2002). Sexton's writing is typically associated with the confessional mode of poetry, which dominated American literature during this period. The mode was first defined in 1959 as autobiographical, taboo-breaking, and therapeutic. As I have shown elsewhere, Sexton expressed reservations about the label and about the possibility of either telling the truth or of curing oneself in poetry: Jo Gill, 'Anne Sexton and Confessional Poetics,' *Review of English Studies* 55 (2004): 425–45.
10. William M. Dobriner, *Class in Suburbia* (Englewood Cliffs, NJ: Prentice-Hall, 1963), 9.
11. Jo Gill, 'Textual Confessions: Narcissism in Anne Sexton's Early Poetry,' *Twentieth-Century Literature,* 50 (2004): 59–87.
12. See Marilyn Chin: 'Poetry has moved to the suburbs . . . I suppose this was first inspired by the confessional poets . . . their poems are self-centered, shortsighted; they don't extend to larger concerns,' cited in K. Sontag and D. Graham (eds.), *After Confession: Poetry as Autobiography* (St. Paul, MN: Gray Wolf Press, 2001), 6.
13. R. E. Gordon, K. K. Gordon, and M. Gunther note that 'salesmen do a good deal of driving, hence are subjected to stresses from this source. Moreover, many of them spend much time in distant travel. This may lead to problems at home.' *The Split-Level Trap* (New York: Bernard Geis, 1960), 92.
14. Diane Middlebrook, *Anne Sexton: A Biography* (London: Virago, 1992); Linda Gray Sexton, *Searching for Mercy Street: My Journey Back to My Mother, Anne Sexton* (Boston: Little, Brown, 1994).
15. Margaret Mead, 'Freedom to Choose,' in Charles M. Haar (ed.), *The End of Innocence: A Suburban Reader* (Glenview, IL: Scott, Foresman, 1972), 18–22.
16. Middlebrook, *Anne Sexton,* 210.
17. Lori Rotskoff, *Love on the Rocks: Men, Women and Alcohol in Post-World War II America* (Chapel Hill and London: University of North Carolina Press, 2002), 2, 8.
18. Ibid., 198, 207.
19. See Elaine Tyler May, *Homeward Bound: American Families in the Cold War Era* (New York: Basic Books, 1999), 21.
20. Lewis Mumford, *The City in History: Its Origins, Its Transformations, and its Prospects* (London: Secker & Warburg, 1961), 512.
21. Anne Sexton, 'The Bar Fly Ought to Sing' in S. E. Colburn (ed.), *No Evil Star: Selected Essays, Interviews and Prose—Anne Sexton* (Ann Arbor: University of Michigan Press, 1985), 6.
22. See Marianne Moore on Lowell's 'Boston-in-its-glory residence' cited in Ian Hamilton, *Robert Lowell: A Biography* (London: Faber and Faber, 1983), 23.
23. Gordon et al, *Split-Level,* 27.
24. Middlebrook, *Anne Sexton,* 229–30.
25. Dobriner, *Class,* 65, 67.
26. Tyler May, *Homeward,* 152.
27. Robert Lowell accounts for parallels between his and Sexton's work in terms of 'similar experience not imitation,' in Saskia Hamilton (ed.), *The Letters of Robert Lowell* (London: Faber and Faber, 2005), 393.
28. Joan Didion, 'Slouching Towards Bethlehem' (1965), in *Live and Learn* (London: Harper Perennial, 2005), 98–9.
29. Gordon et al, *Split-Level,* 60.
30. Sexton, *Complete,* 20.
31. Gordon et al., *Split-Level,* 34.

32. Anne Sexton, letter to Oscar Williams (3 April 1963), Harry Ransom Humanities Research Center, University of Texas at Austin (hereinafter HRHRC).
33. Sexton, *Letters,* 114.
34. Anne Sexton, letter to Fred Morgan (31 March 1966), HRHRC.
35. Sexton, *Letters,* 70.
36. Mumford, *City,* 492. Betty's Friedan's *The Feminine Mystique* confirms the point. Housewives fled to the suburbs with great expectations, only to find themselves 'truly trapped' (London: Pelican, 1982), 216.
37. Middlebrook, *Anne Sexton,* 49, 229.
38. Arthur Furst, *Anne Sexton: The Last Summer* (New York: St. Martin's Press, 2000), viii.
39. W. H. Pritchard, 'The Anne Sexton Show,' *Hudson Review* 31 (1978): 387–92 (390).
40. Sexton had read and annotated Friedan's *The Feminine Mystique.* As her daughter Linda Gray Sexton recalls, Sexton then gave the book to her: 'complete with her scribbled notes across the pages—notes that showed her identification with the problems Friedan described' (*Searching,* 98).
41. Sexton, *Complete,* 116.
42. Mumford, *City,* 485, 486.
43. Anne Sexton, letter to Irene Orgel (6 June 1963), HRHRC.
44. Friedan, *Feminine,* 13, 214–5, 219.
45. Anne Sexton, letter to Tony Hecht (15 September 1961), HRHRC.
46. Gordon et al, *Split-Level,* 29, 7.
47. Anne Sexton, Crawshaw Lectures, HRHRC.
48. Lynn Spigel, *Welcome to the Dreamhouse: Popular Media and Postwar Suburbs* (Durham, NC, and London: Duke University Press, 2001), 32.
49. Sexton, *Complete,* 34.
50. Ibid., 25.
51. The poem anticipates Sylvia Plath's 'Balloons' written some four years later. See Sylvia Plath, *Collected Poems* (London: Faber and Faber, 1981).
52. John Keats, *The Crack in the Picture Window* (Boston: Houghton Mifflin, 1956), xv, 21.
53. Spigel, *Dreamhouse,* 2.
54. Friedan, *Feminine,* 216.
55. Nelson, *Pursuing,* 85.
56. Sexton, *Letters,* 83.
57. Gordon et al, *Split-Level,* 17. In a 'Publisher's Note' to their book we learn that the authors 'surveyed thousands of case histories, making creative interpretations and drawing scientific conclusions about suburban mental health problems . . . they have provided a precise, clear picture of the tremendous emotional stresses that are peculiar to the suburbs' (7).
58. Keats, *Crack,* xii.
59. Sexton, *Complete,* 540.
60. Ibid., 105.
61. Sigmund Freud, 'On Negation' in *On Metapsychology: The Theory of Psychoanalysis* [PFL 11] (Harmondsworth: Penguin, 1991), 437–42.
62. Sexton, *Complete,* 86.
63. Ibid., 384.
64. Sexton, *Letters,* 290.
65. Elisabeth Bronfen, *The Knotted Subject: Hysteria and its Discontents* (Princeton, NJ: Princeton University Press, 1998), 301.
66. Sexton, *Complete,* 173.
67. Ibid., 77.
68. Ibid., 441.

69. Spigel, *Dreamhouse,* 34. See also Jo Gill, 'Anne Sexton and Confessional Poetics,' for an overview of readings of confessional poetry as improper, dirty or poisonous.
70. Sexton, *Complete,* 384.
71. Ibid., 354.
72. Ruth Schwartz Cowan, *More Work for Mother: The Ironies of Household Technology From the Open Hearth to the Microwave* (New York: Basic Books, 1983), 172.
73. Sexton, *Complete,* 155.
74. Anne Sexton, Crawshaw Lectures, HRHRC.
75. Friedan, *Feminine,* 15.
76. Randall Jarrell, *Poetry and the Age* (London: Faber and Faber, 1955), 217.

5 Housewives, Neuroses, and the Domestic Environment in Britain, 1945–70

Ali Haggett

INTRODUCTION

The post-war period has been popularly characterized by its recourse to 'traditional' family values. While the numbers of women in paid employment steadily increased, they were still a minority. For married women, especially middle-class women, it was still seen as more respectable to remain at home.[1] Following the war, families increasingly aspired to the 'male breadwinner' model. The idea that man and wife would undertake complementary roles within marriage formed the basis of William Beveridge's report *Social Insurance and Allied Services* (1942). Beveridge proposed that a man would make insurance contributions on behalf of his wife, 'as for a team, each of whose partners is equally essential,' and thus it was proposed that 'during marriage, most women will not be gainfully occupied.'[2] However, contemporary writers were drawing attention to growing discontent among educated housewives. In 1963, attempting to highlight the so-called 'problem with no name' among American housewives, Betty Friedan wrote the much-publicized text *The Feminine Mystique.* In Britain, Viola Klein, Judith Hubback, and Hannah Gavron all identified a level of confusion surrounding acceptable roles for married women.[3] Since the 1970s, feminist historians have suggested that the lack of opportunities afforded to women and the banality inherent in the domestic role caused symptoms of anxiety and depression in post-war housewives. Correspondingly, they have argued that the primary motive for prescribing psychotropic drugs was to ensure that women 'adapted' to their domestic role.[4]

This chapter explores the key themes that emerged from an oral history project that aimed to explore the recollections and experiences of middle-class women who were married between 1945 and 1970.[5] Feminist authors have routinely argued that the most notable difficulties experienced by married women were related to their roles as homemakers and mothers. However, the evidence provided from this project raises questions about feminist analyses, since it would appear that many women believed that they were undertaking a worthwhile role and often found great satisfaction in it. Although the experiences of marriage, homemaking, and mothering are in many ways interwoven, the interviewees drew clear distinctions between the functional aspects of day-to-day domestic life and the emotional aspects of marriage. Many respondents identified emotional difficulties in the sphere of interpersonal relationships with spouses and other family members as the cause of mental symptoms. Nevertheless, the evidence indicates that even when the need for intimacy and companionship was not met within marriage, women were still able to gain joy and satisfaction from their role as mothers and homemakers.

Judy Giles has recently offered a more productive approach in which she fosters a wider understanding of home 'that neither pathologizes nor pities the millions of women for whom domesticity is a primary concern and an actively created space.'[6] I shall further develop this argument and suggest that future investigation should not focus exclusively on the negative aspects of domesticity, but instead should draw upon and revalidate the voices of those who considered their experiences to be both positive and worthwhile. I will suggest that contemporary feminist social theorists and feminist historians originated from untypical backgrounds that were either highly academic or political, and thus were largely unrepresentative of the average suburban housewife. As Giles observes, 'those who wrote or spoke about suburbia in Britain or America did so from positions outside the phenomenon they so roundly condemned.'[7] This chapter begins with a brief discussion of previous historical accounts before examining in detail the material from the interviews.

As Rhodri Hayward has noted in his contribution to this volume, since the inter-war years, the 'desperate housewife' has become a familiar image, re-emerging under multifarious guises at specific historical moments. From the suburban neurosis that was said to have affected isolated young wives on new post-war housing estates to the darkly comedic television depiction of Wysteria Lane in twenty-first-century American suburbia,[8] the banality of domestic life has invariably been portrayed as pathogenic. Since the 1960s there has been serious academic criticism of the post-war 'domestic dream.' Ann Oakley claims that one of the most important springboards of post-war feminism was 'the actual experiences of people and families, including women feeling over-worked, undervalued, trapped and mistreated.'[9] Germaine Greer went so far as to suggest that 'a housewife's work has no results; it simply has to be done again. Bringing up children is not a real occupation, because children come up just the same—brought or not.'[10] In 1960, Betty Friedan suggested that something was radically wrong with the way that American women were living their lives. In *The Feminine Mystique* (1963), she claimed that women were experiencing 'a strange stirring—a sense of dissatisfaction . . . each suburban wife struggled with it alone . . . as she made the beds, shopped for groceries . . . lay by her husband at night, she was afraid to ask even of herself the silent question "is this all?"' As a result of domestic stultification, Friedan declared that '"the problem that has no name" burst like a boil through the image of the happy American housewife.'[11]

Feminist scholars have suggested that symptoms of anxiety and depression were directly related to the stresses inherent in domestic work and other disadvantageous aspects of the female role:

> The home can become, for the full-time housewife, a setting which, by its peculiar strains, "drives her mad" . . . Doctors act as agents of society and maintain the status quo as far as their female patients are concerned, by adjusting them to their domestic roles . . . In general, they aim to return the patient to their pre-illness condition, but do not consider whether that condition brought about the illness in the first place.[12]

Ancient theories of an alliance between femininity and irrationality have long been challenged. Nevertheless, clinical statistics still suggest that women are more likely than men to experience certain categories of mental illness. There remains discussion about whether this simply reflects the fact that women have always been more likely than men to report symptoms, or, whether there are true differences in health experiences.[13] Key to this debate has been the work undertaken by Walter Gove during the 1970s and 1980s. Gove attempted to show that it was the roles confronting married women that accounted for their higher rates of psychological disorders. His research focused on the domestic aspects of a married woman's life, and he claimed that a number of difficulties associated with the role combined to increase the likelihood of the onset of mental illness. However, Gove's work was based on a number of assumptions. He argued, for example, that 'it seems reasonable to assume that a large number of women find their major instrumental activities—raising children and keeping house—frustrating.'[14] However, he acknowledged in his footnotes that this assumption was based on the writing of authors such as Friedan and Myrdal and Klein, and admitted that he had been 'unable to locate any systematic evaluation of this assumption.'[15] Gove further suggested that, since the housewife's role was 'invisible' and 'unstructured':

> It was likely that she would be able to 'put things off, to let things slide, in sum—to perform poorly. The lack of structure and visibility allows her to brood over her troubles and her distress may thus feed upon itself.'[16]

Gove concluded that the housewife's role was one of 'low prestige . . . being a housewife does not require a great deal of skill, for virtually all women, whether educated or not seem to be capable of being at least moderately competent housewives.'[17] In line with the work of most feminist authors, Gove assumed that the most notable difficulties experienced by married women were related to their role as homemakers and mothers. However, as will become apparent, the women interviewed for this project rarely found serious fault with their domestic role, but often found that difficulties in the marital relationship itself were related to the onset of psychological symptoms.

Writing in Canada during the late 1970s, Ruth Cooperstock agreed with Gove that married women were more likely to receive prescriptions for psychotropic drugs than men.[18] Cooperstock's central contention was that tranquillizer use in women was largely related to difficulties experienced with maintaining the given social role of wife, mother, and house-worker. In her exploratory investigation into tranquillizer use, Cooperstock noted that for women, continued use of these drugs was discussed 'in terms of permitting them to maintain themselves in a role or roles which they found difficult or intolerable without the drug.'[19] However, central to the analysis provided here is the suggestion, as put forward by Ludmilla Jordanova, that we need to move away from academic enquiry that has so often produced one-sided assumptions about power and oppression. Women's mental health may well be *related* to men, children, and family structure; however, we must re-evaluate accounts that brand women as emotional in order that male experts gain 'control.'[20] Furthermore, as Foucault observed, power is not always 'repressive,' but can also be 'enabling.'[21] As the following oral testimony will illustrate, new discourses surrounding the origins and treatment of mental symptoms often allowed women to cultivate new ways of empowering themselves, enabling them to begin new lives and distance themselves from unsatisfactory relationships.

This oral history project firstly expands on previous research in exploring the domestic experience of the interviewees.[22] Respondents were drawn from the National Women's Register, an organisation formerly known as the National Housewives' Register. This group, still active today, originated in 1960 when a housewife, Maureen Nicol, wrote to *The Guardian* suggesting that 'housebound housewives with liberal interests' should form a national register in order that groups could explore interests outside the domestic arena.[23] The women are loosely described as 'middle-class,' either because they were born into a family from a professional or managerial background, or because they were able to aspire to middle-class values following the implementation of the Butler Education Act (1944) and the new opportunities provided by the 11+ exam. Thirty-five women came forward from a wide geographical area over England and Wales. All of the women were married and their dates of birth ranged from 1915 to 1950. All had experience of domestic life during the 1950s and 1960s.[24]

In this instance, the agenda was neither to prove nor disprove feminist hypotheses; instead, the objective was to allow the women themselves to give voice to their own experiences. The technique employed for this project involved long interviews and open-ended questions, the aim of which was to provide an environment in which the women felt comfortable talking about their relationships and the associated subjective feelings. Where necessary, questions were repeated under different guises in order that possible discrepancies in the narrative could be detected. All interviewees were mentally alert and recalled their lives as young wives with clarity. It seems unlikely that they were remembering domestic life with illusory fondness and affection since many of them observed with frequency that aspects of their lives were indeed difficult. However, the women were keen to emphasize that, despite the inherent challenges, they still viewed the role of homemaker as worthwhile. They were questioned in detail about all aspects of domesticity and their responses have been organized around the following themes: practical management of the home; coping mechanisms; and mothering. They were also questioned about the perceived levels of satisfaction/dissatisfaction associated individually with paid employment, child care, and housework, in addition to a general assessment of their role.[25]

An exploration of the experiences of women who were affected by minor psychiatric disorder then follows. A project of this size is not able to offer any definitive conclusions as to the cause of mental illness. However, the objective is to question accounts that have viewed the role of mothering and homemaking itself as necessarily pathogenic. Such accounts have masked the complexities of family life and underplayed the ways in which personal relationships, both past and present, might influence the onset of psychiatric and psychosomatic symptoms. Although the aim is to offer a more balanced approach to the experience of domestic life, it is important to emphasize that this work does not seek to discredit all aspects of feminist research in this field. On the contrary, there is indeed good evidence here to suggest that, although the social and economic structures of society during the period were often advantageous to women during marriage, the reverse was true in separation and divorce. Beveridge's breadwinner model left women economically vulnerable and socially ostracized when the marital relationship became untenable. It is therefore suggested that it was the ongoing difficulties associated with marital discord and the material disadvantages following divorce that were the more probable cause of mental symptoms. Indeed, it appears that satisfactory personal relationships with all members of the immediate family were ultimately the key to a sense of well-being and the ability to cope during adverse circumstances.

DOMESTIC LIFE

In 1963, John and Elizabeth Newson suggested that middle-class mothers might have aspirations to an active intellectual life and that 'for such women, the period when her children are very young may be a time of frustration and despondency.'[26] Evidence from this oral history project does indicate that a level of isolation existed among respondents during these years, particularly for those who moved house regularly in order to follow a husband's career. Certainly, many women felt a desire to participate in intellectually stimulating activities outside the home. Many women found homemaking irritating at times and despite the introduction of household appliances the consensus was that housework remained 'hard work.' However, this appeared unremarkable to the women interviewed and the majority saw their role as less demanding than that of their husband in the working world outside the home:

> 'I think I was fortunate. I never had to work. I was an "at home" wife . . . my husband always had very demanding jobs and he was away a

lot—the stress was more with him than with me. I'd hoped I wouldn't have to work, I didn't enjoy work.'[27]

'I've always been very conscious that I have been fortunate, that I didn't have to work for financial reasons—and the fact that I felt I was doing a worthwhile job.'[28]

'He was my breadwinner. I never went out to work outside the home, it was accepted. As far as I was concerned, that's what it seemed to be, that you gave up work when you had your children—it didn't worry me, I didn't want to, I wanted to be at home with the baby. That was my job. It was my profession.'[29]

'The best aspects of domestic life was doing what I wanted, when I wanted and being with my children constantly until they went to school. [I] considered my life idyllic . . . I felt the role was made for me.'[30]

Although a number of women in this oral history sample described their husbands as 'head of the household,' there is little evidence that the women saw themselves as oppressed. They evaluated their position as part of a team effort. Their responses clearly reflected the practices and beliefs of post-war welfarism. Indeed, many directly acknowledged the advantages of their position and the 'trade off' for less worry and responsibility. Val Parker, for example, moved house frequently because her husband was a member of the armed forces. Naturally, she recalled some difficult times, but also observed that:

'In your home you were secure, you were controlling your own environment . . . when you had to go out to work you had traffic, you had challenges, you had maybe difficult bosses, and so you couldn't just say—well, I'm off for a lie down now! So I did feel that men had much more demands made on them.'[31]

Some respondents were astonished to be asked whether or not they would have liked to work during this period of their lives, since they saw their job at home as 'work.' The consensus was that housework and cooking were still time-consuming, since modern labour-saving technology was expensive and often considered a luxury:

'I didn't have a fridge until 1962 and that was agony in the summer when it was hot. I had a marble—an old-fashioned wash stand on a shelf in the pantry to put all my things on and try to keep them cold. And of course you'd have to go out to the shops more or less every day to get anything that might go off. To keep the milk from going sour, well—it was dreadful.'[32]

Doris Carter noted that many husbands returned home for lunch and therefore some families had their main meal at midday. This entailed shopping and food preparation that would invariably take up most of the morning. Her daughter recalled:

> 'I remember all morning . . . you'd have to go and buy the stuff and have the dinner on the table by 12 o'clock, which is really early. I remember you saying that you'd never get it done on time!'[33]

Jean Hill pointed out that meals were home-cooked as there were no ready-prepared items:

> 'If you think about the food our children ate, it was real food, wholesome food. And you cooked, and you didn't think twice about cooking a meal. . . . you did a pudding, proper dinners and proper puddings.'[34]

The women interviewed recounted a daily routine that included housework, cooking, and washing, with a couple of hours spent 'taking children out' in the afternoon. Cleaning was perceived as something that 'you just got on with,' although a number of women claimed to enjoy it. Eileen Roberts, for example, remembered that: 'I really quite enjoyed being at home and having housework. I enjoyed the housework. I mean, I got fed up obviously, like we all do—but it wasn't a terrible drudge for me.'[35]

While industrious, the women interviewed did not think it necessary to ensure that their houses were immaculate. Angela Holdsworth, writing in 1988, claimed that women increasingly feared the criticism of other housewives. She included oral testimony of women who claimed that the appearance of their homes, their prams and their children had to be 'manicured into order.'[36] However, the majority of women in this project were not aware of social pressure to keep their homes pristine. While it was noted that 'white' nappies were important, by and large other things took priority:

> 'I got satisfaction of having a nice line of washing [but] I'm not house-proud at all! I always had the theory that if you kept the floor clean and tidy, people didn't look higher than that! And if they saw a reasonably clean floor, they missed the fact that everything was a bit dusty and not as it should be . . . I've always enjoyed cooking, so I never minded cooking meals.'[37]

In most cases husbands did not help with the housework. However, many respondents pointed out that, given the long hours they spent at work, it would simply have been illogical to expect men to undertake household tasks. Moreover, some women claimed not to want them to help: 'Well, I never really wanted him to really. Probably because I never expected it.'[38]

It is clear that previous histories have been disproportionately influenced by feminist analyses, which underplay the extent to which women saw their role as acceptable and endurable—and in many cases, desirable. Furthermore, as these accounts illustrate, it did not occur to the majority of women to dwell on 'what might have been,' for this was simply 'what there was':

> 'It sounds weird, but you just got on with what you were doing at the time. I'm sure you know yourself; you are so busy with young children that you don't stand back and get a perspective on it. Things come along so quickly with young children—worrying about schools and keeping them safe and that sort of thing.'[39]

CREATIVE ACTIVITIES AND SUPPORT NETWORKS

Social surveys undertaken by Hanna Gavron, Judith Hubback, and Viola Klein during the post-war period indicated that a significant number of educated, married mothers expressed an interest in going out to work. Extra 'pocket' money for non-essentials was cited as the most common reason; however, many housewives indicated that it would be desirable to meet new people for mental stimulus.[40] Hanna Gavron also commented on the loss of confidence and isolation experienced by mothers of small children.[41] Once again, the evidence from this cohort challenges such findings. While it is clear that a number of women experienced a degree of isolation in their role, the overwhelming majority of respondents made an explicit choice to explore other avenues of creativity that did not necessarily involve paid employment. By focusing upon the ideological debates of the period, historians of domesticity have largely failed to examine the ways in which women exercised their imagination and resourcefulness in the private sphere. Much has been written, for example, about the post-war domestic ideology, the emergence of 'the companionate marriage,' women and work, and the material undervaluation of domestic labour.[42] Although Giles touches on the engagement of American suburban women 'in the micro-politics of suburban life,'[43] few accounts have explored these important avenues of fulfilment in any detail.

As an alternative to seeking paid employment, many respondents interviewed for this project expressed a general preference for activities that would reinforce the beliefs and values that underpinned family life and traditional gender roles. Eileen Roberts, for example, became involved with the Pre-School Playgroup Association and in 1967 opened a playgroup in the basement of her home beneath her husband's general practitioner's surgery. Eileen advocated creative stimulation for women from within the mother/wife role. The experience changed her life:

> 'It was absolutely amazing. It was as much for the mums . . . making them understand that there is a value of being at home . . . I feel very,

very strongly that women should stay at home with children, until they are 5 at least. Where people find staying home with kids "a waste of time" is beyond my thinking, because for me, it's the most important thing you can do. You make or break these people.'[44]

Katherine Stead joined her local branch of the National Women's Register and initiated a babysitting circle. 'I found I needed more stimulation than just reading children's books to them every evening. And we got some more meaty topics—and that was good.'[45] Many of the respondents were members of other organisations such as The Townswomen's Guild and The Inner Wheel. For some, the church provided a social network and support; others met like-minded women through their children. Eileen Bailey joined the local choral society and the drama group of the Women's Institute. Although Eileen confirmed that she had been happy to remain at home full-time, she experienced a troubled marriage and tolerated many years of her husband's adultery. She felt that activities outside the home and her Christian faith enabled her to cope during hard times:

> 'I couldn't have coped if I hadn't had some other interests. And I couldn't have coped if I hadn't been a Christian either. And I know that because I had an inner strength that I couldn't have got from anywhere.'[46]

Not all respondents chose to join outside activities, and some were content keeping themselves usefully entertained at home. Gwen Collins, for example, described herself as 'bookish'—always wanting to read: 'I always had a thing—a bar—against the kitchen window so that I could have a book behind when I was washing napkins and things.'[47] A support network of wider kin did not exist for the majority of interviewees. Most had moved away from relatives, usually as a result of their partner's employment, but on occasions through personal choice. By and large, this was not seen as a cause of inconvenience. In a few cases, a family network did not exist in the first place, as was the case for Margaret Windsor, whose father died when she was ten months old: 'My mother died two years after my first daughter was born . . . and there wasn't a "rest" of the family, because I'd got no siblings.'[48] Provided they had the support of their partners, these women saw coping alone as normal. A recurring feature in the lives of these women was the support of 'one good friend' (or a small group of exclusive friends), with whom it was possible to discuss anything:

> 'The saving grace really has been one good friend . . . she had a large family as well and one day a week we had each other's family. So one day a week we had nine children! But it gave the other a day off. And if things were going wrong, if you were fed up with husbands—anything—you'd pick up the phone. And we had a coded message; we'd pick it up and say "I need a cup of coffee!" And you'd immediately know there was a problem.'[49]

MOTHERING

Contemporary beliefs accentuated the importance of a stable conjugal relationship, and promoted it as the best environment to bring up children. The idea that mothers were the best people to care for and nurture young children was formulated by clinicians such as John Bowlby, Donald Winnicott, and Benjamin Spock, who argued that mother-love in infancy was of paramount importance to the mental health of a child.[50] It is likely that the women interviewed were indirectly influenced by this discourse due to the pervasive way in which subtle messages were conveyed through television, radio and popular culture. Nevertheless, the evidence from this project illustrates that women often bought into these ideals without resentment, and their evidence does not indicate that they believed the idealization of motherhood was contrived as a deliberate plan to limit women's opportunities. Without exception, they placed the care and nurture of their children as their priority in life.[51] It is striking that, given the great diversity of life experiences, similar sentiments were expressed by interviewees. They believed that the labour of childrearing was the most worthwhile task of all and saw themselves in many ways as 'responsible' for the next generation.

> 'Well, a mother's role is really a provider isn't it—a provider of love and everything for their well-being. I always have felt very strongly that it is a parent's duty to bring up their children so that they are equipped to leave home as young adults . . . I'd say that the way we brought our children up, we did to our best . . . how else could we? We had to be true to our beliefs. I wasn't a very introspective mother, or person—consequently it was what I was there for, I was fulfilling my role.'[52]

In 1964 Margaret Lincoln was unexpectedly required to adopt her nephew and niece. Her experience is testimony to the ways in which the familial environment was considered to be of paramount importance to a child's emotional development:

> 'I had to give them a base, to start off with almost eroding what they'd got and put in a new life—very hard work because they actually rebelled. But the social services lady . . . said that "every child needs a frame, and it will knock the frame to find whether it's secure." She said "and you'll be the frame." She said "you'll have to be very firm," and I was. And they've both grown up as they should have done, and not got into any trouble at all.'[53]

When asked what effect this experience had had on her life, she remembered it being hard work. However, she also recalled:

'I'd been married for sixteen years and then I had these two children, and I learned how to be unselfish. Because we'd become wrapped up in one another, you know and I think it taught me to be unselfish. You know, when you've got the flu and you're going around and you have to think of them rather than of yourself—and you're getting up in the middle of the night when one of them's saying "there's a spaceman under the bed" or something [laughing]. All those things are the best.'[54]

Indeed, many respondents commented on how they had been rewarded for their devotion by adult children who expressed appreciation for their parents' commitment. Gwen, for example, was married shortly before the outbreak of war, and had to bring up her first child alone for four years:

'And then [my husband] went away, and I didn't see him for four years. I brought the child up by myself. And one day since, somebody said something to me about this when Martin was there, and he said "yes, but didn't we have a lovely time." And I was really touched by that because I never thought about the child appreciating the mother being there all the time, and playing and reading, and all the things I did with him.'[55]

General acceptance of a woman's ultimate suitability for mothering was conveyed by interviewees among the oral history sample. As a result, many women commented on how fathers were marginal to family life and excluded from many 'hands on' tasks:

'It was 1964 when Elizabeth was born and it was just getting to the stage where men might just occasionally push the pram around the sports field—if pushed.'[56]

'He used to work at home one afternoon a week . . . and that was my afternoon off. He just did things with the babies. It was just the beginning of the hands on fathers, but he had no model for that because he said that his father didn't. He was a loving father, but it just wasn't expected and just wasn't done.'[57]

'You certainly never saw fathers picking up children from school . . . because if you are working you can't do that sort of thing. So it was the normal thing to have to do anyway, for the woman.'[58]

There was thus no sense that these women particularly resented the lack of input from their husbands in this way, as men were expected to act within social norms. Looking back retrospectively, many wives felt that this situation was in fact disadvantageous to men, since they inevitably missed out on much of family life.

EXPERIENCE OF NERVOUS DISORDER

Having been previously preoccupied with the psychoses and other serious forms of mental disorder, during the 1950s and 1960s psychiatrists began to direct attention towards the more minor symptoms observed in relation to anxiety states and depressive disorders. Edward Shorter has argued that 'in their struggle to maintain themselves against non-medical competition, psychiatrists took familiar, real illnesses and expanded their margins.'[59] As has been well documented, there was a corresponding rise in the prescribing of new tranquillizing drugs and antidepressants.[60] However, there was little agreement on diagnostic categories or on the classification of symptoms. Medical debates centred largely around the existence, or otherwise, of two distinct depressive states. The 'endogenous' form of the condition was characterized by early-morning waking, appetite disturbance, and loss of libido. Symptoms were regarded as quite easily recognizable and embodied the more 'classical' aspects of melancholic depression such as feelings of guilt and hopelessness. The other form of the illness was referred to variously as atypical, exogenous, neurotic, or reactive depression. This condition was typified by subtly different symptoms, which usually included anxiety as an additional dimension. Since anxiety came to be seen as a frequent accompaniment to depression, patients were increasingly prescribed tranquillizers alongside antidepressants.[61]

Given the confusion that surrounded the diagnosis of these conditions, women interviewed for this project were asked to include any of the symptoms which might reasonably fall within the term 'affective disorder,' defined here as a mental disorder characterized by the disturbance of mood, thoughts, emotions, or behaviour. When questioned on aspects of psychological ill-health, the most prominent theme to arise from the interviews as a possible cause of symptoms was that of marital discord, followed by negative childhood or adolescent experiences. These themes were by no means mutually exclusive. Indeed, while several respondents located one major set of circumstances as the cause of their problems, they also implied that other aspects of their lives as children could be included as contributory factors. The women were asked whether or not they were afflicted by nervous or emotional conditions and in which ways such conditions presented themselves. They were questioned in detail about their own particular coping mechanisms and any treatment sought for their symptoms. Approximately half of the respondents in this project identified themselves as having suffered from anxiety or depression. Most of these women sought medical advice about their disorder; however, only a small number of these consultations resulted in treatment with psychotropic medications.

Many respondents, while not dissatisfied with their domestic role, experienced marriages that were unhappy. These women were able to link distressing situations with the onset of psychiatric symptoms. Eileen Bailey, for example, 'always wanted to be married with a family,' but indicated early on in the interview that she had 'married the wrong man.'[62] Eileen remained married for twenty-five years and finally divorced her husband following years of his philandering:

> 'It was awful to feel that you couldn't trust him. And I think it happened a lot in the tennis club. And I knew that other people knew and were probably talking about it. And that doesn't make you feel very good.'[63]

At the time, Eileen was not overtly aware of the clinical terms anxiety or depression; however, she remembered things 'getting on top of her' sometimes. This she described as:

> 'Just a feeling. I'd go and see my doctor who knew. And he'd say: "Oh you've got the old trouble again?" . . . When I went to see him it was because I felt "I can't cope any longer." I don't think he gave me anything. But just to talk to someone was nice.'[64]

Eileen remembered that, despite the financial difficulties, after her divorce the 'feelings' soon disappeared: 'They had been caused by the situation and by the time I'd left him, I felt much better.'[65]

Anne and Rose, two friends interviewed together with Jean Hill, remarked that it was not seen as appropriate to discuss marital problems with others. Anne maintained that: 'If you were having trouble in your marriage, you didn't go talking to anyone about it. You know, you suffered on your own.'[66] Jean concurred:

> 'I would go as far as to use the word "ashamed," because you viewed yourself as a failure. You were unaware that other people—you thought all their marriages were wonderful, unless you saw something obviously sticking out like a sore thumb. But everybody was having a "lovely" marriage, so, if you had any problems at all, you didn't tell anybody.'[67]

Nora Kelly moved to Australia with her husband soon after they were married, in order for him to take up a university post. Not only did Nora feel isolated so far away from her family, but, following the birth of her first child, she became resigned to the fact that she had chosen the wrong husband. He was relocated again to America shortly after the birth of their son and Nora made what she felt to be a courageous decision, to return to England as a single parent:

> 'I was actually depressed by the time I'd left my ex-husband because he was an awful person . . . I was with [him] for about six weeks after we arrived in America and then I said "I want to leave you." And I would just burst into tears all the time. And I wonder if then it was the baby blues,

> that we hadn't sort of acknowledged at that time—although it was pretty difficult living with the ex-husband, half the time not speaking.'[68]

Back in England, Nora enrolled at teacher-training college and attempted to juggle single-motherhood with her studies. She talked at length about her experience of obsessive behaviour and depression:

> 'When I started college I was getting anxiety, and I knew I was depressed . . . I'd be going off to college and think "have I got my key?" And I did Geography as a main, and I would think "Oh we're going on a coach, I might be sick on the coach" and all this sort of thing.'[69]

Nora was plagued by these symptoms for many years. She received psychopharmacological remedies from her general practitioner but was unable to remember exactly what she had been prescribed. Although she felt the drugs helped to alleviate the worst of her symptoms, it was with deep regret that she recalled how the situation had taken its toll on her son:

> 'When I was sent out for school practice, I wouldn't get home before James and he used to get home by bus. And he said: "I'd always go and look to see if the suitcases were gone." He always thought I wasn't coming home. I think that's really awful really . . . And I can remember walking along the beach . . . and I just thought: "I want to throw myself into the sea, I want to die" and I just thought: "I can't leave James on his own to go through life with people saying his mother committed suicide."'[70]

Nora was not offered any counselling for her problems; however, she felt lucky to have a doctor who was understanding:

> 'I think for that time, he was very good. He gave me some kind of tranquillizers . . . and he said "I can't even cope with my own kids; I don't know how you are coping with your own and a class-room."'[71]

After approximately six months, Nora reduced her medication by herself; however, her emotional state did not improve until she reached her late forties:

> 'I just weaned myself off them. I didn't really do any follow-up because that was a bus journey the other way and I would have had to take James with me—or have a day off college, and it just—never seemed to have the time to do it.'[72]

What is striking about these accounts is that the mothers were still able to hold on to the joy they experienced in their role as mothers. Nora, for example, remembered that:

'Probably the best memories—just that I was absolutely smitten with James, it was brilliant, despite the other problems. I got fascinated with child-development and thought it was absolutely wonderful.'[73]

Eileen Bailey also asserted that she was happy to be a full-time mother:

'I think deep down I may have been a natural mum. I enjoyed being a mum . . . I think your children need you at all ages. And a lot of people say: "Oh I'll go to work when they go to school" but I think they need you just as much. As they come in the front door: "Mum . . . !" I think once a mother, always a mother.'[74]

Although treatments with new drugs became more familiar, there is little evidence from this oral history project to support Jonathan Metzl's assertion that during the 1950s and 1960s medication was used to reinforce the idea that a woman's desire to leave the home was a 'deep illness.' Metzl contends that representations of psychotropic medications simply reproduced the cultural and social baggage associated with Freudian psychoanalytical paradigms. Consequently, he maintains that drugs were prescribed to women who rejected their maternal duties and thus, 'spread a pathology that was damaging to men.'[75] On the contrary, some of the women interviewed for this project found the reverse to be true. Whilst it was often accepted that the use of psychotropic medications did not provide a permanent solution to the problem, it was not uncommon for women to remark that such treatment gave them clarity of thought and an opportunity to assess their life circumstances with a view to change. One interviewee, Ann Coles, became pregnant while studying for her A' Levels and married 'not very happily' at eighteen. Raised in an orthodox Catholic family, she went on to have five children in quick succession:

'I was nearly nineteen when my daughter was born. I then had a baby every year, for four years—and then there was a gap of less than three years before the fifth one was born . . . I hadn't wanted to get married—I hadn't wanted to get pregnant at that point, and with hindsight, I was depressed. I was pregnant nearly the whole time . . . You know, I felt like for certainly most of the sixties I was just surviving, I was just getting by.'[76]

Not only did Ann have deep regrets about the way in which she became a parent and the lack of control over her fertility, but she also encountered serious difficulties with her husband, who developed psychiatric illness himself:

'He had a personality disorder. And that was part of the problem that brought me to the end of my wits . . . As the years went by, this obsessive behaviour became more compulsive and he would get into cleaning, and

> he'd be on his hands and knees with a tooth brush, cleaning between the tiles. You know, he would take the money from his purse and polish his pennies with Duraglitz. He was really running into trouble. And no-one recognized this, so there wasn't any help.'[77]

When Ann's youngest child was two she received a visit from her health visitor that she recalled as a turning point in her life:

> '[She] recognized that I was depressed and advised me to see my doctor, which I did. And he prescribed antidepressants. And it was when the antidepressants kicked in that I packed my bags and left.'[78]

She described the way in which she felt these drugs enabled her to break free from her circumstances:

> 'It was at that point that I found the wherewithal—it helped me to see through what was stopping me leaving . . . I recognized he was ill, therefore I couldn't leave. So having seen through that, as a result of the antidepressants, I think probably within about a month of starting [them], I left with the children . . . It sort of freed me up in terms of being able to recognize what was keeping me in this situation. And I think, having taken control, and leaving, I was into a new life.'[79]

Ann acknowledged that she has been prone to short periods of depression since, largely she felt due to what her doctor had diagnosed as seasonal affective disorder. However, she maintained that her problems had little to do with motherhood and domestic life. Instead she related them directly to the difficulties in her marriage and the consequences of being unable to control her fertility:

> 'I've never had a planned pregnancy. We were practising Catholics and I suppose the Pope was always sitting on the bottom of the bed. It took me a long time to rebel . . . much later I remarried, and if we had had more children I would have done it very differently. It would have been done very much by choice and I think I would have savoured the experience. There was no savouring the experience, there was only surviving it, and that was to do with my particular circumstances.'[80]

Ann Coles was not the only woman who referred to a husband with psychiatric symptoms. Barbara Vicary felt that her husband was the one to succumb to 'nerves' and 'strain.' Having moved from America to live in London with her English husband, Barbara recounted the ways in which he coped with pressure:

> 'He was starting a company under Wilson's government. It was terrible. We had a garbage disposal strike—the garbage out in London in front

of the nicest buildings. We had an electric strike . . . My husband had a regular strong drink. We didn't keep a "bar" or anything, so he would just keep it in the larder. [My husband] took Valium, and I was very worried about it. And he would take more because of stressful times, and I was worried about the drinking and the Valium.'[81]

Barbara remembered that she had suffered regularly from migraine headaches. She related these to 'stress' but said that she could not rule out the possibility of a hormonal cause. 'Stress' did not appear to be connected to her domestic role and she asserted on more than one occasion that she thought it was important for mothers to stay at home with their children. However, once again, Barbara's testimony reflects a recurring theme of this chapter, since she revealed that she had experienced marital difficulties and ultimately divorced:

> 'I married someone in my class at university, exactly my age, and I don't happen to think that men and women mature in quite the same way. And I think he changed quite a bit. He developed as quite a good businessman but not much else. So I had to fill in with all the love and affection in the family . . . We began to live very separate lives, and they were very full, and they overlapped as long as the children were there.'[82]

After twenty-seven years of marriage, Barbara was finally divorced from her husband:

> 'It was quite horrifying to me . . . and I was very naïve about it, I went to a lawyer that my husband got for me, and he didn't give me very much financially—instead of giving me half. And all that was very hard.'[83]

Of the women interviewed who remained happily married, many also presented anecdotal evidence about friends or relatives who experienced 'nervous breakdown' as a result of unsatisfactory relationships. Betty Sanderson, for example, while never aware of feeling depressed or anxious herself, recalled:

> 'I had a close friend at one point when the children were young who became very nervy—but that was because she discovered her husband was philandering and her marriage was actually starting to break up at this point. I was aware that she was becoming on the point of a nervous breakdown really. But I knew the reason why.'[84]

Margaret Windsor agreed: 'I mean the old terminology was "nervous breakdown"—and that was usually connected with relationship breakdown.'[85] Margaret was interviewed with her friend Doris Carter who was able to relate this to circumstances in her own family:

> 'I think Aunty Gladys was the only one that—yes, she had terrible nerves. And her husband left her with Patricia as a little girl . . . I think it was Albert leaving her.'[86]

In a similar way, Eileen Roberts remembered a woman she knew at her playgroup:

> 'One mum, her husband, he was a teacher, but he got involved with a student and she had a breakdown. He didn't go off, but he was having an affair with this young girl.'[87]

These oral testimonies suggest that, despite adverse circumstances, many women were still able to find contentment and satisfaction from their role as mothers and homemakers. It is certainly true that women encountered significant emotional hardship and economic inequality if their marital relationship broke down; however, previous histories have been disproportionately influenced by the notion that domestic life itself was the cause of emotional disorder.

Not all respondents diagnosed with anxiety or depressive disorders were able to trace the cause to their own marriages. A notable number maintained that their parents' relationship had had a marked influence on them in later life. During a period when divorce was socially ostracized and difficult to obtain, it is not surprising that some women witnessed difficult or tense relationships between their parents. Others recalled specific incidents or traumatic experiences that were to affect them later in adulthood. A small number of interviewees remarked that they were influenced by their own relationship with their parents. These accounts support the contention that domesticity had little to do with neuroses, since these women often remembered the onset of symptoms occurring long before they were married.

Frances Wilson, for example, experienced a 'breakdown' by the time she took her A' Levels. To Frances, there were clear and straightforward reasons for this.

> 'I was a scholarship pupil at a direct grant school . . . it was an absolute revelation, but I was unhappy because I had to conceal my home background. At one point, we were homeless and living in a homeless hostel . . . so self-esteem was low by the time I left school. I'd collapsed by the time A' Levels came, and had a nervous breakdown . . . we were living in this one room and my parents were terribly unhappy, and I think what happened to me—which was really an adolescent anxiety state—was a perfectly natural, normal response to incredible stress . . . living in one room with my parents constantly quarrelling.'[88]

Frances recounted a story of resilience and a long struggle with minor mental conditions, culminating much later with the diagnosis of depression.

However, she was keen to assert early on in the interview, that: 'I can explain why, and it had nothing to do with domesticity.'[89] When asked how she felt about domesticity and her role as a mother, Frances affirmed:

> 'Domesticity suited me very well. I was content with that. And of course the children just made it so super. Family life was good. I have to say that although I'd had very poor parenting myself, from somewhere or other I'd got a good idea of what I wanted. And although nobody had told me that shouting was bad for self-esteem, in here [pointing to her head] I knew it was. And I never shouted at them. I never said shut-up to them.'[90]

Judith Morgan was another interviewee to recall that her upbringing and events from her childhood had affected her emotional security in later life. Judith's parents were both in the teaching profession and she felt that undue pressure was put upon her to succeed. Judith maintained that her mother's desire for academic achievement also had a negative effect on her:

> 'I always felt she was a bit before her time. My friend's mothers didn't go out to work . . . and I learned by her mistakes . . . I felt I couldn't divide my time up—not that I couldn't—I didn't want to. So it certainly made me very aware when I had children of my own. She never actually had time for us.'[91]

Judith developed symptoms of anxiety during her adult life; however, she believed that this was due to the fact that her mother was anxious and overprotective. She believed that these traits were consequently projected onto them as children:

> 'I am convinced, having had psychiatric help, that it actually has rubbed off—that you know, you're not born with fear, it's something that you learn. I think when somebody's constantly putting that in your face, then you are going to pick it up at some point . . . And funnily enough, a lot of the fears diminished after her death—as if she had sort of held me for many years.'[92]

Judith's mother was agitated and apprehensive about all aspects of life and was prone to making telephone calls expressing concern about normal daily events:

> 'I travelled endlessly when I was teaching, and it worried her. I would get endless phone calls where she would say "do you have to go there? The weather's not very good—can you not go?" That was very difficult to come to terms with because it filtered into your existence the whole time.'[93]

Her mother's anxiety is interesting in itself since, to Judith, there appeared to be no obvious cause. She maintained that it had little to do with domestic life since her role as a teacher was central to her life. Moreover, it appeared to be unrelated to her career as the symptoms continued into old-age. However, during the interview it became clear that Judith's parents experienced difficulties in their marriage:

> 'It was very volatile. Very, very volatile. My father drank quite a lot in the early stages of the marriage which my mother wasn't happy about. And he became belligerent and aggressive. And so there were times when he used to hit her about. And I remember this as a young child, and being very upset by the fact that there was this sort of unease all the time. And he was going to leave, but he never did—so there was this unrest. And they bickered and quarrelled and fought until their dying day. We were just brought up on that which is not nice . . . I often used to think "why don't they get divorced. You know, surely it must be easier than all this agro." But I don't think it was done. I didn't know any of their generation or anyone within the family who got divorced.'[94]

As children, the older women in this cohort were often witness to traumatic war-time events, some of which were to make a significant impact on them in future years. Judy Giles has observed that for many women during this period, hopes and aspirations for the future were framed by the knowledge that they had survived where so many others had not.[95] Eileen Roberts attended a school in London where six teachers and thirty-nine children were killed during a bombing raid. Her best friend was buried under debris for three days. She asserted that 'you just don't get over anything like that.'[96] She also remarked that the strain had badly affected relationships within her family:

> 'My father, because of the war, became very religious . . . he became very strict—Baptist. I wasn't evacuated. My father wouldn't let me go to be evacuated, because of this religious thing—we went into the air-raid shelter, and then he decided that no, we weren't going to do that. If we were going to get killed, we were going to get killed and that was that. So we slept in the house all the time—right through the blitz . . . you just don't get over anything like that really.'[97]

Eileen intimated that the war had affected her father's psychological health. His behaviour became erratic and normal family activities were suddenly banned: 'We weren't allowed to go to the pictures; he threw my mother's make-up away; he used to read the bible to us every night—a complete change.'[98] She remembered her mother and father shouting at each other and found this 'distressing.' Eileen thought it possible that her family were predisposed to depressive disorders:

> 'If I look back, I'd probably always suffered from depression—but it wasn't acknowledged you see. Nobody talked about it, there was little understanding of these conditions . . . I mean Dad was a depressive. I just think it's familial and that's the way you are.'[99]

In Eileen's case, the onset of anxiety and depression was clearly unrelated to domestic life since she remembered feeling unwell before her marriage and the birth of her children:

> 'I was like this when we lived in Luton, when I was travelling up to London—I couldn't keep awake, and I'd get into the office and I'd start typing, and I'd go into the cloakroom and I'd sit down and go to sleep.'[100]

Eileen and her husband had always wanted a large family and had chosen to have five children. She was strongly of the opinion that there was great value in being at home with them.

Respondents thus shared the perception that some individuals might be predisposed to mental illness; however, many also indicated that environmental factors could trigger illness. When asked to comment on the cause of their illness, women referred to traumatic events and dysfunctional relationships, and not to aspects of domesticity and mothering. Some of the women interviewed vividly recalled that the onset of symptoms was before marriage, and others remarked that husbands were more likely to be predisposed to anxiety and depression due to the pressures they experienced at work.

CONCLUSION

This chapter has suggested that historians have disproportionately emphasized the negative aspects of housework and mothering. Consequently, they have often failed to foreground the possible links between mental illness and other situational circumstances—in particular, relationship breakdown. It has been suggested that it would be productive to move beyond a feminist analysis and place these findings within the context of their time, acknowledging both the disadvantages and advantages of women's role in the home. Giles argues that much of the feminist historiography has accepted Friedan's narrative unquestioningly.[101] Indeed, this approach has permeated the whole of society to the extent that a number of respondents initially assumed that the prime objective of this research would be to illustrate discontent and disillusion among women of this period. Betty Sanderson, for instance, was concerned that she 'hadn't been a very good person' to interview, since she was unable to provide any real discontent with her role. This was also exemplified in the testimony of Barbara Rogers, who recalled: 'I had people saying I had wasted my education, but I never felt guilty about staying at home and felt it was the right thing to do at the time.'[102] The hopes and aspirations conveyed by these women must be understood as the product of a specific historical moment,[103] and thus, it is possible that given the different opportunities that emerged during the late 1960s and early 1970s, some women may have made different choices. However, this should not detract from the experience of many who look back on their lives as happy and successful. Indeed, Gwen Collins aptly noted, 'Well we weren't trying to "find ourselves" or whatever it is you've got to do—"find your identity," or whatever you've got to do today!'[104]

These findings would certainly suggest that Judith Hubback might not have been speaking on behalf of the majority of married women when she claimed in 1957 that 'brains are a distinct handicap to a woman's prospect of happiness and contentment.'[105] The present findings differ substantially from those highlighted by feminist scholars. It is suggested here that the ideas emanating from these authors originated not from the experience of the average suburban housewife, but rather that they were formulated by a unique group of women who were largely unrepresentative of married women. The biographies of both contemporary sociologists of the 1950s and 1960s and later academics suggest that they emerged from untypical backgrounds that were either highly academic or political.[106] Betty Friedan claimed that her feminism had its roots in suburban captivity; however, Daniel Horowitz and Judy Giles have recently shown convincingly that, to the contrary, her experiences as a labour journalist and her involvement with the Popular Front played a significant role in fostering her feminism.[107] Ann Oakley, daughter of social policy theorist Richard Titmuss, pertinently admitted that 'feminism has never been a mainstream or a fashionable political belief. You have to be a bit of an outsider to be a feminist. That describes me exactly.'[108] However, she still identifies the roots of her feminism in her experiences as 'a conventional suburban housewife.'[109] A Mass Observation investigation undertaken in 1957 into 'The Housewife's Day' perhaps more accurately describes the milieu in which post-war women found themselves:

> 'It is fashionable to look on housewives as an under-privileged group, overworked, underpaid and undervalued—legitimately dissatisfied with their lot . . . to the contemporary eye, her domestic day of varied, overlapping activities may look muddled and wasteful. That she should prefer it that way is a point rarely considered.'[110]

It is thus possible that for Ann Oakley and other feminist theorists the experience of being a suburban housewife had been shaped by factors that were unrepresentative of most middle-class wives and that resulted in an alternative evaluation of the role. Future investigation, therefore, should not only consider the negative aspects of domesticity, but also draw upon and validate the voices of those who considered their experiences positive and worthwhile.

NOTES

1. Angela Holdsworth, *Out of the Doll's House* (London: BBC, 1988), 29.
2. William Beveridge, *Social Insurance and Allied Services,* (London: HMSO, 1942), paragraphs 107, 111.
3. Hannah Gavron, *The Captive Wife* (London: Routledge, 1966); Judith Hubback, *Wives Who Went to College* (London: William Heinemann, 1957); Viola Klein, *Britain's Married Women Workers* (London: Routledge and Kegan Paul, 1965).
4. Ruth Cooperstock and Henry L. Lennard, 'Some social meanings of tranquilizer use,' *Sociology of Heath and Illness,* 1 (1979), 331–47.
5. The oral history element comprises two chapters of my doctoral thesis, in which oral testimony is supported by a wide range of documentary sources from Mass Observation and the women's periodical press. The research project also examines representations of women in pharmacological advertising for drugs prescribed for anxiety and depression, and suggests that, in contrast to the findings of feminist theorists, women were not a deliberate target in advertising images.
6. Judy Giles, *The Parlour and the Suburb: Domestic Identities, Class, Femininity and Modernity* (Oxford: Berg, 2004), 144.
7. Ibid., 148.
8. *Desperate Housewives,* Channel 4 Television.
9. Ann Oakley, *Gender on Planet Earth* (Cambridge: Polity, 2002), 116.
10. Germaine Greer, *The Female Eunuch* (London: Flamingo, [1970], 1999), 312.
11. Betty Friedan, *The Feminine Mystique* (London: Penguin, [1963], 1992), 13, 19.
12. Agnes Miles, *Women and Mental Illness* (Brighton: Wheatsheaf, 1988), 47, 12.
13. This debate is addressed in detail in: Miles, *Women and Mental Illness;* Elaine Showalter, *The Female Malady* (London: Virago, 2001); Jane Ussher, *Women's Madness: Misogyny or Mental Illness?* (Hertfordshire: Harvester Wheatsheaf, 1991); Hilary Graham, *Hardship and Health in Women's Lives* (Hertfordshire: Harvester Wheatsheaf, 1993); and Catherine Niven and Doug Carroll, *The Health Psychology of Women* (Switzerland: Harwood, 1993).
14. Walter R Gove and Jeannette F Tudor, 'Adult sex roles and mental illness,' *American Journal of Sociology,* 78 (1973), 812–35.
15. Ibid., 814.
16. Ibid., 815.
17. Ibid.
18. Ruth Cooperstock, 'Sex differences in psychotropic drug use,' *Social Science and Medicine,* 12B (1978), 179–86.
19. Cooperstock and Lennard, 'Some social meanings of tranquillizer use.'
20. Ludimilla Jordanova, 'Mental illness, mental health: changing norms and expectations,' in *Women in Society: Interdisciplinary Essays* (London: Virago, 1981), 102, 112.
21. Michel Foucault, *The Will to Knowledge: The History of Sexuality: 1* (London: Penguin [1976] 1998), 94.
22. Here, the boundaries of research have been expanded to include not only domesticity and mothering, but also the experience of relationships and mental ill-health.

23. See Betty Jerman, *The Lively Minded Women: The First Twenty Years of the National Housewives Register* (London: Heinemann, 1981).
24. In total twenty-nine women were interviewed and a further six women who were unable to meet for interview sent written testimonies. Pseudonyms have been used to protect anonymity.
25. The format of the interviews was loosely based on those developed for research by Ann Oakley and others, in order that comparisons and contrasts could be drawn between research projects. See in particular: Ann Oakley, *The Sociology of Housework* (Oxford: Blackwell, 1985); and Melanie Henwood, Lesley Rimmer and Malcolm Wicks, *Inside the Family: Changing Roles of Men and Women* (London: Family Policy Centre, 1987). For discussion of the merits and difficulties associated with the practice of oral history, see: Robert Perks and Alistair Thomson (eds.), *The Oral History Reader* (London: Routledge, 1989); Raphael Samuel and Paul Thompson (eds.), *The Myths we Live By* (London, Routledge, 1990); and Sherna Berger Gluck and Daphne Patai, *Women's Words: The Feminist Practice of Oral History* (London: Routledge, 1991).
26. Gavron, *The Captive Wife,* 61.
27. Chris Richards was brought up in London and married in 1949. She moved to Scotland with her husband and had two children. Interviewed with her friend Margaret Lincoln on 6th September 2004.
28. Betty Sanderson was born in Sussex in 1929. She married in 1955 and had three children. Interviewed on 3rd September 2004.
29. Frances Wilson was raised in London and married in 1960. She had two children. Interviewed on 11th April 2005.
30. Written testimony of Barbara Rogers. Barbara was born in Lincoln and married in 1962. Even though she had gained a degree at university, she 'chose to stay at home for almost 20 years' and considered herself 'privileged to have been able to do it.'
31. Val Parker was born in 1935. Both her father and her husband were in the army, therefore she moved home frequently. She married in 1955 and had two children. Interviewed on 2nd November 2004.
32. Edna Goodridge was born in Birmingham in 1925. She was married in 1950 and had two children. Interviewed on 4th January 2005.
33. Doris Carter was born in 1915 in Essex. She was married in 1945 and had one daughter in 1951. Interviewed with three friends and her daughter on 18th January 2005.
34. Jean Hill was born in Middlesex in 1933. She married in 1955 and had two children. She also had two still-born children. Interviewed with two friends on 24th September 2004.
35. Eileen Roberts was born in Lewisham in 1929. She was married in 1949 and had five children. Interviewed on 17th January 2005.
36. Holdsworth, *Out of the Doll's House,* 29.
37. Katherine Stead was born in 1937 in London. She married in 1958 and had five children. Interviewed on 30th November 2004.
38. Christine Calderwood was born in Nottingham in 1937. She was married in 1960 and had two children. Interviewed on 5th October 2004.
39. Val Parker.
40. Klein, *Britain's Married Women Workers,* 37.
41. Gavron, *The Captive Wife,* 111.
42. See for example: Elizabeth Wilson, *Only Half Way to Paradise: Women in Post-War Britain 1945–1968* (London: Tavistock, 1980); Penny Summerfield, 'Women in Britain since 1945; Companionate Marriage and the Double Burden,' in James Obelkevich and Peter Catterall (eds.), *Understanding*

Post-War British Society (London: Routledge, 1994); Jane Lewis, *Women in Britain Since 1945* (Oxford: Blackwell, 1992); Mary Abbott, *Family Affairs: A History of the British Family in 20th Century England* (London: Routledge, 2003); Ann Oakley, *Woman's Work* (London: Penguin, 1974) and *The Sociology of Housework* (Oxford: Blackwell, 1985).

43. Judy Giles, *The Parlour and the Suburb*, 150.
44. In later years Eileen Roberts went on to become a teacher, and the Pre-School Playgroup Association was the topic of her dissertation at university.
45. Upon moving to a new area, Katherine later founded her own group of NWR.
46. Eileen Bailey was born on the Isle of Sheppey in 1922. She married in 1943 and had three daughters. Interviewed on 30th November 2004.
47. Gwen Collins was born in Cardiff in 1919. She married in 1940 and had three children. Interviewed on 18th January 2005 with two friends: Doris Carter and Margaret Windsor.
48. Margaret Windsor was born in Stockport in 1933. She was married in 1953 and had two children.
49. Katherine Stead.
50. John Bowlby, *Maternal Care and Mental Health* (Geneva: WHO, 1951) and *Child Care and the Growth of Love* (Middlesex: Pelican, 1853); D. W. Winnicott, *The Family and Individual Development* (London: Tavistock Publications, 1965) and *The Child and the Family: First Relationships* (London, Tavistock Publications, 1957); Benjamin Spock, *Baby and Child Care* (London: Bodley Head, 1955).
51. With the exception of Faith Lawson, who chose not to have children, and Ann Shepherd, who was unable to.
52. Betty Sanderson.
53. Margaret Lincoln was born in Drayton Bassett in 1930. She married in 1951 and adopted her nephew and niece, ages 5 and 7, in 1964. For financial reasons she continued to work following the adoption. However, she was always home for the children after school and stressed the importance of being at home to care for them when they were ill.
54. Ibid.
55. Gwen Collins.
56. Christine Calderwood.
57. Diane Braithwaite was born in New York in 1937. She married an Englishman in 1962 and came to Coventry. She had two children.
58. Katherine Stead.
59. Edward Shorter, *A History of Psychiatry: From the Era of the Asylum to the Age of Prozac* (Canada: John Wiley, 1997), 292.
60. David Healy, *The Antidepressant Era* (Cambridge, MA, and London: Harvard University Press, 1997); David Healy, *The Creation of Psychopharmacology* (Cambridge, MA, and London: Harvard University Press, 2002); Christopher M. Callahan and German E Berrios, *Reinventing Depression: A History of the Treatment of Depression in Primary Care 1940–1970* (Oxford: Oxford University Press, 2005).
61. The classification, causes, and treatment of affective disorder are examined in full in Ali Haggett, 'Housewives, neuroses and the domestic environment, 1945–70,' PhD thesis, University of Exeter, 2007.
62. Eileen Bailey.
63. Ibid.
64. Ibid.
65. Ibid.
66. Anne Shepherd was born in Clevedon in 1938. She married in 1960 but was unable to have children.

67. Jean Hill.
68. Nora Kelly was born in 1936 in Oxford. She married in 1961 and had two children.
69. Ibid.
70. Ibid.
71. Ibid.
72. Ibid.
73. Ibid.
74. Eileen Bailey.
75. Jonathan Metzl, *Prozac on the Couch* (Durham, NC: Duke University Press, 2003), 74, 81.
76. Ann Coles was born in Cardiff in 1944. She married in 1962 and had five children. Interviewed on 16th November 2004.
77. Ibid.
78. Ibid.
79. Ibid.
80. Ibid.
81. Barbara Vicary was born in Illinois in 1931. She moved to England with her husband in 1963 and had two children. Interviewed on 14th October 2004.
82. Ibid.
83. Ibid.
84. Betty Sanderson.
85. Margaret Windsor.
86. Doris Carter.
87. Eileen Roberts.
88. Francis Wilson.
89. Ibid.
90. Ibid.
91. Judith Morgan was born in 1943 and thus her perspective was as a child of the 1950s. She married and raised a family in the 1970s.
92. Ibid.
93. Ibid. Judith gave up her teaching when her first child was born. She worked part-time as an illustrator until the children were older.
94. Ibid.
95. Giles, *The Parlour and the Suburb,* 161.
96. Eileen Roberts.
97. Ibid.
98. Ibid.
99. Ibid.
100. Ibid.
101. Giles, *The Parlour and the Suburb,* 155.
102. Barbara Rogers.
103. Giles, *The Parlour and the Suburb,* 48. Giles illustrates how 'home' meant (and means) different things to different women; thus, the desires represented by home are differentiated historically and socially (159–61).
104. Gwen Collins.
105. Hubback, *Wives Who Went to College,* 156.
106. Viola Klein, for example, born in 1908, attended the Sorbonne. She lost both parents in concentration camps. Alva Myrdal was engaged with the women's movement and worked as Secretary to the Swedish Government Commission on paid work. Judith Hubback was educated at Cambridge and married the son of Eva Hubback—joint founder of The Townswomen's Guild.

107. See Daniel Horowitz, *Betty Friedan and the Making of the Feminine Mystique: American Left, the Cold War and Modern Feminism* (Amherst: University of Massachusetts Press, 2000).
108. www.AnnOakley.co.uk/AOFAQs.htm.
109. Ann Oakley, a guest speaker on 'Thinking Allowed,' BBC Radio Four, 22 June 2005.
110. Mass Observation, (1957), New Series 54, 'The Housewife's Day.'

6 'I Thought You Would Want to Come and See His Home':[1]

Child Guidance and Psychiatric Social Work in Inter-War Britain

John Stewart

INTRODUCTION

This chapter examines child guidance in the inter-war period and its perspective on, and engagement with, the home life of its child 'patients.' Concern with the home derived in part from child guidance's organisational structures and the respective roles of those who carried out its work, in part from the psychiatric model employed, which emphasised the need to understand the whole child and his or her environment, and in part from an increasing emphasis on the child's relationship with its parents in the domestic setting. While child guidance was in principle a clinic-based form of psychiatric medicine, it was through observation and treatment in the home that mental maladjustment was to be tackled.

The present chapter is intended as a contribution to the important, but as yet imperfectly understood, international movement for child guidance. Historians such as Margo Horn, Theresa Richardson, and Kathleen Jones have analysed child guidance in its American homeland, although they pay relatively little attention to its international dimensions.[2] British child guidance has been less well served, although important contributions have been made by Harry Hendrick and Deborah Thom for England, and by Lynn Abrams for Scotland.[3] This bears out Roger Cooter's recently made point about the limited historical writing on children's medical welfare.[4] The present chapter is thus part of a broader project that seeks to address these gaps in the historiography and to provide a more detailed and nuanced account of child guidance than previously by analysing how different practices and philosophies took root in different parts of Britain.[5] As will be evident even from this chapter, the project has identified a wide range of rich, but previously unexploited, archival material from important centres such as Birmingham and Glasgow.

Finally, this chapter seeks to contribute to the history of social work, a field of welfare provision seriously under-researched and little understood.[6] The inter-war period was crucial in this history because of the impetus to professionalisation provided by the training and practice of psychiatric social workers, a profession that emerged after 1918 in an organic relationship with child guidance. Moreover, the latter's increasing emphasis on the home afforded significant opportunities for psychiatric social work and its claims to 'scientific' knowledge and observation.

CHILD GUIDANCE

What was child guidance and what did it seek to achieve? Although it had deep historical roots, the movement is generally agreed to have begun in the United States in the immediate aftermath of the First World War. Child guidance was part of the broader, and self-consciously international, concern for 'mental hygiene.' As Mathew Thomson has suggested, the latter derived from 'an expansion of interest' during the inter-war era in the 'prevention of mental disorder' and the 'promotion of environmental conditions to encourage positive mental health among the normal population.'[7] As we shall see, child guidance was to be concerned with the environment and the 'normal' child. We should note also the idea of mental hygiene as a form of preventive medicine and of mental health being something that, in modern conditions, could be hard to maintain. As the Institute of Medical Psychology wrote to British local authorities in the early 1930s: 'Post war conditions have induced and increased the incidence of nervous disorders; that increase is likely to be maintained unless co-ordinated action is taken to get at the root of the problem.'[8] Here children had a key role to play. A report on the Liverpool clinic by a member of its medical staff claimed that child guidance was 'particularly valuable as a key to mental hygiene in that, at an early age, slight abnormalities are often easily corrected.' In turn, this would avert 'the grosser forms of problem.'[9] Good mental health in childhood was, in other words, the key to good mental health in later life.

Central to the development of child guidance, in the United States and subsequently in Britain, was the New York-based philanthropic organisation the Commonwealth Fund. In Britain, the fund operated through its 'English [sic] Mental Hygiene Program.'[10] The fund was keen to promote a medicalised approach to child mental and emotional well-being, and it is this medical model—the classic, or American, model—on which I focus. This was adopted by most child guidance clinics in England and by some of the leading clinics in Scotland as well as being adopted more or less intact in continental European countries such as the Netherlands.[11] Adopting such an approach had a number of important implications for the way in which child guidance was organized and sought to achieve its aims.

First, much emphasis was placed on teamwork through co-operation between psychiatrists, psychologists, and psychiatric social workers.[12] Nonetheless, the medically qualified psychiatrist was the lead figure. Child guidance was thus to be a branch of medicine and not of education or psychology, despite the claims made by members of these professions, most notably in Scotland.[13] But even here, certain key clinics adhered to the American model. The reports of the Notre Dame Clinic in Glasgow, for instance, routinely described the children referred to it as its 'patients.' These patients manifested their problems as 'symptoms' in turn brought about by 'aetiological factors.' What they required, therefore, was 'diagnosis' and 'treatment.'[14]

Secondly, the child guidance team was to be located not in schools or as attachments to the justice system. Rather, child guidance was the provenance of the clinic. The idea of a 'clinic' itself attested to the medicalised approach to child guidance. The clinic, though, was not just a particular building. As one early publication by the London Child Guidance Council put it: 'A Child Guidance Clinic is not primarily a "place," though, of course, it must have a location: it is primarily a *specially trained staff*.'[15] This alerts us to a central theme of this chapter, that much 'child guidance' was actually carried out in the home, rather than the clinic, by psychiatric social workers. It is also worth mentioning that many child guidance practitioners sought to spread the movement's message through popular publications such as *Mother and Child*. Founded in 1930, and so an almost exact contemporary of the founding of British child guidance, this journal carried articles by psychiatrists and psychiatric social workers for its lay readership. In 1937, for instance, Douglas MacCalman, the psychiatrist and leading exponent of child guidance, wrote on 'Familiar Problems of Child Upbringing.'[16]

Thirdly, child guidance sought to deal not with the abnormal, the mentally defective, or problems that were primarily educational. Rather, it dealt with the 'normal' child. Any children, so the argument went, might find themselves in circumstances that could cause emotional or psychological upset or damage. Such problems—usually referred to as 'maladjustment'—might manifest themselves in a range of ways, from 'difficult' behaviour through to bed-wetting or stammering. Although its leading proponents undoubtedly promoted a medicalised version of child guidance, they also acknowledged that difficulties 'medical, psychological, social, educational, familial, and personal' could, in varying degrees and combinations, be involved.[17] The Medical Director of the Birmingham clinic, C. L. C. Burns, remarked that it was 'often said that there are really no problem children but only problem parents.' This was indeed a major theme in child guidance work. Nonetheless, Burns continued that this was 'an exaggeration of the truth' as there were 'many other factors besides the parents in the production of neurosis or behaviour disorder in children.'[18] Maladjustment thus had multiple causes and the child in its totality—from its physical health through its measurable intelligence to the emotional landscape of its home—had to be examined. As another psychiatrist prominent in the movement, R. D. Gillespie, remarked, the 'antithesis between Mind and Body may be an interesting philosophical problem' but it had 'no place' in a child guidance clinic.[19] This was therefore a consciously holistic approach, in keeping with an inter-war movement in Western medicine that sought to move away from purely 'scientific' understandings of health and disease.[20]

Unless properly treated, the problems that any child might encounter would not only cause unhappiness in childhood, but would also work against proper adjustment and social integration in adulthood. As MacCalman observed: 'the normal child has to bear vast personal and environmental strains if he is to grow up to healthy adulthood. We err too much on the side of expecting him to be able to meet these difficulties.'[21] Gaining and maintaining good mental health during childhood and adolescence was not, in other words, easy. The London Child Guidance clinic issued a flyer seeking financial support, which asserted that: 'Learning to Drive is child's play, compared with—Learning to Live!.' Pursuing the motoring metaphor, it continued that 'a crash may mean stealing, violence, rudeness or truancy, and a breakdown is tragic.' Whatever happened, childhood was a 'nervous time, anyway, especially for parents.'[22] Averting mental ill-health was thus as important as averting any other disease. Dr William Moodie, Medical Director of the London Child Guidance Clinic, remarked that 'the unstable child of to-day is the neurotic adult of tomorrow—a disturbing element in the community, unhappy and inefficient in himself and a source of misery to those with whom he associates.'[23]

Who then were the children who attended child guidance clinics? The Dundee clinic in a 9-month period in the mid-1930s dealt with 78 cases, the majority of whom were between 2 and 16 years old. Their 'maladjustments' could be placed in various categories, most notably behaviour difficulties such as stealing and truancy, habits such as stammering and masturbation, and 'undesirable character traits and faulty social adaptation' such as moodiness and timidity.[24] Clearly, this was not an exact science and categories and their contents varied across locations. Nonetheless, this, and other similar evidence, bears out Thom's broad conclusion about the clientele of British clinics.[25] The British experience in turn roughly replicates the experience of the United States, where, for instance, a 1930s textbook on child guidance broke down problems into three categories: socially unacceptable behaviour; personality problems; and 'bad' habits.[26]

If such problems resulted in a child being referred to child guidance clinics, what happened to them once actually there? As one of its annual reports explained, on arrival at Notre Dame each 'patient' was examined physically to 'eliminate the possibility of bodily disease.' The psychologist would then 'estimate the patient's intellectual endowment and this method of attacking an intellectual problem.' The third member of the team, the psychiatric social worker, was charged with making 'numerous visits to the home, in order to view the child in relation to the emotional life of the family.' When all data had been gathered, a case conference was held at which information was pooled 'and interpretation of the problem is suggested and a plan of treatment is decided.' If, during the course of treatment, new information came to light, then further case conferences would be convened. No case was to be closed 'unless there is lack of co-operation on the part of the parents or complete disappearance of the symptoms originally complained of and the personality difficulties subsequently uncovered.'[27]

The demand for child guidance increased dramatically in the inter-war period. At the end of the 1920s there was only one clinic that specifically designated itself as dealing with 'child guidance.' Ten years later there were nearly fifty clinics in England and Wales and around thirteen in Scotland.[28] London, which had the first designated clinic, had nine recognised institutions by 1939.[29] Individual clinics reported steady rises in patient numbers. Liverpool, for instance, had 47 cases referred in 1930 and 103 the following year. By 1935 this had risen further, to 166; and in the last full year of peace to 268.[30] Many clinics complained of inadequate income and resources, and, although other factors were involved, rising demand prior to 1939 contributed to the embedding of child guidance in the post-war welfare state.

BRITISH CHILD GUIDANCE AND PSYCHIATRIC SOCIAL WORK

While psychiatrists were undoubtedly the occupational group with the highest status in the 'classic' child guidance team, psychiatric social workers had considerable scope to influence the information given about the child, or more accurately the child and its home and family circumstances, to the case conference. It also fell largely to the psychiatric social worker to 'interpret' the psychiatric diagnosis to children and their families. As Thom remarks, this meant that although in theory psychiatric social workers had little formal power, in practice 'their recommendations could affect the future of a child radically.'[31] However, child guidance, through the medium of the psychiatric social worker, became less concerned with the child per se. Rather the emphasis was on the child in its domestic setting and, thereby, on the parents.

Jones has analysed this trend in the United States.[32] One authority cited is Helen Leland Witmer, a perceptive analyst of child guidance, its history, and its practitioners. In an important work published in 1940 she acknowledged the shift towards treatment on the part of the psychiatric social worker, utilising the insights of psychiatry in case-work practice. Famously, Witmer observed that child guidance clinics had come to recognise that 'parents as well as their children were their patients'—hence the dictum 'for every problem child a problem parent.'[33] These remarks find a British echo in Moodie's brusque observation that: 'Parents often feel that they are the cause of their children's difficulties, and in so far as they are responsible for their training and upbringing, this is true.'[34] This, of course, has to be qualified in the light of the range of factors identified earlier—not least by Dr Burns—in the creation of maladjustment. Nonetheless, it does point to the issue of parental responsibility, something also highlighted by other chapters in this volume.[35]

In the United States the practice of psychiatric social work contributed to the tensions between the three main professional groups involved in child guidance. But by the same token, advocates of child guidance based on psychiatry had explicitly supported the employment of psychiatric social workers and, crucially, the latter were also to have dedicated training programmes. Daniel Walkowitz observes that the period of the 1920s was, in the United States, a 'significant historical "moment" in the production of social workers' professional identities.'[36] The same can be said of Britain. In both countries, moreover, psychiatric social work played a key role in this professionalisation—in Britain, for instance, through the creation of the Association of Psychiatric Social Workers (APSW).[37] This body was in close contact with, and modelled on, its American counterpart. British psychiatric social work undoubtedly developed its own practices and philosophies. But at least in its early days it was strongly influenced by the American experience and emerged, as in the United States, in an organic relationship with child guidance.

In the late 1920s, leading members of the Child Guidance Council, a body set up to promote the development of child guidance in Britain, travelled to the United States to examine American practice and philosophy. The report that they produced on their return stressed 'the necessity for an adequate staff of specially trained social workers, as they are an indispensable part of the Clinic.' All the successful clinics visited used social workers, and it thus appeared impossible 'to treat the maladjusted child without their assistance.'[38] One member of this visiting group was the social worker Miss St Clair Townsend. She produced a further report devoted solely to psychiatric social work, the rapid growth of which in the United States was 'one of the most striking facts in the history of Mental Hygiene work' in the last ten years. She attributed this primarily to the work of the National Committee for Mental Hygiene and to the instruction given at Smith College.[39] It was at the latter that Mary C. Jarrett, the leading figure in the development of American psychiatric social work, had set up a training course in 1918.[40]

The first course in psychiatric social work in Britain was created at the London School of Economics (LSE) in 1929. It was financially underwritten by the Commonwealth Fund as part of its English Mental Hygiene Program. The first generation of British psychiatric social workers and the LSE course tutors were taken to America to observe child guidance in practice, again with Fund support. The extent to which British psychiatric social workers fully bought into American practices and theory is a complex issue not dealt with here.[41] It is worth noting, though, that those British social workers who visited Smith College would have been exposed not simply to American ideas, but also to those emanating from Continental Europe. Jarrett was keen to utilise contacts with psychiatric clinics in Berlin and Vienna.[42] More generally, it is also notable that one of the declared aims of the APSW was 'to contribute towards the general purposes of mental hygiene.'[43]

For present purposes, however, what is important is that the profession emerged alongside child guidance, and that it had both psychiatric and social work dimensions. A sense of what the training of psychiatric social workers involved can be gained from the 1929 LSE syllabus. Apart from their practical placements—which could take place at, inter alia, the London Child Guidance Clinic—trainees had a total of sixty hours of lectures over the academic year, of which seventeen were to be devoted to psychiatry, twelve to psychology, seven to mental deficiency, six to general psychology, five to abnormal psychology, four to social casework, three to the administration of the Mental Deficiency Acts, and two each to the administration of mental hospitals, social case report presentation, and social work.[44] To be accepted on this course, applicants were expected to have prior social work experience.

Psychiatric social work training thus consisted of a rather uneasy mix between, on the one hand, 'traditional' social work concerns such as casework, and, on the other, new analytical and 'scientific' approaches such as psychiatry. Roy Lubove has argued that in America this raised the critical question that, if psychiatric knowledge was fundamental to social work, how then were psychiatric social workers to be distinguished from the psychiatrist and psychotherapist? The obvious answer here, at least for Lubove, was 'the social worker's inferior training.'[45]

But of course this was not how psychiatric social workers perceived their role. In the United States Jarrett had forcefully, and successfully, argued the case for specialised training with explicitly psychiatric and psychological foundations. This would give the psychiatric social worker the ability to both gather relevant data and interpret the outcome of the case conference.[46] As such, she (since social work was at this point predominantly a female occupation) would employ 'scientific' method and insights. Comparable arguments were made by British psychiatric social workers and their supporters. Dr Moodie stressed that social work investigation into a child's environment was 'no matter of question and answer.' Rather, it was 'scientific observation, with the co-operation of parents and guardians.' Such 'scientific observation' was of vital importance if the social worker was to give the psychiatrist information appropriate for diagnosis.[47] Miss Goldberg, addressing a London child guidance conference in 1939, claimed that the 'psychiatric social worker is in a unique position to act as interpreter as she has knowledge of both the family background of a child and the nature of clinic treatment.' Using the analogy of translating foreign languages, she continued that 'the social worker's interpretative task is twofold: 1. The interpretation of clinic treatment to the family. 2. The interpretation of family attitudes to the therapist.'[48] The social worker's role in both diagnosis and treatment was crucial.

PSYCHIATRIC SOCIAL WORKERS IN THE HOME

Such statements about the role of social workers bring out the centrality of the home to child guidance and to the part therein of the psychiatric social worker. It was in the home that a child's mental and emotional problems often started, from where crucial information could be gathered, and in which some measure of treatment could be effected. Given child guidance's holistic approach, this is unsurprising. Moodie told a Liverpool audience in 1933 that there was an 'epidemic of what people call freedom' but which was, in fact, licence. This disturbing situation arose because of the failure of guidance in the home and at school.[49] Beatrice Robinson, a social worker at one of the London child guidance clinics, told readers of *Mother and Child* that only a 'superficial observer' could see the child and his environment as separate and distinct from one another. Any such 'sharp dividing line' vanished 'when we study the relationships which the child constructs with those around him.'[50]

In her home visits, then, what more explicitly was the social worker's role? Writing in the journal *Mental Hygiene,* the APSW chair, Miss M. A. Lane, suggested that there was 'no doubt that the material gathered from interviews with relatives and friends and from observations of the patient's home' was best obtained by a social worker. Her particular training and experience enabled her 'to evaluate the facts and understand the significance of what she learns from them.' Psychiatrists appreciated such 'social history.' More than this, though, the social worker had a crucial role in explaining both illness and treatment to family members and in this way 'she may be able to adjust the social environment to the patient's needs.'[51]

Bridget Yapp, another psychiatric social worker who also wrote extensively on the subject, likewise argued that it was 'often impossible' for psychiatrists and psychologists to gain an adequate picture of family circumstances 'solely by interviewing the child's parents and others concerned with him, inside the clinic.' Rather, social workers sought to visit the home even before a clinic visit. The relationship with the parents was crucial, and the social worker aimed to establish that the clinic existed 'to help parents and not merely to interfere, as is sometimes suspected'—a revealing comment on contemporary suspicions of both social workers and psychiatry. Parents might be initially hostile but, Yapp continued, generally realised that a 'child's difficulties cannot be understood without the fullest possible knowledge of the circumstances of his life, including the sort of home in which he lives.' So, she claimed, the social worker was often greeted with expressions such as: 'I thought you would want to come and see his home.'[52] The subordination of the clinic, purportedly the locus of child guidance, is notable here.

The engagement of parents in this manner was seen as a positive aspect of child guidance work. Another social worker, Pauline Shapiro, asserted that her colleagues acted as a 'friend and confidante of the parents' a point also made, in identical language, by Moodie. Indeed Moodie, revealingly, also suggested that because of this relationship parents would confide more easily in the social worker than in the psychiatrist.[53] At Notre Dame in Glasgow, meanwhile, it was claimed that a monthly visit by the social worker 'and the time spent quietly discussing things in the home atmosphere, has proved of more value than a weekly visit paid by the parents to the Clinic.' Once again, the downgrading of the clinic's role is notable. The aim of social work was to 'establish friendly relations with the parents.' Rather disingenuously, it was then argued that there was 'no idea in the visiting of any inspection of, or inquiry into, home conditions or family circumstances.' As will become apparent, this was true only insofar as the socio-economic environment was played down as a contributory factor to the child's problems. The social work department's principal role was thus 'to help the Team to assess the contribution made by the social environment to the problem, and, as far as possible, to adjust unfavourable conditions.'[54]

But how was this to be achieved? First, the psychiatric social worker fed information about the home environment into the case conference, thereby significantly shaping diagnosis. A 1933 report from the Edinburgh Catholic Child Guidance Clinic gives us some insight into the ascribed causes of child mental ill-health, and the important point here is how often 'the home' was seen as the fundamental causal factor. Of the eleven children treated for 'backwardness,' for example, psychological tests had shown 'poor mental ability' in over half. In three cases, however, the trouble was 'partly accounted for by unhappy home conditions.' In another diagnostic category, 'nervousness,' in all cases the condition was again mainly due to 'unhappy home conditions.' Of the children who were 'difficult at home,' meanwhile, nearly all had been 'wrongly handled at home.'[55]

Given the economic problems of inter-war Britain, it is inevitable that occasional reference was made to socio-economic circumstances. In Liverpool, for instance, the child guidance clinic's social worker observed that her cases were mixed in terms of social class. Of those from the poorest parts of the city, she continued, 'I am sure that the fundamental problem in most instances is that of unemployment, poverty and material deprivation generally, and with these the Clinic is not designed to cope.'[56] Nonetheless, it is clear that when child guidance workers used the expression 'environment' they were not generally concerned with socio-economic explanations for child 'maladjustment.' As another Notre Dame report put it, in nearly every case seen 'environment played a large part in the production of symptoms.' What this implied for treatment was that 'in many cases the re-adjustment of the environmental factors resulted in the adjustment of the problem.' And of these environmental factors 'the most important was found to be the emotional relationship between the child and its parents' since 'the child tends to mirror the attitude of its parents.' Picking up on the issue of 'bad handling,' the report continued that if parental attitudes were abnormal 'either in the direction of over-domination or over-protection, the child is found to suffer.' Parents were consequently made to realise this and to change attitudes so that, in turn, the child might make a 'satisfactory re-adjustment.' Hence in the majority of cases treatment involved 'the adjustment of the parent-child situation and . . . the alleviation of physical disorders which were found to be playing a part in the production of symptoms.'[57]

At least in the first of these—the 'adjustment' of the parent–child relationship—the social worker played a key role. In a further British report on American child guidance from the late 1920s it was noted that recommended treatment most frequently engaged with 'the child's home life and environment; here, the supervision is undertaken by the social worker.' In consequence, it was generally the case that treatment that had 'begun by seeking to modify the behaviour of a child has developed into trying primarily to modify the behaviour of his parents.'[58] In fact by the late 1930s it was recognised in the United States that modifying parental behaviour of itself raised important philosophical issues in psychiatry, given that they were not, in the first instance, the 'patients.'[59] But at least initially the British approach seems to have followed the early American pattern.

Shapiro, for instance, argued that adjustment was 'often effected by means of the social worker' through her ability to discuss with the parents the psychiatrist's advice and 'by making suggestions for putting it into practice.' Shapiro illustrated her point through the case of 'Hilda,' a four year old brought to a clinic as a result of temper tantrums and attacks on her baby sister, for which she was severely punished by her mother. Hilda was found to be physically healthy and of above average intelligence. The social worker discovered, though, that the child had been spoiled by her father since birth and it was he to whom she appealed when punished by the mother. The psychiatric diagnosis was thus that Hilda was 'normal,' and that it was the parents who needed to change. Shapiro observed that the social worker, as an 'experienced and impartial "onlooker"', was able to understand the attitudes of both parents. She could thus be of 'immediate assistance' in reassuring the mother that Hilda was 'normal' and in alerting the father to the 'dangers' of over-indulgence. The social worker also arranged for Hilda to enter the local infants' school, and in so doing briefed the teacher on the child's home situation.[60]

Here we see both aspects of the social worker's role in practice—supplying crucial information and interpreting the consequent diagnosis. All this was done as an 'impartial' observer, a testament to the social worker's 'scientific' training. Shapiro's observations also raise, however, questions about what exactly went on in the domestic discussions when the social worker came to call; and, in turn, what was the actual content of child guidance, particularly in the home setting. On the first of these we can make only general observations. Of course, it is now virtually impossible to reconstruct these conversations of over half a century ago.

On the other hand, there is evidence of what would not have been discussed. In important respects, British and American experience almost certainly diverged here. Many child guidance practitioners argued for openness with children on sexual matters. But this was problematic. In 1930 the psychiatrist at London's Maudsley Hospital, Dr Mapother, wrote to the Commonwealth Fund outlining possible obstacles to British acceptance of child guidance. Among these was 'a marked tendency to suspicion of what is vaguely called Psycho-analysis of the Child.' This, he continued, was construed as meaning 'detailed psychological investigation, and perhaps particularly such investigation of sexual matters . . . I have heard it said that the party of suspicion is largely a Roman Catholic one.'[61]

Mapother overstated the case, but his remarks draw attention to two issues, namely, the role of Roman Catholic child guidance clinics and the association of psychoanalysis with sexuality. Regarding the former, one of the most successful clinics in Britain was based at the Catholic teacher training college, Notre Dame, in Glasgow. While in many respects a pioneering institution, it also had a clear and specific Catholic agenda that, for example, did not allow social workers or psychiatrists to raise matters such as birth control with their patients' parents. It is notable too that Notre Dame, like other Roman Catholic clinics, would only employ Catholic social workers and would ideally have liked to engage a Catholic psychiatrist, a situation that in fact prevailed at its smaller counterpart in Edinburgh. The intersection of religious belief and child guidance was important in Scotland and almost certainly so in other centres with large Catholic populations, for instance, Liverpool.[62]

As to psychoanalysis and sexuality, it was certainly not the case that 'problems' such as masturbation were ignored or neglected by child guidance workers. The psychiatrist R. G. Gordon, by the late 1930s Medical Director of the Child Guidance Council, wrote in *Mother and Child* that 'irrational disapproval' by parents of their child's habit of masturbating could lead to unhealthy feelings of guilt and shame—'not a very good preparation for the parent of the next generation.'[63] But whether for this, or indeed any other, 'problem,' one course of 'treatment' was avoided. As Moodie forcefully put it: '*The psycho-analytic method is never employed in a Child Guidance Clinic.*' The child requiring treatment was 'always extremely conscious of, and acutely worried by his own abnormal thoughts.' But he would engage with a trusted adult 'and this discussion, which need only follow the lines of an ordinary commonsense conversation, is all that is required.' In the great majority of cases, therefore, 'no discussion of the child's thoughts is necessary or advisable.'[64] With the benefit of hindsight, this was perhaps an unfortunate approach. In the 1980s the internationally famous psychiatrist John Bowlby, recalling the early history of the child guidance movement in which he himself had played an important part, expressed his regret over 'our complete ignorance of either the occurrence or the ill-effects of physical and sexual abuse.'[65]

From the perspective of the psychiatric social workers, there are suggestions, albeit elusive and tantalizing, in the Commonwealth Fund files that some British trainees who paid educational visits to the United States were extremely uncomfortable with the sexual nature of the information to which they were exposed. A report on one of these, for example, discussed a British student's dealings with a patient whose problems, so it appeared, arose out of the 'marital disharmony' of his parents. It was further remarked that both parents seemed more concerned with discussing their own problems 'than in telling about the patient.' The trainee had admitted 'some sensitivity about intimate information on marital situations' and had been 'at first rather overwhelmed by the frankness of these parents.' She had, the report concluded, 'discussed her own problems and is handling same. It is too early to gauge results.'[66] In this context a comparison of materials written by and for British psychiatric social workers with their American counterparts is instructive, with the latter being much more inclined to employ the language and concepts of psychoanalysis and to discuss sexual issues.[67]

For at least some British social workers it would appear that, for religious or cultural reasons, one important aspect of psychiatric theory was out of bounds. The unwillingness of psychiatrists themselves to engage with such matters further reinforced this position. Graham Richards observes that while sex was undoubtedly one reason for British inter-war interest in psychoanalysis, it was 'equally a source of cultural resistance.'[68] As far as psychiatric social workers were concerned, therefore, their role in the home was not to delve deeply into the minds of individual family members, far less to attempt to uncover any hidden sexual 'causes' of maladjustment. The implication is thus that what they did talk about on these home visits was a watered down, 'practical' version of psychiatry almost certainly accompanied by more 'traditional' social work practices such as 'practical' advice on household and family organisation.

CONCLUSION

Child guidance started off as a clinic-based form of preventive medicine based on the scientific claims of medicine and, especially, psychiatry. In practice, however, its focus came to be on the home and the dynamics of familial relationships. By the late 1930s this was more or less openly recognised in Britain as in the United States. As MacCalman put it: 'we do know . . . that parent-child relationships play a huge part in the production of nervous and behaviour disorders.' 'Is it a visionary dream,' he continued, 'to believe that a vast system of parent education could be organized?'[69] Although none of this was necessarily incompatible with a more clinic-based approach, the structures and holistic philosophy of child guidance also required a central role for the psychiatric social worker and her interventions in the home. As we have seen, the child's 'environment' referred primarily to the emotional landscape of the home and not its socio-economic circumstances. In this respect, the British experience again mirrored that of the United States.[70]

In training and practice, though, many British social workers shied away from the more controversial and challenging aspects of contemporary psychiatric theory. Given the limited nature of the British profession's training and the cultural and other constraints within which it operated, it seems reasonable to argue that a movement that sought to present itself as scientific and clinic-based actually was, in practice, simply a new form of home-oriented social casework. This was despite the repeated claims to 'scientific' training and modes of observation by its supporters. Nonetheless, even such relatively modest levels of scientific training undoubtedly had a major influence on the professionalisation of social work. British psychiatric social work, after the Second World War, successfully embedded itself in the welfare state and for a time enjoyed considerable professional prestige, not least through the intellectual standing of the *British Journal of Psychiatric Social Work*.[71]

As to the 'patients,' it can be argued that the child moved from being, at first, at the centre of the picture to, by the end of the 1930s, an individual located firmly in a particular version of its 'environment' that focused on the home and the familial relationships it encompassed. Although evidence is hard to obtain, it is not unreasonable to assume that at least some children benefited from their visits, however brief, to the clinic and to subsequent social work intervention. Equally, some parents almost certainly found the advice reassuring in the face of their children's apparently unfathomable behaviour. Of course, psychiatric theory claimed to be non-judgemental, and we have seen how psychiatric social workers laid great emphasis on their detached, 'scientific' approach.

What is further apparent, however, is that by the outbreak of the Second World War child guidance was not about the child per se. Rather, it was about parents and their purported shortcomings. Not for the first time in British welfare history, the child slipped from view, to be replaced by an attitude that, implicitly if not explicitly, 'blamed' parents for children's mental or emotional 'ill-health.' All this was, furthermore, to have resonances beyond the inter-war era. These can be seen in, for example, Bowlby's post-war theories and in the conclusions drawn from the wartime evacuation surveys, which also had a notable input from individuals involved in child guidance. Child and family policy in the welfare state, it might thus be argued, drew at least some of its inspiration and ideas from the curious history of child guidance and psychiatric social work in the 1930s and their associated fixation on the home.

ACKNOWLEDGEMENTS

I am grateful to the Wellcome Trust for its support of my research on child guidance; to the Rockefeller Archive Center, New York, for two grants enabling me to work at the Center on the records of the Commonwealth

Fund; and to the staffs of the archives and libraries cited in the notes. I would also like to thank the Stein Rokkan Center, Bergen, for a Visiting Fellowship in November 2005 that allowed me to make important strides in the researching and writing of this chapter.

NOTES

1. W. M. Burbury, E. M. Balint, and B. J. Yapp, *An Introduction to Child Guidance,* (London, Macmillan: 1945), 100.
2. M. Horn, 'The Moral Message of Child Guidance, 1925–1945,' *Journal of Social History,* 18 (1984): 25–36; M. Horn, *Before It's Too Late: The Child Guidance Movement in the United States, 1922–1945* (Philadelphia: Temple University Press, 1989); T. R. Richardson, *The Century of the Child: The Mental Hygiene Movement and Social Policy in the United States and Canada* (Albany: State University of New York Press, 1989); and K. W. Jones, *Taming the Troublesome Child: American Families, Child Guidance, and the Limits of Psychiatric Authority* (Cambridge, MA: Harvard University Press, 1999).
3. L. Abrams, *The Orphan Country: Children of Scotland's Broken Homes from 1845 to the Present Day* (Edinburgh: John Donald, 1998); H. Hendrick, *Child Welfare: Historical Dimensions, Contemporary Debate* (Bristol: The Policy Press, 2003); D. Thom, 'Wishes, Anxieties, Play and Gestures: Child Guidance in Inter-War England, in R. Cooter (ed.), *In the Name of the Child* (London: Routledge, 1992), 200–219.
4. R. Cooter, 'In the Name of the Child Beyond,' in M. Gijswit-Hofstra and H. Marland (ed.), *Cultures of Child Health in Britain and the Netherlands in the Twentieth Century* (Amsterdam: Rodopi, 2003), 287–96, at pp. 288–9.
5. J. Stewart, 'Child Guidance in Inter-War Scotland: International Influences and Domestic Concerns,' *Bulletin of the History of Medicine,* 80:3 (2006): 513–39.
6. For a recent contribution, see M. Payne, *The Origins of Social Work: Continuity and Change* (Basingstoke: Palgrave Macmillan, 2005).
7. M. Thomson, 'Mental Hygiene as an International Movement,' in P. Weindling (ed.), *International Health Organisations and Movements, 1918–1939* (Cambridge: Cambridge University Press, 1995), 283–304, at p. 283.
8. Central Library, Manchester: Local Studies and Archives, 'Minutes of the Public Health Committee, Corporation of Manchester, 14th April 1931,' letter, 23rd March 1931, from the Institute of Medical Psychology.
9. Liverpool Record Office, H360.5 QUA, Dr M. Barton Hall, 'Liverpool and Mental Hygiene,' *The Liverpool Quarterly,* 1:6 (1933): 10.
10. On the Fund, see A. McG. Harvey and S. L. Abrams *'For the welfare of mankind': the Commonwealth Fund and American Medicine* (Baltimore, MD: Johns Hopkins University Press, 1986).
11. H. Oosterhuis, 'Insanity and Other Discomforts: A Century of Outpatient Psychiatry and Mental Health Care in the Netherlands, 1900–2000,' in M. Gijswijt-Hofstra, H. Oosterhuis, J. Vijselaar, and H. Freeman (eds.), *Psychiatric Cultures Compared: Psychiatry and Mental Health Care in the Twentieth Century* (Amsterdam: Amsterdam University Press, 2005), 73–102, at p. 79.
12. On American psychiatric social work see R. Lubove, *The Professional Altruist: The Emergence of Social Work as a Career, 1880–1930* (Cambridge, MA: Harvard University Press, 1965), Chapters 3 and 4; and J. M. Gabriel, 'Mass-Producing the Individual: Mary C. Jarrett, Elmer E. Southard, and the Industrial Origins of Psychiatric Social Work,' *Bulletin of the History of Medicine,*

79:3 (2005): 430–58. For a history of the British profession by an 'insider' see N. Timms, *Psychiatric Social Work in Britain (1939–1962)* (London: Routledge and Kegan Paul, 1964). For an important recent engagement with the history of psychiatric social work, see V. Long, 'Changing Public Representations of Mental Illness in Britain, 1870–1970,' unpublished Ph.D. thesis, University of Warwick, 2004, Chapter 3.

13. Stewart, 'Child Guidance.'
14. Glasgow City Archives, Mitchell Library, Glasgow (hereafter, Mitchell Library), Corporation of Glasgow, D-TC 7/7/13, *Notre Dame Child Guidance Clinic: Annual Report, 1993–34* (Glasgow: Notre Dame Child Guidance Clinic, 1934).
15. The Wellcome Library for the History and Understanding of Medicine, Archives (hereafter, Wellcome Archives), Robina Scott Addis Papers, PP/ADD/C.3/9, leaflet *The London Child Guidance Council* (n.p., 1929), 6—emphasis in the original.
16. D. R. MacCalman, 'Familiar Problems of Upbringing,' *Mother and Child,* 8:3 (1937): 90–1. See also C. Urwin and E. Sharland, 'From Bodies to Minds in Childcare Literature: Advice to Parents in Inter-war Britain,' in Cooter (ed.), *In the Name,* 174–99, although this chapter does not mention *Mother and Child.*
17. University of Liverpool, Achives and Special Collections, Papers of Professor Sir Cyril Burt (hereafter, Burt Papers), D.191/20/1; The Child Guidance Council, *The Child Guidance Council* (Child Guidance Council, 1929), 6.
18. Birmingham City Archives, BCC/BH 1/1/1/36, 'City of Birmingham Education Committee. Child Guidance Clinic. Report of the Medical Director, 1936–1938,' p. 3.
19. Library of the Wellcome Unit for the History of Medicine, Oxford, WX 28 FE5.2 Lon Guys, *Report of the Institution and Development of the Child Guidance Clinic at Guy's Hospital London, 1930–1936* (n.p., n.d.), 16.
20. C. Lawrence and G. Weisz, 'Medical Holism: The Context,' in C. Lawrence and G. Weisz (ed.), *Greater Than the Parts: Holism in Biomedicine, 1920–1950* (New York: Oxford University Press, 1998), 1–22.
21. D. R. MacCalman, 'The Management of the Difficult Child,' *Journal of the Royal Institute of Public Health and Hygiene,* 1:2 (1937): 93–96, at p. 93.
22. Wellcome Archives, John Bowlby Papers, PP/BOW/C.3/1, London Child Guidance Council, undated flyer.
23. University of Manchester: The John Rylands University Library (hereafter, Rylands Library), Store (Med.Pam.2)/87.28i, W. Moodie, *The London Child Guidance Clinic: A Survey* (London: London Child Guidance Clinic, n.d. but 1935 or 1936), Foreword.
24. Dundee City Archives, City of Dundee, *Report of the Medical Officer of Health for the Year Ending 31st December, 1937* (Dundee, 1938), 15.
25. Thom, 'Wishes,' 215.
26. Cited in Horn, 'Moral Message,' 27.
27. Mitchell Library, Corporation of Glasgow, D-TC 7/7/13, *Notre Dame Child Guidance Clinic: Annual Report, 1933–34* (Glasgow: Notre Dame Child Guidance Clinic, n.d. but 1934), 5–6.
28. Modern Records Centre, University of Warwick, Archives of the Association of Psychiatric Social Workers, MSS.378, 20/5, undated (but ca.1940) list of child guidance clinics recognised by the Child Guidance Council and represented on the Scottish Council for Mental Hygiene.
29. See London Metropolitan Archives, 22.06, Education Committee Minutes, 'Report of the General Sub-Committee 14th September and 9th and 23rd November, 1943' for a complete list.

30. University of Liverpool, Archives and Special Collections, E X 65: 39, The Liverpool Child Guidance Council, *Report for the Year 1939* (Liverpool: The Liverpool Child Guidance Council, n.d., but 1940), 11.
31. D. Thom, 'The Healthy Citizen of Empire or Juvenile Delinquent?: Beating and Mental Health in the UK,' in Gijswit-Hofstra and Marland (ed.), *Cultures of Child Health*, 189–212, at p. 199.
32. Jones, *Taming*, 77–83.
33. H. L. Witmer, *Psychiatric Clinics for Children, With Special Reference to State Programs* (New York: The Commonwealth Fund, 1940), 345; also quoted in Jones, *Taming*, 174.
34. Moodie, *The London Child Guidance Clinic*, 6.
35. See the chapters by Sarah Hayes and Mark Jackson in this volume.
36. D. J. Walkowitz, 'The Making of a Feminine Professional Identity: Social Workers in the 1920s,' *American Historical Review*, 95:4 (1990): 1051–75, at p. 1052.
37. Long, 'Changing Public Perceptions,' 131, 134–5.
38. Burt Papers, D.191/20/1/7, 'Report Presented to the Child Guidance Council by the Signatories, Who Visited the United States to Enquire into the Working of the Child Guidance Clinics,' (no date, but late 1920s), 5.
39. Burt Papers, D.191/20/1/9, Miss St Clair Townsend, 'Report on Psychiatric Social Work,' (no date, but late 1920s), 1.
40. Gabriel, 'Mass-Producing,' 441.
41. For preliminary observations see Stewart, 'Child Guidance'; and idem, 'An "Enigma to Their Parents": the Founding and Aims of the Notre Dame Child Guidance Clinic, Glasgow,' *The Innes Review*, 57: 1 (2006): 54–76.
42. E.A. Danto, *Freud's Free Clinics: Psychoanalysis and Social Justice, 1918–1938* (New York: Columbia University Press, 2005), 205–6.
43. Quoted in Long, 'Changing Public Perceptions,' 133.
44. Archives of the London School of Economics and Political Science, British Library of Political and Economic Science, Central Filing Registry/514/1/A, Letter from Child Guidance Council to LSE, 3rd June 1929.
45. Lubove, *Professional*, 117.
46. Gabriel, 'Mass-Producing,' 439.
47. Rylands Library, Store (Med. Pam. 2)/87.29, William Moodie, *Child Guidance by Team Work* (London: Child Guidance Council, 1931), 2–3.
48. The Child Guidance Council, *Proceedings of the Child Guidance Inter-Clinic Conference of Great Britain 1939* (London: Child Guidance Council, 1939), 98.
49. Rockefeller Archive Center, New York, Commonwealth Fund Archives, Series 16, English Mental Hygiene Program (hereafter, CF), Box 6, Folder 58, cutting, 28th January 1933, *Liverpool Post and Mercury*.
50. B. H. Robinson, 'The Difficult Child: A Medical, Psychological and Sociological Problem: III The Function of the Social Worker,' *Mother and Child*, 1:7 (1930): 249–52, at p. 249.
51. M.A. Lane, 'The Place of the Social Worker in Mental Health,' *Mental Hygiene*, V, 4 (October 1939): 132–6, at pp. 132–3.
52. Burbury, Balint, and Yapp, *Introduction*, 99–100.
53. Rylands Library, Store A 141639, P. C. Shapiro, *How Child Guidance Contributes to Mental Health* (London: Child Guidance Council, 1933), 6–7; Moodie, *Child Guidance by Team Work*, 5.
54. Mitchell Library, Corporation of Glasgow, D-TC 7/7/13, *Notre Dame Child Guidance Clinic: Annual Report, 1935–36* (Glasgow: Notre Dame Child Guidance Clinic, 1936), 9–10.
55. CF Box 6, Folder 60, Letter from Lady Margaret Kerr, Edinburgh, to Child Guidance Council, 30th June 1934, to which is attached 'Edinburgh Child Guidance Clinic: Report for year January 1933 to December 1933.'

56. University of Liverpool, Archives and Special Collections, EX 65: 33, The Liverpool Child Guidance Council, *Report for the Year 1933* (Liverpool: The Liverpool Child Guidance Council, 1934), 23–4.
57. Mitchell Library, Corporation of Glasgow D-TC 7/7/13, *Notre Dame Child Guidance Clinic: Annual Report, 1933–34* (Glasgow: Notre Dame Child Guidance Clinic, 1934), 11–12.
58. Burt Papers, D.191/20/1/8, 'Report of C. Spearman on the Clinics for Maladjusted Children in the United States and Canada,' (n.d. but late 1920s), pp.2–3.
59. Witmer, *Psychiatric Clinics,* Ch.12.
60. Shapiro, *How Child Guidance Contributes,* 6–7.
61. CF, Box 22, Folder 249, letter, 25th September 1930, Mapother to Barry Smith, Commonwealth Fund.
62. Stewart, 'An "Enigma to Their Parents"'; idem, 'Child Guidance.'
63. R. G. Gordon, 'The Dangerous Age of Childhood,' *Mother and Child,* 9:3 (1938): 80–5, at p. 83.
64. Moodie, *Child Guidance by Team Work,* 4–5, emphasis in the original.
65. Wellcome Archives, John Bowlby Papers, PP/BOW/C.5, copy of *The Child Guidance Trust: Newsletter No.3* (June 1987), with article by Bowlby entitled 'A Historical Perspective on Child Guidance,' 2.
66. CF, Box 19, Folder 211, Institute for Child Guidance, Field Work Report—New York School, Winter Quarter—March 1929.
67. Compare, for instance, L. M. French, *Psychiatric Social Work* (New York: The Commonwealth Fund, 1940), or Witmer, *Psychiatric Clinics,* with Burbury, Balint, and Yapp, *An Introduction.*
68. G. Richards, 'Britain on the Couch: The Popularization of Psychoanalysis in Britain, 1918–1940,' *Science in Context,* 13:2 (2000): 183–230, at p. 191.
69. MacCalman, 'The Management,' 95.
70. Jones, *Taming,* 202 and passim.
71. Payne, *Origins,* 192; Long, 'Changing Public Perceptions,' Chapter 3.

7 Rabbits and Rebels

The Medicalisation of Maladjusted Children in Mid-Twentieth-Century Britain

Sarah Hayes

INTRODUCTION

On 17 December 1927, in an article in *The Lancet,* Dr. E. A. Hamilton-Pearson, chief physician at the Children's Department of the Tavistock Clinic for Functional Nervous Disorders in London, highlighted the findings of a Home Office investigation that had been running for seven years and that was aimed at seeking scientific explanations for the causes of juvenile delinquency. Hamilton-Pearson stated that the study had been 'undertaken in no narrow psychological spirit, but with the object of exploring all factors, physical as well as psychological and environmental.' In particular he emphasised one key finding:

> An environment characterised by a harsh unbending discipline may produce a *psychological rabbit* or *a rebel* against any form of authority. In one type the conflict resulting from non-adaptation remains un-resolved, a collecting point for irresolutions, *a neurosis.* In another type, the conflict is resolved in action which is at variance with accepted standards, *a delinquency.* [1]

This statement neatly expresses three crucial elements of contemporary formulations of child behavioural disorders. First, it suggests that by the late 1920s a medical model had been developed in Britain relating to children whose behaviour was considered to be socially problematic. As Hamilton-Pearson succinctly suggested, this model consisted of two polarised categories of children: psychological 'rabbits' and delinquent 'rebels.' Secondly, this model was built around the concept of 'non-adaptation,' more commonly expressed as 'maladjustment,' according to which the environment was considered to be a crucial aetiological factor. Finally, deviation from 'accepted standards' was a primary criterion in the identification of children considered to be in need of medical intervention.

This chapter examines the ways in which medical conceptualisations of maladjustment evolved and became established in Britain in the early decades of the twentieth century, and the manner in which social concerns about behavioural and emotional difficulties in children led not only to their evaluation and categorisation, but also to subsequent intervention by specialist medical professionals. It also explores the development of theories about the aetiology of maladjustment, notably theories that sought to identify the relative influence of hereditary and environmental factors on the emotional and behavioural development of children. The first section focuses on the process by which the notion of the social 'rebel' became increasingly medicalised during this period, reflecting the changing ways in which medical professionals identified and defined maladjustment. Following scientific studies into the causes of criminality, shifting medical, judicial, and educational perceptions of delinquency resulted in the classification of delinquent children as 'pre-psychotic.' Professional medical intervention was considered necessary as a preventative measure to protect society from the potential dangers of untreated psychotics. Secondly, the chapter explores the emergence of the concept of the 'psychological rabbit' and shows how medical and social fears concerning the 'pre-neurotic' child shaped approaches to 'delicate' children as the growing influence of psychoanalytic theories placed increasing emphasis on the wider social problems caused by unrecognised and unresolved neuroses.

These developments were greatly influenced by the work of the American psychiatrist William Healy (1869–1963), and British psychologists Cyril Burt (1883–1971) and John Bowlby (1907–1990). These figures have been the subject of continued historical analysis for many decades, largely through their contributions to the development of professional interest in the role of the domestic environment in the aetiology of child behavioural problems. However, historians have overwhelmingly chosen to focus on one particular element of their work: the ways in which professional attention increasingly highlighted the role of parents, specifically mothers, in seeking explanations for maladjusted behaviour in children. Whilst this was undoubtedly a key feature of theoretical developments during the inter-war period, it fails to fully represent the complexities of contemporary notions, and therefore presents a restricted image of professional approaches to maladjusted children. This chapter aims to show how professional consideration of 'good' or 'bad parenting' was far more complex than historians have acknowledged. Poor parenting and mothering was only one of a range of factors identified within the domestic environment that could lead to maladjustment.

In addition, this chapter highlights ways in which medical notions of 'environment' changed significantly within this period. In the mid and late nineteenth century, professionals dealing with child health and welfare were concerned with environmental factors defined exclusively in economic terms, emphasising in particular the effects of financial deprivation on the physical health of the nation. In the early decades of the twentieth century, this focused shifted significantly to a new consideration of the significance of a child's home and educational environment, concentrating on domestic, familial, and social relationships, and to an emphasis on the importance of this external social environment on maintaining the stability of the internal emotional environment of all individuals.

CONCEPTUALISATIONS OF MALADJUSTMENT: THE 'INTERNAL ENVIRONMENT'

The term *maladjusted* was applied throughout the twentieth century to an individual (child or adult) who had failed, in one way or another, to adapt to socially dominant standards of behaviour. The concept of a maladjusted child had become firmly established in Britain by the end of the 1920s, particularly following the emergence of the Child Guidance Movement from 1927 onwards in Britain. Subsequently this category of child became the focus of interest for a wide range of agents, including medical professionals, educationalists and the State, leading to the recognition of maladjustment as a statutory 'handicap' in 1944. Much of the literature relating to the history of maladjustment locates the origins of the condition firmly within the inter-war period and associated exclusively with child guidance, citing the 1920s as the decade when the term first appeared.[2] However, it was clearly not a totally new concept in the twentieth century. The idea of mental adjustment was first conceived in the mid–nineteenth century in the context of the emergence of evolutionary science and empirical psychology. Recognition of maladjustment was based on growing realisations that mental health was largely dependent on an individual's ability to adjust mentally and emotionally to his external surroundings. For example, in 1855 the English philosopher Herbert Spencer (1820–1903) wrote:

> Mental life consists initially in the continuous adjustment of internal relations to external relations, of the individual organism to its material and social environment.[3]

Spencer's *Principles of Psychology* introduced the idea that social life could be analysed scientifically. He argued that human life was built around social conflict, in particular the continual fight for limited resources, and that only those individuals who were physically and mentally adjusted to their environment would survive, a theory of the 'survival of the fittest' that preceded Darwin's *Origin of the Species*.[4] Emphasis on the scientific study of the human mind and human behaviour, which emerged in the middle decades of the nineteenth century, led to a new understanding of the significance of internal adjustment. This notion was reinforced in other areas of scientific investigation. Physiologist Claude Bernard (1813–1878) was particularly prominent in promoting the concept of the importance of the 'internal environment of the organism' in this period.[5] Most importantly, new concepts of the internal environment revealed the implications that the failure to adjust might have on an individual's physical and mental state. This became a key factor in developing conceptions of mental illness and psychiatric medicine throughout the late nineteenth century and early twentieth centuries. The relationship between internal psychological stability and insanity was further reinforced by the work of psychiatrist Charles Mercier (1852–1919), who argued that sanity or insanity was dependent on the 'stability or instability of the highest nervous arrangements,' determining the ability of an individual to adjust to external stresses.[6] The realisation that mental problems could arise through an inability to adjust to external factors marked the beginnings of a significant move away from established assumptions that madness and lunacy were inherent, inherited, and incurable.[7]

Whilst theories emphasising the importance of internal adjustment were driving the emergence of psychology from within the established discipline of philosophy in the second half of the nineteenth century, these new psychological approaches began to be applied in other areas. Most notably, in the later decades of the nineteenth century, these ideas were increasingly incorporated into the judicial and education systems. The medical model of maladjustment that became established in Britain in the early 1920s evolved from concerns around three specific types of children in the late nineteenth century. From the 1880s onwards, doctors warned of problems with overly nervous or 'delicate' children, the judicial system raised fears about criminal or 'delinquent' children, and educationalists were concerned with those considered educationally subnormal, officially categorised as 'dull and backward' children. Commentators distinguished between the 'socially disturbed,' including such groups as juvenile delinquents, and the 'emotionally disturbed,' including neurotic and psychotic children who may or may not behave anti-socially.[8] By the early decades of the twentieth century, common factors had been identified across each of these types of problem child, bringing professional approaches to the three different categories together, and resulting in the creation of a new model of maladjustment. Scientific investigations into the aetiology of child behaviour problems soon concluded that the common factors shared by these groups were to be found in the children's domestic and social environments.

'DELINQUENT REBELS' AND THE DOMESTIC ENVIRONMENT

The medical model of the delinquent 'rebel' has a long history. Concerns about juvenile delinquency were clearly not new in the 1920s. Since the mid-nineteenth century, there had been growing concerns amongst both professionals and lay philanthropists about increasing numbers of children entering the criminal justice system. Officially, the term 'juvenile delinquent' was used to refer to children who had appeared before a court of law as a result of criminal activity. Socially, the term was used more loosely to refer to any child who displayed challenging or difficult behaviour within the child's home, school, or community. The medical model of delinquency became established through international interest in seeking scientific explanations for criminality. Delinquent children were those who, by committing crime, had failed or refused to meet social expectations of behaviour. These expectations were framed around specific, and highly gendered, categories of behaviour. Delinquent behaviour was perceived in two ways, with acts labelled either criminal or immoral. Boys were most commonly labelled as delinquent predominantly as a result of aggressive behaviour, stealing in the form of petty theft or burglary, and truancy. Girls, however, were most likely to be labelled delinquent through sexual behaviour that was deemed inappropriate, such as forming relationships with older men or keeping undesirable company. This discrepancy was highlighted in the earliest medical studies of delinquency. For example, a comparative survey carried out in Chicago in 1916 noted that 70% of male delinquents were arrested for theft, as opposed to 30% of females. However, 73% of female offenders were found guilty of sexual offences, compared to only 4.5% of males.[9] Female delinquents were most often charged with prostitution, but others appeared in court for 'exhibitionism,' 'extreme obscenity,' and 'the grave misdemeanour of deliberately teaching bad sex knowledge.'[10] Female delinquents were also associated particularly with lying and the making up of 'false and dangerous accusations' or 'secretiveness.' These girls were perceived as transgressing the idealised 'accepted standards' of behaviour for women defined by established domestic ideologies, which valued qualities such as modesty, morality, and respectability.[11] Notions of delinquency were therefore framed around socially constructed expectations of behaviour dependent on biological sex.

Until the mid-nineteenth century, any child who was accused of criminal behaviour was treated in the same way, and within the same system, as adult offenders. In the second half of the nineteenth century, approaches to juvenile criminals began to change. Through the work of key individuals, in particular in Britain the teacher and philanthropist Mary Carpenter (1807–77), growing recognition of the complexities of dealing with child criminals resulted in a re-evaluation of the treatment of young offenders by both magistrates and police.[12] The first significant step in the medicalisation of delinquency was the intervention of magistrates requesting the involvement of medical professionals in the judicial process. This initially occurred in the United States, where, in the first two decades of the twentieth century, the criminal actions of children began to be interpreted medically as symptoms of deeper internal emotional problems. This new approach evolved largely through the work of psychiatrist William Healy (1869–1963). In 1909, Healy founded the Juvenile Psychopathic Clinic, attached to the Chicago Municipal Court, at the behest of Judge Meritt W. Pinckney of the juvenile court.[13] This clinic was established with the aim of employing medical and psychological approaches to research and dealing with the reasons for repeated criminal behaviour, and followed previous models established by psychologists Wilhelm Wundt (1832–1920), James Cattell (1860–1944), and Lightner Witmer (1867–1956).[14] After successful work in Chicago, Healy was invited to set up a similar clinic in Boston, opened in 1917, by Judge Harvey H. Baker. Healy's subsequent work with recidivist juveniles presented to the courts led him to challenge the established beliefs of the 'Progressive Child Savers' who promoted welfare legislation and philanthropic funding to alleviate the economic poverty that they believed to be the overriding factor in creating juvenile delinquents.[15] Healy believed that criminality was the result of buried emotional factors that created psychological conditions such as emotional maladjustment and mental abnormalities, resulting from mental conflicts and 'bad habits of mind.'[16] He emphasised particularly that the emotional and behavioural problems of these children arose as a result of the inter-play of many complex factors, explaining 'the anatomy of delinquency' using medical rhetoric and physiological terms to describe behaviour. Healy's stated aim was to understand 'the relationship of mental life to conduct,' placing it in the context of 'the complexity of human nature in relation to complex environmental conditions.'[17]

Healy, together with psychologist Augusta Bronner (1881–1966), carried out extensive comparative studies in the hope of identifying common influential factors. They established an original methodology based on a 'triple team' consisting of psychiatrist, psychologist, and a new form of medical professional, a psychiatric social worker. The aim was for the team to work together to assess all areas of the child's life, including physical health, mental and emotional state, intelligence level, and domestic environment. Healy and Bronner were, therefore, among the first to actively explore the role of the domestic environment in the aetiology of emotional and behavioural problems in children. Assessment of the child's domestic environment was carried out by a female psychiatric social worker, whose role was to visit the child's home, interview the child's parents, and gauge such factors as the condition of the home, number of siblings, and nature of the parent/child relationship.[18] The social worker's report, based on a subjective middle-class opinion of the home and the parents, was considered of crucial importance in aiding the subsequent psychiatric diagnosis.

Healy was one of the first to identify the implications of family relationships, observing that 'the problem of crime must hark back to parental guardianship,' but acknowledging the complexities of issues that affected this factor.[19] In considering the environmental background of each child, Healy considered three elements: 'home conditions', 'family relationships', and 'bad companionship.'[20] Within the category of 'home conditions,' the dominant factor appeared to be 'extreme lack of parental control,' noted in 46% of the delinquents. This had occurred in some cases because of parental negligence, the type of behaviour that would be identified in later studies as 'bad parenting.'[21] However, in many cases lack of control occurred not as the result of deliberate neglect by uncaring parents but because of domestic pressures, such as the economic need for both parents to work, or practical difficulties in coping with large families. Poverty was considered a factor in only 24% of cases, a figure that challenged established views of the aetiology of delinquency.

Whilst prioritising the significance of environmental factors, however, Healy concluded that ultimately, delinquency had a 'many sided aetiology' with 'combined types of causations.'[22] He considered that environmental factors might not always be the overriding determinant, as delinquents often came from families where no other siblings were offenders, despite sharing the same environmental conditions. This observation relied on the belief that siblings within a domestic unit received the same style and quality of parenting, an assumption that Healy never questioned. However, this anomaly led him to seek further explanations for delinquent behaviour. He suggested that:

> A mental process immediately precedes conduct . . . whatever influences the individual towards offence must first influence the mind of the individual. To ascertain the driving forces which make for social offence is to get at the mental mechanisms antecedent to the behaviour in question.[23]

Healy concluded that mental mechanisms were unique to each individual and 'social and biological backgrounds must take second place to these causative factors of delinquency.'[24] Healy thus challenged established notions of 'general causation' that were popular within psychological thinking at the time, locating the motivation for delinquent behaviour in the mind of the individual. This was significant in placing responsibility for anti-social behaviour with the individual, rather than seeking to blame hereditary factors, parental neglect, or poverty.

One significant aspect of Healy's work was his emphasis on the fact that many delinquent adolescents had begun their criminal careers at a very young age and that professional, specifically psychiatric, intervention was crucial at as early a stage as possible.[25] Healy's findings were reinforced by other contemporary research into the causes of criminality, in particular that of psychiatrist Bernard Glueck (1884–1972), who carried out a detailed study into the background of prisoners in Sing Sing Prison in 1917. He argued that individuals who had committed minor offences, such as pilfering, in childhood were likely to continue as repeat offenders into adulthood. In addition, Glueck identified a psychopathic delinquent type:

> unstable individuals who from early childhood show psychopathic traits such as impulsiveness, irritability and emotionalism. They are in frequent conflict with the school authorities on account of an inability to adapt themselves to the required regime.[26]

Glueck stressed the importance of emotional stability and adaptation, linking 'emotionalism' with potential psychiatric illness and concluding that delinquency was 'the direct result of physical or social maladjustment.'[27]

The linking of delinquent behaviour to psychopathic personality types reshaped the view of delinquency, raising the possibility that problems in children were indicative of incipient mental illness. The medical model of delinquency thus rapidly shifted from 'pre-criminal' to 'pre-delinquent' to 'pre-psychotic.' As Margo Horn has pointed out, these studies 'paved the way for emphasis on intervention during childhood.'[28] The recognition and treatment of maladjustment was increasingly seen, therefore, as being of crucial importance in the long-term prevention of crime and the maintenance of social stability.

The role of the social and domestic environment in the aetiology of maladjustment became a major focus following the publication in 1915 of Healy's seminal book *The Individual Delinquent*, which set out the findings of five years' work at the psychopathic clinic. Healy's ideas were disseminated and adopted by professionals working with delinquent children throughout the world. Leading professionals dealing with behaviourally problematic children in Britain, within both the judicial and medical arenas, were aware of Healy's work in the United States and were incorporating his ideas into their own work from 1915 onwards. In England, for example, the leading expert in this field was considered to be psychologist Cyril Burt (1883–1971). Burt cited both Healy and Bronner throughout his work, with their theories of the multi-factional nature of maladjustment clearly framing the formulation of his own ideas and reinforcing medical approaches to criminality. This is evident in one of Burt's earliest statements regarding delinquency: 'A crime . . . is only a symptom. It is a mental symptom with a mental origin.'[29] Regarding the management of child criminals, he further stated that the 'aim must not be punishment, but treatment.'[30] Burt subsequently became one of the primary agents in developing Healy's medical model of the delinquent 'rebel' in Britain. In 1925, Burt published an account of his own work with juvenile delinquents in London, *The Young Delinquent*. This book was well received and, like Healy's earlier publication, proved highly influential in shaping approaches to child criminals in Britain. Furthermore, Burt felt that his own survey was of greater relevance than Healy's in representing 'the ordinary city delinquent' rather than the older, hardened recidivists of the Chicago Psychopathic Clinic.[31]

Historians have consistently criticised Burt's work for emphasising the hereditary nature of behavioural problems in children, linking difficulties to inherited intelligence levels.[32] However, analysis of this work shows that Burt developed an acute awareness of the influences of a number of significant environmental factors. Whilst Burt devoted a section of thirty pages to hereditary factors, referring to certain children as inherently 'immorally deficient,' a much longer chapter was concerned with the complex influence of the external domestic and social environments.[33] The significance of environmental factors, and in particular the home, was ultimately the dominant message of Burt's work, although some contemporaries (like later historians) chose to focus exclusively on Burt's interest in heredity.[34] Others, however, did note his prominent argument for the significance of environmental factors. For example, Dr. R. Evelyn Lucas, a Rockefeller Medical Fellow working at the Maudsley Hospital, challenged an earlier review of Burt's book: 'Surely no one who has read Burt's careful and thorough work can fail to appreciate the very great stress which he lays on environmental conditions of every type.'[35]

Burt's theories in *The Young Delinquent* also illustrate the ways in which the definition of 'domestic environment' underwent a significant shift in the early decades of the twentieth century. In considering 'home circumstances,' Burt explored the input of poverty, overcrowding, and 'absence of facilities for recreation.' However, he challenged the established economic interpretation of environment, which carried with it an inherent assumption that poverty itself, defined by Burt as 'economic stress,' caused behavioural problems and crime. He stated, for example:

> All attempts to rectify environmental factors should proceed from one prime consideration: how have they affected the delinquent himself? Time, money and labour are constantly lavished upon an effort to ameliorate material conditions which, however much they may shock the cultivated visitor, however sordid and unsanitary they may seem, have yet, no real psychological connexion with the child's misconduct.[36]

Burt concluded that if 'the majority of delinquents are needy, the majority of the needy do not become delinquents.'[37] He observed that there were 'as many virtuous children in the tenements of Hoxton as in the mansions of Mayfair.'[38] These comments illustrate the ways in which, by the mid 1920s, the notion of the domestic environment had begun to encompass both psychological and material elements. Burt suggested that it was 'relative' rather than 'absolute' poverty that led to delinquency, poverty induced by 'extravagant wants as much as by an insufficient income.'[39] Like Healy, Burt concluded that factors other than economic hardship were more significant, ranking poverty as one of the least significant factors in the aetiology of delinquency.

Burt's main methodology in seeking to explain anti-social behaviour in children was the comparative study of delinquent versus non-delinquent school children. The scientific observation and comparison of children, in terms of physical growth, perceived intelligence, and behaviour, had historical precedents in the child study movement of the late nineteenth century. Child study had developed as a trend amongst Victorian scientists to examine, observe, and compare behaviour in children, and was founded predominantly on the work of British psychologists Francis Galton (1822–1911) and James Sully (1843–1923), and the American psychologist G. Stanley Hall (1844–1924).[40] Quantitative comparison of children resulted in the establishment of idealised 'scientific' standards of 'normal' and 'abnormal' children, assessed in terms of intelligence, temperament, and behaviour. In the inter-war period, comparison studies of children by sex, class, and intelligence became a key tool in theoretical and policy development. This approach was supported by the Board of Education, which granted Burt permission to carry out psychometric testing in a number of different schools. Burt subsequently explored a comprehensive range of influential factors—hereditary, environmental, psychological, and physical—constructing a list of fifteen influences that he considered to be of significance in the aetiology of delinquency.[41] Environmental factors featured prominently in this list. Burt identified two specific areas of concern under the title of environment, defined as 'the home' and 'outside the home.' In doing so he raised awareness of a range of issues that could be significant in the aetiology of maladjustment. Heading the list as the most influential factor of all, in Burt's opinion, was 'defective discipline.' In some cases, he accredited weak discipline either to 'moral or intellectual weakness' or to 'physical weakness.' However, in a significant number of cases, he noted that this was due to 'the absence of parent at work,' again acknowledging the stress placed on families by external pressures, rather than by deliberate parental neglect.[42]

Familial relationships were also a prominent feature of Burt's approach, evident in his investigation into 'defective family relationships' as a significant factor in the aetiology of delinquency, a detail rarely mentioned in historical analyses.

> Many outbreaks of juvenile crime arise ultimately out of the emotional relations subsisting between the child himself, and the various members of his family . . . Nearly every tragedy of crime is in its origin a drama of domestic life.[43]

Rather than focusing on bad parenting, Burt identified a much more significant problem, the 'broken home.' This he defined as households experiencing 'prolonged absence from parents.'[44] Others compared the 'disturbed home,' where one or both parents were missing, with the 'normal home,' defined as 'both child's own parents present.'[45] Contemporary awareness of the problems caused by the absence of one or other parent from the family unit was an issue that has been largely neglected by historians, but was a factor that featured prominently in professional explanations for delinquency in the early and mid twentieth century. Healy and Bronner, for example, noted in 1916 that one parent was absent in over 50% of the families studied.[46] A range of professional and State investigations presented several key reasons why prolonged parental absence might occur, highlighting the complexities of family circumstances. Firstly, following a noticeable peak in Home Office figures on delinquency in the closing years of both the First and Second World Wars, many professionals highlighted the negative psychological effects on children of prolonged absences of fathers, and increasing demands on mothers, due to conscription.[47] This was considered particularly with regard to boys who had been 'left too much to their own devices' with greater opportunities for 'misapplied energy.'[48] Even in peacetime, fathers could be absent for long periods due to employment. The importance of the presence of the father in the home was frequently highlighted by experts throughout the mid-twentieth century, but contemporary focus on the significance of fathers is often ignored in historical preoccupations with the role of mothers.

A second factor that was found to impact significantly on the emotional well-being of children was the death of a parent. Problems arose, however, not only from the immediate loss of the parent and the resulting grief, but from the substantial changes that occurred in family structure. In particular, the introduction of a new parenting figure in the household began to be recognised as a significant element in the aetiology of maladjustment. Burt was amongst the first to acknowledge this: 'Inquiring into domestic circumstances of case after case, the investigator cannot fail to be struck with the marked recurrence of one suggestive item—the presence of a foster parent.'[49]

Burt defined the term 'foster parent' as stepmothers, stepfathers, grandmothers, aunts or 'a guardian or recipient related neither by matrimony or by blood.'[50] He argued that step-parents, and stepmothers in particular, were more likely to display impatience, indifference, jealously and hostility. Burt's surveys suggested that problems occurred particularly when the step-parent had children of his or her own from previous relationships.[51] This factor was highlighted in later child guidance studies. In 1936, for example, Muriel Barton-Hall and Fred Hopkins, psychologists working at the Liverpool Child Guidance Clinic, observed that 'mild forms of behaviour disturbance which would be understood by the child's own parents are less readily tolerated by the substitute parents.'[52] Emanuel Miller, Director of the East London Child Guidance Centre, also suggested the possible significance of the grandmother as a 'hidden potent force in family affairs,' highlighting the complexities of family dynamics and presenting a precursor for family therapy.[53]

Finally, maladjustment could occur when a parent or child needed hospital treatment. The frequency and nature of treatment of many infectious diseases meant that family members admitted to hospital might be absent from the domestic environment for substantial periods of time. Stays of several months or, particularly in cases of tuberculosis, even years were common. In other cases, parents might be incarcerated in asylums or prisons. The full emotional impact of long-term separation of the child from its parents was not recognised until the 1940s, when the medicalisation of delinquency was taken a stage further by psychiatrist John Bowlby (1907–1990).[54] Bowlby carried out a detailed study of a group of child criminals referred to him by the courts for pilfering. In seeking to understand the motivation of these children, he noted that a significant proportion of these adolescents had been separated from their mothers at an early age, as a result of the death of the parent, the breakup of the family, or through hospitalisation. This realisation formed the basis for the formulation of his seminal theory of 'maternal deprivation,' which subsequently dominated medical and governmental approaches to maladjusted children in the following decades. Underlining the significance of the domestic environment, Bowlby published the results of the study in 1944 in a paper entitled 'Forty-four juvenile thieves: Their characters and home lives.'[55]

Notions of the home and the domestic environment, however, encompassed many factors other than just parenting. The position of the child in the family was considered to be of significance, for example, with professionals noting that the eldest child in particular was more susceptible to maladjustment than younger siblings, with the 'only child' being considered at even greater risk of developing behavioural problems. This issue featured prominently amongst psychoanalytic explanations of maladjusted behaviour. Maladjustment in eldest children was seen to arise most frequently as a result of feelings of jealously on the arrival of younger siblings, whilst problems in only children were explained, in psychoanalytic opinion, as arising through 'over-fussy' mothering.[56]

Another factor considered to be important was the influence of a child's wider social environment. Burt, for example, argued that the social environment was, in many cases, of greater significance than any other. Again, this element of Burt's work is rarely mentioned in historical accounts, but he strongly suggested that 'Influences that affect him (the delinquent) beyond the circle of his family life may at times be the sole factors in his delinquency.'[57] He identified specific areas where problems might occur:

> Outside of the child's home, these are the chief conditions that make for juvenile delinquency—unemployment, uncongenial school or work, defective or excessive facilities for leisure hour amusements, the influence, deliberate or unintentional of adult friends and strangers, and above all, the influence of associates of the child's own age. None is so powerful as the last.[58]

Burt considered the influence of 'school-fellows, work-fellows or play fellows . . . of the same age and sex' to be significant in 18% of his cases. He also recognised that this factor was the most difficult for parents to deal with, challenging the assumption later made of parental neglect and 'bad parenting' as the defining factor in delinquency.

Burt was also one of the first to note the potential influence of the rapidly growing media in shaping children's behaviour in the 1920s. He observed that 'I have noted an excessive passion for the cinema among over 7% of my delinquent boys . . . and in a few cases have had to rank it as the principal cause of crime.'[59] In raising awareness of the 'Power of the Pictures,' he argued that the cinema, still a novelty in the mid 1920s, was potentially harmful, firstly as a 'faculty of imitativeness,' secondly in providing a standing temptation to steal money for admittance, and finally in presenting 'wild emotionalism' and 'immoral frivolity and vice' as 'the normal characteristics of the everyday conduct of adults.'[60] This factor featured highly in Burt's aetiological list, above that of defective family relationships. It was not only

Burt who considered that the cinema could have significant effects on children's moral perceptions. Other psychologists also started to investigate this possibility in this period. In the United States, for example, L. L. Thurstone concluded from his investigation in 1931 that 'motion pictures can be used to affect the social attitudes of school children and that these effects can be objectively measured.'[61] In Britain, this line of research was continued into the 1940s by Dr. W. D. Wall. His survey of 2,058 adolescents in Birmingham led him to argue that adults, in the context of both home and school, were failing to provide children with the basic social skills that were of primary importance in desired social integration, and that the behaviour of a significant number were consequently being shaped by cinematic example:

> For very many the screen is the only source of information on many topics about which adolescents are avid for information. On whole areas of human life—on how to behave, on the relationship between people, on how to make the most of ones' physical self, on the techniques of social intercourse, on the coin of light conversation our school curricula are silent. The emotional and social education of the growing youth is left to the vivid realism of the screen.[62]

Finally, an environmental factor that was considered by many professionals to be of major significance in the aetiology of maladjustment was the classroom. Following the introduction of compulsory education with the Education Act of 1876, all children of school age were expected to conform to a range of daily educational demands. Burt revealed the problems of the 'one size fits all' approach inherent in the system, as the issue of problematic children within the education system increasingly became the subject of professional attention. He stated:

> The strain of sitting for four or five hours a day over lessons for which he has neither taste nor ability is apt to induce in an active frame a vigorous recoil.[63]

Burt's concerns regarding the high burden of expectation placed on children within the classroom environment were echoed by several prominent educationalists at the time, for example, by Maria Montessori, who warned of the problems, both physical and emotional, of children being forced to sit at desks for hours at a time.[64]

Within the classroom, professional attention initially focused on the problems of mental deficiency and feeble-mindedness. However, fears around children identified as 'mentally deficient' soon shifted to concerns over the 'mentally unstable.' Initially, this label was applied primarily to children identified as delinquent, prompting a desire to identify potential delinquents. Sources show that attempts were actively being made by the State to identify pre-delinquent children through the education system, emphasising 'the importance of getting hold of the delinquent or potential delinquent at as early an age as possible.'[65] Reporting to the Central Association for Mental Welfare in July 1922, for example, Dr. Hughes, the School Medical Officer for Stoke on Trent, stated:

> The juvenile delinquent is found not so much among what is called the mental deficient children in the legal sense, as among the temperamentally unstable child. It is the temperamentally unstable child we want to get hold of.[66]

In describing the methods employed to identify such children, Dr. Hughes stated:

> The second method I tried was sending out special forms to the Head teachers, giving just a few indications of what I regarded as likely symptoms.[67]

This comment illustrates that the view of delinquency as a symptom of a medical condition needing professional intervention was framing approaches within the education system well before the establishment of child guidance in England. Notions of the 'pre-delinquent' or 'pre-psychotic' child, central to the work of the child guidance clinics in the United States at this time, were already at the forefront of professional attention within an educational context in Britain by the early 1920s.

By the end of the 1920s, the model of the delinquent 'rebel' had developed further with the emergence of psychoanalysis as a primary tool in the understanding and treatment of maladjusted children. Initially, the psychoanalytic approach developed around considerations of the internal emotional environment, ignoring theories into the significance of the external environment. The main agent in this development in Britain was Austrian analyst Melanie Klein (1882–1960). Klein developed a technique of analysing children through interpretation of play, and identified the role of unconscious aggression in promoting anxiety in young children. She argued that play highlighted unconscious 'phantasies' that could give rise to feelings of extreme guilt, anxiety, and disappointment in even very young children, manifesting in angry, aggressive, and sadistic behaviour, together with problems such as wetting and soiling. This was an important theory in seeking to explain troublesome behaviour in delinquent 'rebel' children. She went on to identify the complex interplay between a child's internal fantasies and real experiences, and the ways in which the development of a child's internal world, expressed through play, gave insight into its external relationships. Klein's theories, however, met with hostility from many of her contemporaries, with one key criticism being her lack of acknowledgment or investigation into the possible significance of the home environment or familial relationships on a child's behaviour. This issue was taken up and developed by one of Klein's pupils, John Bowlby, whose work was to prove of major significance in the development of the medical model of maladjustment, with a professional dominance spanning over fifty years.

The psychoanalytic model of maladjustment acknowledged and reinforced the notion of the aggressive, anti-social and disobedient behaviour of delinquent 'rebels' as a key symptom of internal emotional conflict. Throughout the 1930s and 1940s, psychoanalytic theory dominated approaches to the assessment and management of delinquent children. It also became a primary factor in the conceptualisation and identification of a second category of maladjusted child, the psychological 'rabbit.'

PSYCHOLOGICAL 'RABBITS' AND THE EDUCATIONAL ENVIRONMENT

Whilst notions of juvenile delinquency and psychotic rebels were formulated around scientific, medical, and finally psychoanalytic explanations of behaviour, the concept of a maladjusted 'rabbit' developed following longstanding concerns with children who were considered to be overly nervous or emotionally 'delicate.' In the late nineteenth century, a significant rise in professional and State interest in the overall health of children resulted in new ways of thinking about the well-being of children. Initially, attention focused on physical and mental development.[68] However, following growing interest in the emerging discipline of psychology, professionals within the medical, judicial, and educational spheres began to place importance on moral, temperamental and emotional development. These elements became incorporated within medical notions of normal or abnormal child mental health, highlighted particularly in professional conceptualisations of the delicate child. Mirroring the development of scientific theories on the aetiology of criminality, increasingly professional attention moved from hereditary notions of 'pre-disposition' to physical or mental illness to a focus on the effects of the child's social and domestic environment on emotional health.

A delicate child was considered to be particularly vulnerable or pre-disposed to disease or illness. Initially, the term encompassed children who were in poor physical condition, for example, malnourished or anaemic.[69] Most importantly, the condition was seen as a degenerative process, which, if left unattended, would result in 'a delicacy of the whole system' leading to 'functional derangement.'[70] The possibility of degeneration emphasised, and provided justification for, the importance of professional medical intervention as a preventative measure. Initially, the classification of 'delicate' was assessed predominantly in the context of infectious or contagious diseases, particularly tuberculosis. Whilst historians, such as Linda Bryder, have focused on children who were considered physically delicate, few have highlighted the fact that, from the late nineteenth century onwards, children were also being seen as delicate in terms of susceptibility to mental problems resulting from nervous or emotional disorders.[71] Concerns around this type of child emerged largely from the work of the Child Study Movement. In addition, those working in the fields of neurology and physiology increasingly highlighted the dangers of 'nervous disease' in children. Emphasis on this aspect of physiological health became a prominent feature of Victorian medical practices following the publication of *A Practical Treatise on Nervous Exhaustion (Neurasthenia)* in 1880 by American neurologist George M. Beard (1839–1883).[72] The application of the term 'nervous' has been examined in historical studies of medical approaches particularly to women in this period.[73] However, it also became a primary consideration in framing approaches to children at this time, particularly amongst the middle classes, becoming an influential factor in late nineteenth-century debates about the development of children's brains. The condition of a child's mind thus became linked with physiological concerns. Several prominent medical professionals, inspired by the work of Charles Mercier, insisted that problems within the nervous system could adversely affect mental state. Emotionally delicate children were considered to be particularly susceptible to nervous conditions. The emergence of scientific child study can be placed within the context of Victorian preoccupation with neuroses, and fears amongst nineteenth-century doctors and psychologists that children in particular were prone to nervous exhaustion, through over-stimulation. Subsequently, worries that brain exhaustion could cause long-term damage to children's mental health became widespread within Victorian society, reinforced by doctors such as asylum psychiatrist James Crichton-Browne (1840–1938).[74] The medical model of the 'nervous child' developed further in the inter-war period, following the work of Dr. Hector Cameron (1878–1958), who emphasised the preventative nature of intervention in childhood and argued that psychological approaches should be applied increasingly in nurseries and schools.[75]

The work of the Child Study Movement appealed particularly to teachers, who were represented significantly amongst the membership. Approaches to child behaviour, framed by psychological theory, were subsequently disseminated throughout the education system by liberal educationalists keen to promote child study teachings. Psychological approaches were increasingly introduced as a means of understanding and managing problems in the classroom. Following the introduction of compulsory education, behaviourally problematic children became a prominent concern for the Home Office and the Board of Education. Particularly significant were children considered to be underachieving academically. The introduction of the Mental Deficiency Act in 1913 and the Elementary Education (Defective and Epileptic Children) Act in 1914 led to the removal of many children classified as mentally subnormal or feeble minded into colonies or segregated institutions. Others were identified as delinquent. However, a large number of children remained who, according to their I.Q. assessments, were not mentally deficient, but were considered 'educationally subnormal' and officially categorised as either 'dull' or 'backward.'

It became increasingly clear that academic achievement was not solely dependent on a child's intelligence level, but could be affected by other factors. This realisation was reinforced by the work of U.S. psychologist Lightner Witmer (1867–1956) who was one of the first to apply the notion of maladjustment to children who were underachieving, but not delinquent. In 1896, Witmer, following the example of Wilhelm Wundt's experimental clinic in Leipzig, opened the first psychological clinic dealing specifically with problems of maladjustment at the University of Pennsylvania in Philadelphia.[76] Witmer recognised that many educational problems were not the result of pre-determined and fixed hereditary factors, but could be explained by either physical problems or environmental influences. Witmer focused on developing a psychological approach to education which placed emphasis on the differing needs of individual children, In Britain, the practice of educational psychology developed by Witmer, and also G. Stanley Hall, was promoted primarily by Cyril Burt, and became formally validated by the State when Burt was appointed the first official educational psychologist by London County Council in 1913.[77]

Burt's contribution to the treatment of behaviourally problematic children is most frequently located in an educational context. Initial attention had focused on the problems raised with the presence of mentally deficient and feeble-minded children who could not learn. However, following the removal of these children from mainstream schools under the terms of the Elementary Education Act of 1914, educational attention shifted to other children who were equally problematic within the classroom environment, through either disruptive behaviour or low academic achievement. Maladjusted children were prominent within this category of child, particularly since in many cases their I.Q. ratings, the definitive tool for categorisation, were significantly higher than average. Burt highlighted the problems arising from 'functional nervous disorder' and 'psycho-neurosis' in school children in 1925, identifying two categories, 'neurasthenia' and 'anxiety states.'[78] He argued that whilst these forms of neuroses were clearly apparent in overly introverted children, they could also be present as an unrecognised cause of delinquent behaviour.[79] In both cases, psychoneurosis could result in low academic achievement, with children categorised within the education system as backward or educationally subnormal. In 1937, he investigated the aetiology of backwardness in more detail, highlighting a range of environmental factors in both the school and the home that could lead to low academic achievement.[80]

Medical focus on overly nervous school children was reinforced by the child guidance movement. Child guidance became formally established in Britain with the opening of the East London Child Guidance Clinic on 21 November 1927. This clinic, located at the Jewish Free School, Bell Lane, Spitalfields, operated under the direction of psychiatrist Emanuel Miller (1893–1970).

A year later, the London Child Guidance Clinic opened at Tudor House, Canonbury Place, Islington. The British Child Guidance Council was formed shortly after. The aim of child guidance in Britain was 'to explore the evil (of maladjustment) at its roots, to destroy the causes rather than to prune the diseased branches of established neuroticism.'[81] Fears over both delinquency and neuroticism continued to shape professional approaches to maladjustment within this model.

In 1921, Healy's methodologies came to the attention of the influential philanthropic Commonwealth Fund of America and were subsequently used in the establishment of the first Child Guidance Clinics throughout the United States. As Margo Horn has shown, the attention of the child guidance clinics quickly moved from dealing primarily with the criminal behaviour of juvenile delinquents to incorporating a large number of children displaying a wide range of habits and behaviours that were not criminal, but of concern or irritation to adults around them. This shift of attention resulted in the medicalisation of a range of behaviours that were newly interpreted as outward symptoms of deeper internal problems, indicative of either an existing or a potential psychiatric condition that needed medical intervention and treatment. Within the child guidance model of maladjustment, symptoms considered indicative of internal conflict were categorised in three ways: first, 'undesirable habits' such as thumb sucking, nail biting, masturbation, stammering, and, most commonly, enuresis or bed-wetting; secondly, 'personality traits' such as over-sensitivity, apathy, and excessive imagination or lying; and finally, 'undesirable behaviours' such as disobedience, bullying, temper tantrums, defiance, and immoral sexual behaviour.

Accounts of work carried out at clinics both in Britain and in the United States show that children were presented at a clinic usually displaying only one of these symptoms, but that frequently the medical professionals would further identify other less obvious problems. Discovery of previously unnoticed problems, missed by the untrained parental eye, would validate the diagnosis of an underlying medical condition, identified as either neurosis or psychosis, and the need for professional intervention and psychiatric treatment. With this new emphasis on the complexities of diagnosis, the medical model of the delinquent child became encompassed within a new broader model of maladjustment, as delinquency increasingly became seen as only one outward sign amongst many of internal emotional conflict. Horn has noted that a shift of attention occurred within Commonwealth Fund clinics, from juvenile delinquents to mildly problematic, predominantly middle-class, children, as work with this second group was more likely to attain positive results of successful 're-adjustment' than the deeply ingrained, challenging, and often un-resolvable problems of working-class immigrant child criminals. Increasingly these behaviours were emphasised as indicative of future, rather than existing, neurotic or psychotic illness, emphasising the notion of the 'pre-psychotic' or 'pre-neurotic' child, with ever-increasing importance placed on the social and emotional origins of mental illness. Psychiatric intervention in childhood was seen as a crucial preventative measure in maintaining the mental health of the nation.

With the arrival of child guidance in Britain in 1927, the child guidance model of the maladjusted child was adopted, incorporating the psychological 'rabbit' alongside the delinquent 'rebel.' Emphasis on the potential problems of 'pre-neurotic' children was further reinforced by the advent of psychoanalysis. Melanie Klein, for example, suggested that excessive obedience and passivity could also be an indication of maladjustment in the form of neurosis that, without specialist psychoanalytic intervention, would otherwise have remained undetected. Klein believed that guilt and anxiety, whilst frequently manifesting as aggressive behaviour, could be an unrecognised problem in apparently well-behaved and docile children.

> In small children, too, an over-strong rejection of reality (often disguised under an apparent docility and adaptability) is, therefore, an indication of neurosis and only differs from an adult neurotic's flight from reality in its form of expression.[82]

Studies in the problems of neurosis in small children was carried further by Klein's student, John Bowlby. Bowlby began his medical training in 1929, just at the point when child psychiatry and child psychoanalysis were emerging as specialised professional fields. Qualifying in 1933, Bowlby initially trained in adult psychiatry at the Maudsley Hospital in London, and in 1936 was employed at the London Child Guidance Clinic.[83] After qualifying in psychoanalysis in 1937, he began training as a child analyst under Melanie Klein. Bolwby began to challenge Klein's theories, questioning one of her main premises, that unconscious fantasy was the overriding factor in determining emotional problems rather than real experience and trauma. His clinical work highlighted cases where, in his view, the role of the parents was clearly significant in the problematic behaviours of overly nervous children. This view was enforced particularly by two psychiatric social workers at the London Child Guidance Clinic, Molly Lawden and Nancy Fairbairn, who, following the American model, reported on visits made to the child's home, their domestic environment, and also observed the relationships and interactions among child, parents, grandparents, and siblings. As Bowlby described:

> It was these two who first introduced me to the notion that unresolved conflicts from the parents' own childhood play a large part in causing and perpetuating the problems of their children.[84]

Bowlby explained this in psychoanalytic terms as 'transgenerational transmission of neurosis,' articulating his findings in a paper presented to the British Psychoanalytic Society in 1939.[85] His work with both delinquent and neurotic children led Bowlby to redefine the model of maladjustment that had been established by the child guidance clinics and that had dominated approaches to problem children throughout the 1920s and 1930s. Bowlby set out a detailed analysis of 'personality types,' dividing the population into two basic categories: 'emotionally normal' and 'unstable.' Unstable personalities were further divided into eight subcategories: obsessive/perfectionist; inhibited/nervous; hysterical; cheerful manic; aggressive manic; affectionless thief; schizoid types—hysterical, solitary, or obsessional; and finally, epileptic.[86] The simple polarised medical concept of maladjusted 'rabbits and rebels' consequently became a far more complex model defined using detailed psychiatric terminology, seeing maladjustment as a sign of mental abnormality.

The increasingly complex model of maladjustment that developed from the 1940s, whilst being welcomed by medical professionals, was met with a greater degree of scepticism and hostility by others involved in the day-to-day management of maladjusted children. Although child guidance clinics were overwhelmingly seen as the main agents dealing with these children, by the 1940s the most challenging cases were being managed by privately run residential homes or schools. These homes were initially established by key individuals who were prominent in promoting alternative forms of education, most notably Homer Lane (1875–1925), A. S. Neill (1883–1975), Dr. Frederick Dodd (1892–1950), Otto Shaw (1908–1976), and David Wills (d.1981). These authors challenged the established educational approach to children, particularly the unrealistic expectations placed on children who were unable to cope with the social and educational environments in which they were placed, but also began to contest the increasingly complex psychiatric models of maladjustment that were being developed by the medical profession, presenting by contrast a much more pragmatic and simplified view of maladjustment. Frederick Dodd, for example, defined a maladjusted child simply as one 'unable to cope with the circumstances with which faced.'[87] The most forceful view was put forward by A. S. Neill, who challenged the belief that maladjusted children were psychologically abnormal, but said they were simply 'angry 'cos of lack of love mostly.'[88] David Wills emphasised the social environment in his definition, drawing on Bowlby's earliest work, stating:

> A maladjusted child is one whose capacity to make relationships, and thus to identify and acquire moral standards, has failed to develop owing to early deprivation or maltreatment.[89]

The key aim of the alternative educationalists was to provide a 'protected environment in which to act out anti-social impulses,' thus reinforcing the belief that 'nurture' rather than 'nature' was the most significant factor in the aetiology of maladjustment.[90]

CONCLUSION

In 1938, Noel Harrison, psychologist at the London Child Guidance Clinic, gave a lecture to a group of students in which he concluded that the maladjusted child was 'the square peg in the round hole.'[91] By the late 1930s, therefore, it is evident that a medical model of maladjustment had become established around the notion of children who did not fit. In particular, they did not fit the behavioural expectations that society placed on them, especially within an educational environment that demanded long hours of concentration and obedience, together with uniform targets of academic achievement. Many could not match the social expectations of middle-class parents who desired the 'ideal child,' in keeping with prevailing domestic ideologies. Their behavioural and educational problems could not be understood within established medical models of deviancy and inherited sub-normality. The medical model of maladjustment therefore was a means of presenting a scientific explanation for a range of behaviours and undesirable habits in children. Whether in the form of the worried parent presenting the child to a child guidance clinic, the teacher faced with an under-achieving or disruptive child in the classroom, or the psychiatrist identifying potential neurotics or psychotics, intervention became justified in order to prevent future problems for society.

By the end of the 1930s, the general consensus amongst professionals dealing with behaviourally problematic children was that the domestic environment was a primary factor and that 'maladjustment starts at home.'[92] However, most acknowledged the aetiological complexity of maladjustment, emphasising five particular factors in the aetiology of the condition: familial relationships; conscious and unconscious parental behaviour; the place of the child in the family; economic pressures (though not necessarily poverty); and, most significantly of all, the broken home. Thus, while psychoanalytic focus increasingly highlighted the role of parents' behaviour in the causation of behavioural and emotional problems in children, a range of other environmental factors was also considered to be significant in the aetiology of maladjustment. Extensive effort was put into scientific and medical studies seeking to identify common denominators in the external environments of the children being investigated, demonstrating considerable understanding, rather than condemnation, of the daily problems faced by parents.

NOTES

1. E. A. Hamilton-Pearson, 'Child Delinquency,' *The Lancet* (17 Dec. 1927): 1312.
2. For example, George Behlmer, *Friends of the Family* (Stanford: Stanford University Press, 1998), 164, and Nikolas Rose, *The Psychological Complex: Psychology, Politics and Society in England 1869–1939* (London: Routledge & Kegan Paul, 1985), 164.
3. Herbert Spencer, *Principles of Psychology*, I (London: Williams & Norgate 1855), 293.

4. Charles Darwin, *On the Origin of Species* (London, 1859).
5. For more details of Bernard's work, see Jerome Tarshis, *Claude Bernard; Father of Experimental Medicine* (New York: Dial Press, 1968).
6. Charles Mercier, *Sanity and Insanity* (London: Walter Scott, 1890), 141.
7. The belief that insanity was inherited and therefore inherent and untreatable underpinned psychiatric practice throughout the nineteenth century, reinforced by the work of leading psychiatrists such as Henry Maudsley (1835–1918) and Alfred Tredgold (1870–1952). Long-term incarceration in asylums was common practice, but the apparent failure of the asylums and psychiatry to help these cases was seen as proof that most forms of mental disorder were incurable—Roy Porter, 'Mental Illness,' in Roy Porter (ed.), *The Cambridge Illustrated History of Medicine* (Cambridge: Cambridge University Press, 1996), 297.
8. Maurice Bridgeland, *Pioneer Work with Maladjusted Children* (London: Staples, 1971), 32.
9. William Healy and Augusta Bronner, 'Youthful offenders: A comparative study of two groups, each of 1,000 young recidivists,' *American Journal of Sociology,* 22, 1 (July 1916): 38–52.
10. Ibid., 42.
11. For an account of the establishment of gendered domestic ideologies, see Leonore Davidoff and Catherine Hall, *Family Fortunes: Men and Women of the English Middle Class, 1780–1850* (London: Routledge, 1987).
12. J. Manton, *Mary Carpenter and the Children of the Streets* (London: Heinneman, 1976).
13. Kathleen Jones, *Taming the Troublesome Child* (Cambridge, MA: Harvard University Press, 1999); Margo Horn, *Before It's Too Late* (Philadelphia: Temple University Press, 1989); and A. M. Harvey and S. L. Abrams, *For the Welfare of Mankind: The Commonwealth Fund and American Medicine* (Baltimore, 1986).
14. Thomas Leahey, *A History of Psychology: Main Currents in Psychological Thought* (6th ed., Upper Saddle River, NJ: Pearson Prentice Hall, 2006).
15. Jones, *Troublesome Child,* 57.
16. William Healy, *The Individual Delinquent* (Boston: Little, Brown, 1915), 32.
17. Ibid., 21, 4.
18. Healy stated that the psychiatric social worker must always be female in order to establish a particular type of relationship with the child that was necessary in the diagnosis process—Ibid., 36. See also the chapter by John Stewart in this volume.
19. Ibid., 4.
20. Healy and Bronner, 'Youthful offenders,' 50–2.
21. Psychoanalyst Susan Isaacs, in particular, placed great emphasis on the role of the parents in her influential work throughout the 1930s and was critical of neglectful parenting. See for example, Susan Isaacs, *The Psychological Aspects of Child Development* (London, 1935).
22. Healy, *Individual Delinquent,* 18.
23. Ibid., 28.
24. Ibid., 30.
25. Healy's study included children as young as 8 or 9 years of age—Healy and Bronner, 'Youthful offenders,' 40.
26. Bernard Glueck, 'Types of delinquent careers,' *Mental Hygiene,* 1 (1917): 185.
27. 'Director's Special Report on Delinquency,' (26 June, 1920), 3, Commonwealth Fund file CW.
28. Horn, *Before It's Too Late,* 21.

29. Cyril Burt, *The Young Delinquent* (London: London University Press, 1925), 4.
30. Ibid., 611.
31. Ibid., 606.
32. This aspect of Burt's work is particularly emphasised by biographer L. S. Hearnshaw, *Cyril Burt, Psychologist* (London: Hodder & Stoughton, 1979), and in the critique of Burt's work by Stephen Jay Gould, *The Mismeasure of Man* (London: Pelican, 1981), 234–320.
33. Burt, *Young Delinquent*, 62–206.
34. For example, E.M.L., 'Review of The Young Delinquent,' *Economica*, 16 (Mar. 1926): 102.
35. R. Evelyn Lucas, 'Social capacity in delinquency,' *The Lancet* (18 Dec. 1926): 1292.
36. Burt, *Young Delinquent*, 118.
37. Ibid., 143.
38. Ibid., 187.
39. Ibid., 143.
40. For more on the Child Study Movement in Britain see Lyubov Gurjeva, 'Everyday Bourgeois Science: The Scientific Management of Children in Britain, 1880–1914' (PhD diss., University of Cambridge, 1998).
41. Burt, *Young Delinquent*, 606.
42. Ibid., 65.
43. Ibid., 124.
44. Ibid., 64.
45. For example, Muriel Barton-Hall and Fred Hopkins, 'Parental loss and child guidance,' *Archives of Disease in Childhood*, 11, 64 (Aug. 1936): 187–194.
46. Healy and Bronner, 'Youthful offenders,' 51.
47. The figures for delinquency peaked at 51,000 cases in 1917, compared to 37,500 in the pre-war period. In 1921, it fell again to 30,000—Victor Bailey, *Delinquency and Citizenship* (Oxford: Clarendon Press, 1987), 17.
48. Anon., 'Juvenile Crime and the War,' *Justice of the Peace*, 80 (17 June 1916): 261–2.
49. Burt, *Young Delinquent*, 93.
50. Ibid., 93.
51. Ibid., 94.
52. Barton-Hall and Hopkins, 'Parental loss and child guidance,' 193.
53. Miller quoted in George Renton, 'The East London Child Guidance Clinic,' *Journal of Child Psychiatry* (1978): 311.
54. Harry Hendrick has been one of the few historians to highlight this issue. See Harry Hendrick, 'Children's Emotional Well-being and Mental Health in Post-Second World War Britain, 1940s–1950s: The Case of Unrestricted Hospital Visiting,' in Marijke Gijswijt-Hofstra and Hilary Marland (eds.), *Cultures of Child Health in Britain and the Netherlands in the Twentieth Century* (Amsterdam-NewYork: Rodopi, 2003), 213–42.
55. John Bowlby, 'Forty-four juvenile thieves: Their characters and home lives,' *International Journal of Psychoanalysis*, 25 (1944): 207–28.
56. Donald Winnicott, 'A Note on Normality and Anxiety (1931),' in *D. W. Winicott: Collected Papers* (1958), 3–21; Susan Isaacs, *The Psychological Aspects of Child Development* (London, 1935).
57. Burt, *Young Delinquent*, 128.
58. Ibid., 186.
59. Ibid., 142.
60. Ibid., 149.

61. L. L. Thurstone, 'Influence of motion pictures on children's attitudes,' *Journal of Social Psychology,* 2, 2 (1931): 304.
62. W. D. Wall and W. A. Simson, 'The effects of cinema attendance on the behaviour of adolescents as seen by their contemporaries,' *British Journal of Educational Psychology,* 18 (Feb. 1948): 61.
63. Burt, *Young Delinquent,* 181.
64. Maria Montessori, *The Montessori Method,* translated by Anne Everett George (New York, Frederick A. Stokes Co., 1912), 7.
65. Dr. Hughes, 'Report of a conference on mental deficiency—Afternoon session,' *Reports of the Central Association for Mental Welfare* (26/27 July, 1922): 57.
66. Ibid., 57.
67. Ibid.
68. Bernard Harris, *The Health of the Schoolchild: A History of the School Medical Service in England and Wales* (Buckingham: Open University Press, 1995); Jane Lewis, *The Politics of Motherhood: Child and Maternal Welfare in England, 1900–1939* (London: Croom Helm, 1980).
69. Anon., 'The Subnormal School Child,' *The Lancet,* 210, 5441 (10 Dec. 1927): 1245; Lewis Williams, 'Open-air schools and residential schools for defective children,' in T. N. Kelynack, *Defective Children* (London, 1915), 357.
70. Anon., 'The subnormal school child,' *The Lancet,* 210, 5441 (10 Dec. 1927): 1245.
71. Linda Bryder has highlighted the ways in which children could be categorised as 'pre-tuberculous' and removed from their home environment even though they had no sign of the disease: Linda Bryder '"Wonderlands of buttercups and daisies": tuberculosis and the open air school movement in Britain, 1907–39,' in Roger Cooter (ed.), *In the Name of the Child: Health and Welfare 1880–1940* (London, 1992), 72–95.
72. On Beard, see Trevor Turner, 'The early 1900s and before,' in Hugh Freeman (ed.), *A Century of Psychiatry: Vol. I* (London: Mosby-Wolfe, 1999), 3–29.
73. For example, see Nancy Tomes, 'Historical perspectives on women and mental illness,' in Rima D. Apple (ed.), *Women, Health and Medicine in America* (New York: Garland, 1990), 143–72.
74. In 1884, Crichton-Browne carried out a survey of fourteen London elementary schools to investigate the detrimental effects of educational pressures on the mental health of children: James Crichton-Browne, 'Report upon the alleged over-pressure of work in public elementary schools,' *Parliamentary Papers,* LXI (1884), 56.
75. Hector Cameron, *The Nervous Child* (London: Oxford University Press, 1919).
76. Wundt's clinic, established in Leipzig in 1879, provided a model that was copied around the world. Witmer spent a short period studying under Wundt in Leipzig in 1888. See Paul McReynolds, *Lightner Witmer: His Life and Times* (Washington: American Psychological Society, 1997).
77. G. Sutherland and S. Sharp, '"The fust official psychologist in the wurrld": aspects of the professionalisation of psychology in early twentieth century Britain,' *History of Science,* 18 (1980): 181–208.
78. Burt, *Young Delinquent,* 581.
79. Ibid., 581.
80. Cyril Burt, *The Backward Child* (London: University of London Press, 1937), 110–34.
81. Noel Burke and Emanuel Miller, 'Child mental hygiene—Its history, methods and problems,' *British Journal of Medical Psychology,* 9 (1929): 218.
82. Melanie Klein, *The Psycho-Analysis of Children* (Berlin, 1932), 12.

83. Jeremy Holmes, *John Bowlby and Attachment Theory* (London: Routledge, 1993).
84. John Bowlby, 'Early Days at the London Child Guidance Centre,' *Child Guidance Trust Newsletter* (June 1987).
85. John Bowlby, 'The influence of the environment in the development of neuroses and neurotic character,' *International Journal of Psycho-Analysis,* 21 (1940): 154–78.
86. John Bowlby, 'Diagnosis and psychopathology,' *Personal Papers of John Bowlby,* Wellcome Library PP/BOW/C.3/6.
87. In preparing his book on work carried out with maladjusted children, Maurice Bridgeland asked several key individuals for their own definition of 'maladjusted.' Following the death of Dr. Dodd, his wife quoted his words in personal correspondence to Maurice Bridgeland—Bridgeland, *Pioneer Work,* 30.
88. This was A. S. Neill's response to Bridgeland's question, quoted from personal communication—in ibid., 30.
89. David Wills quoted in Bridgeland, ibid., 30.
90. Ibid., 32.
91. Noel G. Harrison, 'Lecture Notes,' *Child Guidance Correspondence* (1938), Wellcome Library PP/NGH/11.
92. Otto Shaw, *Maladjusted Boys* (London, 1965), 25.

8 *'Allergy con amore'*
Psychosomatic Medicine and the 'Asthmogenic Home' in the Mid-Twentieth Century

Mark Jackson

INTRODUCTION

In March 1962, *The Times* newspaper reported the strange case of a man whose asthma had apparently been cured by the death of his wife. According to his general practitioner, the patient had quite suddenly developed asthma at the age of forty-five, but clinical tests had revealed no evidence of allergy to the familiar array of immediate environmental triggers, such as pollen and dust. However, a clue to the possible emotional and domestic origins of his illness emerged when it became apparent that the man had 'never had an attack of asthma' since the death of his 'formidable and overpowering wife.' With little hint of irony, the report concluded that the patient 'had obviously been allergic to his wife.'[1]

The implicit, and moralising, link between emotional tension and asthma evident in *The Times* report was echoed in other popular representations of asthma and allergy during the 1950s and 1960s. In *Allergy,* a play first performed in 1966, for example, the Scottish playwright Cecil Philip Taylor (1929–81) explored the manner in which emotional stress could precipitate allergic skin complaints. One of the play's central characters, Christopher, develops a 'very nasty, ugly red rash' whenever he contemplates committing adultery with Barbara; in response to concerns that the rash might be infectious, he insists that it is merely an allergy 'to adultery.'[2] At around the same time, as Jo Gill argues elsewhere in this volume, the American confessional poet Anne Sexton (1928–74) captured the emotional desolation of suburban marriage by referring to a married couple as 'two asthmatics whose breath sobs in and out through a small fuzzy pipe.'[3] Links between asthma and sexual passion also appeared in newspaper cartoons from this period. Reg Smythe's Andy Capp cartoon in the *Daily Mirror* in March 1958, for example, not only suggested symptomatic similarities between certain emotions (notably love) and asthma but also hinted at a possible causative relationship between the two states.[4]

These popular cultural images of asthma and other allergies as the products of particular emotional states were paralleled, and perhaps legitimated, by prominent medical preoccupations with the psychological determinants of allergic diseases in the post-war period. Although scientific understandings of the material causes and immunological mechanisms of allergy had developed rapidly during the early twentieth century, interest in the emotional triggers of asthma, hay fever, and eczema persisted. Indeed, during the middle decades of the twentieth century, allergists and other physicians on both sides of the Atlantic regularly attempted to identify not only the psychological contours of the 'allergic personality,' but also the emotional, rather than merely material, elements of domestic life that could precipitate asthma attacks in vulnerable individuals. During the 1940s, 1950s, and 1960s, the 'asthmogenic home'[5] became both an aetiological explanation for asthma, particularly in children, and a site for clinical investigation and psychological intervention.

The aim of this chapter is to explore and explain the clinical dimensions and popularity of psychosomatic approaches to asthma in the middle decades of the twentieth century. The first section sets out earlier, traditional approaches to asthma, which, while recognizing the immediate biological causes of the condition, nevertheless acknowledged the role of emotions as triggers of asthma attacks and construed asthma as a form of hereditary neurosis. In addition, this section will trace the persistence of such accounts following the substantial reframing of asthma and hay fever as allergic phenomena in the first decades of the twentieth century. Focusing on the work of Helen Flanders Dunbar (1902–59), Erwin Pulay (b. 1899), John Freeman (1876–1962), and many other allergists and physicians, the second section explores the proliferation of psychological theories of asthma during the 1940s and 1950s, linking developments particularly to the rise of psychosomatic medicine in this period and to novel concerns about the emotional, as well as material, hazards posed by modern homes and families. In the process, I argue that psychodynamic theories of asthma became popular in the mid-twentieth century not only because, by playing on prevalent fantasies of the 'good mother,' they sustained implicitly conservative attempts to reinforce gendered notions of domesticity, but also because, at the same time, they legitimated nascent radical, holistic, and ecological critiques of biomedical reductionism that emerged predominantly in the forms of social or psychosocial medicine in the post-war period.

ASTHMA AND THE ALLERGIC PERSONALITY

The term *asthma* has a long history, stretching back to ancient medical texts. In Hippocratic, Galenic, and Chinese traditions, asthma constituted merely a generic form of dyspnoea, that is, difficulty breathing or shortness of breath. Typified by panting or wheezing, or what the Roman stoic philosopher Seneca referred to as 'a sort of continued "last gasp"', asthma was most commonly attributed to humoral imbalance.[6] Over subsequent centuries, treatises by physicians tended to confirm traditional uses of the term, but also began to challenge ancient accounts of the condition. During the seventeenth century, for example, studies by the Belgian Jan van Helmont (1577–1644) and two English doctors, Thomas Willis (1621–75) and John Floyer (1649–1734), not only focused attention on the lungs as the organic seat of the disease but also identified particular environmental triggers of asthma, such as dust, feathers, tobacco smoke, and certain foods, as well as speculating on the possible familial distribution of asthma. In addition, these authors recognized the ability of both exercise and emotions to trigger asthma attacks.[7]

During the late eighteenth and early nineteenth centuries, the introduction of novel diagnostic techniques, such as percussion of the chest, auscultation with a stethoscope, and spirometry, and the emergence of a more scrupulous pathological anatomy facilitated the gradual differentiation not only between 'asthma' as a distinct condition of the lungs and the more general symptom of dyspnoea, but also between the renal, cardiac and bronchial forms of asthma regularly described in medical treatises.[8] As clinical confidence in locating asthmatic symptoms in the lungs grew during the nineteenth century, medical authors restricted the use of the term asthma to the bronchial form, which was often found in conjunction with hay fever.[9] Increased medical interest in bronchial asthma during the late nineteenth century also generated new understandings of the aetiology and pathogenesis of asthma, which came to be regarded, much like hay fever, as a form of 'hereditary neurosis' in which 'tonic contraction of the circular fibres' resulted in obstruction of the smaller bronchi.[10]

As asthma and hay fever became more closely linked as analogous forms of neurosis, the social characteristics of asthma were transformed. According to some eighteenth-century authors, such as the Scottish physician John Millar (1733–1805), asthma was primarily a disease of artisans. During the nineteenth century, however, asthma and hay fever came to be regarded by clinicians on both sides of the Atlantic as predominantly 'aristocratic diseases,' or as manifestations of what George Beard (1839–83) referred to as neurasthenia or American nervousness,[11] rarely found in either municipal or charitable hospital wards but regularly diagnosed and treated by physicians privately attending the educated, intelligent élite.[12] In both cases, the social contours of the disease may well have dictated the preferences of doctors and their patients for climate therapy (or 'hay fever holidays' as they were known in the United States) in seaside resorts or continental mountain retreats, affordable only by the rich and generating, in the process, a brand of health tourism.[13]

In the early twentieth century, approaches to asthma were in many ways transformed by the work of a young Austrian paediatrician, Clemens von Pirquet (1874–1929). Drawing on his observations of incubation times in children with infectious diseases and in those undergoing serum therapy at the Universitäts Kinderklinik in Vienna, in 1906 von Pirquet introduced the term *allergy* to denote any form of altered immunological reactivity.[14] Although von Pirquet's formulation of allergy was not immediately accepted by his colleagues, in the early decades of the twentieth century altered immunological reactivity was rapidly implicated in the pathogenesis of hay fever, asthma, urticaria (or nettle-rash), eczema, food idiosyncrasies, supersensitivity to aspirin and other drugs, reactions to bee stings, infectious diseases such as tuberculosis, and a variety of diffuse clinical manifestations including rheumatism, eclampsia, migraine, and epilepsy. In this way, gradual adherence to Clemens von Pirquet's language of allergy or altered reactivity established the foundations both for the construction of a novel category of disease and for the growth of a new medical specialty.[15]

However, it is important to recognize that, although altered immunological reactivity was implicated in many pathological processes, von Pirquet's notion of allergy did not precipitate any clear, or immediate, revolution in theories of disease. On the contrary, well-established, alternative explanations of asthma and hay fever persisted. In addition to studying the role of pollen, local irritation of the nasal or bronchial mucous membranes, bacterial infections, and heredity, for example, a number of writers also continued to stress the nervous origins and class distribution of both conditions. In the eighth edition of his book on the principles and practice of medicine, published in 1914, a Canadian physician and Regius Professor of Medicine at Oxford, Sir William Osler (1849–1919), echoed the views of several nineteenth-century authors when he suggested that there was 'in the majority of cases of bronchial asthma a strong neurotic element.'[16] At around the same time, the American paediatrician W. C. Hollopeter echoed Osler's thoughts (as well as reiterating earlier formulations of the disease) by insisting that the predominance of asthma amongst 'the better educated classes and those of fair social position' supported the assertion 'that the disease is essentially a neurosis.'[17] Some years later, Sir Humphry Rolleston (1862–1944), Regius Professor of Physic at Cambridge, objected to the manner in which preoccupations with hypersensitivity often excluded consideration of the effect of 'reflex causes acting on an irritable nervous system,' pointing out at the same time that the efficacy of adrenalin in treating asthma attacks was probably related to its ability to stimulate the sympathetic nervous system, thereby 'abolishing the dominance of vagotonia.'[18]

More particularly, in the present context, medical writers also continued to emphasize and investigate the emotional determinants of asthma. In an address on asthma presented to a regional meeting of the British Medical Association in 1921, for example, Arthur Hurst (1879–1944), the founder of the British Society of Gastroenterology, discussed cases of 'hysterical and emotional asthma,' in which 'an idea or an emotion' or, on occasions, 'any little excitement, business worry, or annoyance' might precipitate an asthma attack in patients with 'an irritable bronchial centre.'[19] Hurst's approach found general acceptance. As Humphry Rolleston pointed out in 1927, Hurst's description of asthma as 'the reaction of an over-excitable bronchial centre to blood borne irritants and to peripheral or psychical stimuli' carried the distinct advantage of including cases bought on by emotions as well as those precipitated by other mechanisms.[20]

Similar preoccupations were evident in the contemporaneous studies of North American allergists. In 1929, for example, Horace Baldwin, working in the Asthma Department of the Cornell Clinic at Cornell University Medical College in New York, published the results of 'continued observation of twenty-five patients' attending the clinic. His survey of the various stimuli involved led him to conclude that, in addition to the role of specific proteins and respiratory tract infections, asthma was triggered in thirteen of the patients by the 'influence of psychoemotional states such as nervous strain and nervous fatigue, depressions and worry.' The cases that Baldwin cited to support this assertion were instructive. For some patients, asthma attacks were precipitated by the strain of caring for dying relatives; in another case, a patient whose asthma was stimulated by 'argumentation and aggravation' improved when the 'whole family gradually adopted tacitly a program of quiet and compromise.' In his final example, which prefigured the domestic circumstances alluded to in *The Times* many years later, Baldwin suggested that an attack could be provoked by depression or excitement as well as by 'the nervous strain felt by the patient over increasing incompatibility with his wife.'[21]

Clinical interest in the emotional and psychological determinants of asthma and hay fever was especially evident in studies carried out by Erich Wittkower (1899–1983) into what he termed the 'allergic personality.' Wittkower was a German physician who had come to England in the early 1930s to work at the Tavistock Clinic in London and who later became professor of psychiatry at McGill University in Canada and president of the American Psychosomatic Society. Shortly after his arrival in London and with the support and collaboration of John Freeman, director of the world's largest allergy department at St. Mary's Hospital in London, Wittkower set out 'to investigate the mental make-up' of hay fever patients attending Freeman's clinics. As Wittkower acknowledged, as the result of widespread recognition of the role of emotions in triggering asthma and hay fever, allergic diseases had often been 'the subject of studies demonstrating the interplay of mind and body.' 'In these conditions the emotional origin of single attacks is generally admitted,' he wrote, 'but it is still a controversial subject whether, or to what extent, asthma, migraine and urticaria can be considered as part manifestations of a general psychopathological constitution.'[22]

Having reviewed previous literature on the role of 'nervous temperament' in the aetiology of allergies, Wittkower exposed 55 patients from Freeman's clinic (as well as a similar number of control cases) to an extensive psychological examination, in order to collect information about the 'psychological make-up' and 'personality structure' of hay fever patients in particular, and to 'elucidate the psychodynamics of allergic diseases in general.' With regard to hay fever, Wittkower identified various factors in childhood that might precipitate the development of hay fever:

> the data in general seem to indicate that the early development of the hay-fever patients studied was influenced by various adverse circumstances, which were liable to render their adjustment to life more difficult than that of the control group of patients examined for comparison. In contrast to the control group, the hay-fever patients frequently come from small families in which 'nervousness' is common. Often they are 'delicate' children or have been treated as such. A fair number of them are 'only' children. In a majority of these their impressions of childhood are unpleasant.[23]

Wittkower's tentative assumption from the statistical evidence 'that hay-fever patients are ill-equipped for life and therefore liable to maladjustment' was apparently supported by personal accounts of the patients. Although he recognized the possible sources of error in retrospective studies of childhood experiences using adult patients, his interviews suggested that most patients with hay fever had been 'shy, self-conscious and hypersensitive children.' Although outwardly polite and well-mannered, many patients had been as children 'openly disobedient, stubborn, obstreperous, cantankerous and given to fits of temper.' In contrast to the 'easy-going, carefree, happy-go-lucky type of children predominantly encountered among the control group, the hay-fever patients were serious children, disinclined to associate with others, wrapped up in their own minds and exceedingly ambitious.' Such qualitative evidence led Wittkower to conclude that, in the particular context of hay fever, 'Almost uniformly the character traits pointing to an emotional maladjustment are more frequent and more pronounced in the hay-fever group than in the control group.'[24]

Significantly, neither the medical nor the social impacts of these personality traits ceased with the onset of adulthood. On the contrary, Wittkower's studies suggested that emotional maladjustment in childhood bestowed hay fever patients 'with qualities of character likely to render adjustment and integration within society difficult' throughout their lives. In addition to demonstrating incomplete adjustment in their sexual life (an issue that was to figure strongly in later formulations of the psychodynamic origins of asthma), adult hay fever patients apparently displayed the same character qualities that they had in childhood 'often in an accentuated form':

> More than half of the hay-fever patients, in contrast to a few of the control group, were shut-in, self-absorbed, self-centred, unsociable, and eclectically sociable. They felt lonely, imperfectly understood, isolated, aloof, detached, outside of everything. Unable to cope with the business of their life they turn away from reality and take refuge in a dream world of their own. Most of them are extremely sensitive, abnormally tender, constantly wounded—the 'mimosa-like natures' of Kretschmer.[25]

Wittkower's assessment of the personality of hay fever patients was supposedly transferable to patients with other allergic conditions, such as asthma, urticaria, and migraine. While he acknowledged that the precise nature, direction, and biological mechanism of the link between constitution, emotions, and allergies was still unclear (but possibly mediated by the autonomic nervous system), Wittkower suggested that the 'allergic tendency may be regarded as a part manifestation of an inherited organ inferiority which long before the actual onset of allergic symptoms prepares the soil for the development of a neurotic constitution in the sense of Adler.'[26] Although Wittkower appeared to prioritize hereditary over environmental factors in the generation of the allergic personality, his preoccupations with early childhood experiences, with sexual adjustment, and with the emotional contours of patients and their families provided a crucial framework for subsequent psychodynamic interpretations of the role of home and family life in the aetiology of asthma.

THE 'ASTHMOGENIC HOME'

For most allergists attempting to establish the theoretical and practical parameters of their discipline during the first few decades of the twentieth century, Wittkower's analysis of the allergic personality proved relatively marginal. Although most allergists and other physicians readily accepted both the role of emotions in triggering asthma and the possibility of a constitutional predisposition to allergies, their clinical interest was more acutely absorbed by the problems of identifying the immediate material determinants of allergies, such as pollen, dust, certain foods, and animal dander (referred to collectively as allergens), elucidating the immunological mechanisms and mediators of allergic reactions, and more accurately diagnosing and treating a spectrum of allergic diseases. Thus, in the allergy clinic at St. Mary's Hospital, Freeman and his colleagues were largely preoccupied with refining the diagnosis of allergies by applying purified allergen preparations to the skin and conjunctiva of patients, or with perfecting the therapeutic technique of allergen desensitization that had been developed by Freeman and his early collaborator at St. Mary's, Leonard Noon (1877–1913).[27]

In addition, it is noticeable that some contemporary allergists distanced themselves from the inferences that could be drawn from Wittkower's psychological approach to asthma and hay fever. In an extensive account of research being carried out at the Asthma Research Clinic at Guy's Hospital in London during the 1930s, for example, a feature in *The Times* suggested that psychological, rather than biological, explanations for the apparent worsening of asthma at home, and its improvement away from home, should be accepted only with caution, noting in particular that troubled domestic circumstances could not be readily implicated in the aetiology of the condition.

> It is difficult to explain such cases except in terms of psychology, but the possibility exists that a chemical and not a psychological explanation ought to be looked for. There may be houses, or even districts, the atmosphere of which is charged with some "allergic substance," capable of producing asthma. Parents' quarrels seem to have played no part in causing the disease, because in none of the cases studied was there any evidence of marital disharmony. The comment is made: "This is an interesting point, because in child guidance clinics, problem-children often appear to result from strife in the home."[28]

During the 1940s and 1950s, however, psychodynamic accounts of asthma, in which emotions and psychological traits played a critical role, became more commonplace in both medical and popular literature. In some cases, psychodynamic approaches shaped contemporary formulations of the aetiology and pathogenesis of asthma; in others, they initiated or legitimated novel approaches to treatment, most notably the use of hypnosis or relaxation to reduce allergic sensitivity or the rising reliance on removing asthmatic children from their homes and placing them in residential open-air schools. In both cases, psychodynamic interpretations of the asthmatic persona fixed clinical attention on the emotional factors in early childhood or the psychological constraints of domestic life that might be contributing to the frequency and severity of asthma attacks in both children and adults. Increasingly, asthma was regarded as the product of a particular, and by inference pathological, domestic and familial environment.

The proliferation of psychodynamic interpretations of asthma and other allergies in the post-war years was largely stimulated and encouraged by the emergence, and growing popularity, of psychosomatic medicine in that period. Supported financially partly by the Josiah Macy Jr. and Rockefeller Foundations and partly by the National Research Council, psychosomatic medicine emerged initially in North America during the 1920s and 1930s. The contours of psychosomatic medicine at that time were shaped by a number of distinct, but interlocking, clinical and scientific traditions, most notably the theoretical and practical dimensions of Freudian psychoanalysis, attempts to develop a brand of clinical holism that effectively resisted the biological reductionism and specialization sweeping through modern medicine, and the physiological studies of Walter Cannon (1871–1945) and others into the impact of emotions (such as fear and rage) on the autonomic nervous system and hormonal regulation.[29] In 1939, leading proponents of psychosomatic medicine, such as the Hungarian-born psychoanalyst Franz Alexander (1891–1964) and the American psychiatrist Helen Flanders Dunbar (1902–59), founded a new journal, *Psychosomatic Medicine,* dedicated to reforming 'medicine by scientifically reintegrating the "mind" into medicine.'[30] Three years later, they established the American Society for Research in Psychosomatic Problems, later named the American Psychosomatic Society.[31]

Although the field of psychosomatic medicine was, from the start, fragmented by disputes about whether the relationship between mind and body in disease was one of causation or correlation,[32] there were also significant points of agreement between different proponents. Most medical commentators, for example, focused their research on a narrow range of what appeared to be paradigmatic psychosomatic diseases: asthma; essential hypertension; rheumatoid arthritis; peptic ulceration; ulcerative colitis; hyperthyroidism; and neurodermatitis.[33] Under the guiding intellectual and entrepreneurial hand of Hans Selye (1907–82), these pivotal psychosomatic diseases, often referred to by Franz Alexander and his colleagues as the 'magic seven,'[34] later became those linked most clearly to biological formulations of stress.[35] In this context, it is worth noting that advocates of psychosomatic medicine, at least in the early years of this society, also largely agreed that the impact of psychological insult was mediated through somatic mechanisms (whether hormonal or neurological), thereby eschewing what they regarded as an artificial divide between psychiatry, on the one hand, and somatic medicine, on the other. In addition, it is clear that early formulations of psychosomatic medicine were heavily influenced by psychoanalytical approaches to mental and physical health, with the result that many leading figures in the field focused predominantly on the impact of emotional, and often explicitly sexual, factors in early childhood and on the psychological dynamics of the family and the home.

These preoccupations are particularly evident in the extensive technical and popular writings of Helen Flanders Dunbar. Born in Chicago in 1902, Dunbar graduated in philosophy, divinity and medicine before training as a psychoanalyst and setting up practice as a psychiatrist and analyst in New York. Although her professional reputation was challenged by a high-profile case in which one of her patients died in the early 1950s and although she herself died relatively young in 1959, Dunbar's impact on the field of psychosomatic medicine was immense. During the 1930s, Dunbar pioneered an extensive study of the familial, social, economic, and emotional backgrounds of 1,600 patients, the results of which led her to formulate the notion of an 'accident-prone' personality. During the same decade, she became the first chief editor of *Psychosomatic Medicine* and, subsequently, a founding member of the American Psychosomatic Society.[36] She published widely, not only scientific and clinical studies of the impact of emotions on the body, which, like Selye's studies of stress, were heavily influenced by the physiological researches of Walter and Ida Cannon,[37] but also popular books on the relationship between mind and body.[38]

According to Dunbar, the roots of many diseases were to be traced back to childhood experiences, the results of which 'may be reaped years later and turn out to be the fundamental or contributing causes of an illness.' These experiences, she argued in 1947, were generally more important than hereditary factors and constituted what she referred to as 'the delayed-action mines of childhood, planted either in the shock of some single incident or in the steady friction of a conflict between mind and environment.' In these circumstances, the role of the physician was to 'locate these mines before their final, disastrous explosion.'[39] Significantly, according to Dunbar, allergies offered a prime example of these psychosomatic processes in operation. Pointing out that conventional clinical approaches to allergies, such as identifying and avoiding specific allergens, had led to an inappropriate 'subordination of the emotional factor' by clinicians and as a result often proved unsuccessful, she argued conversely that in many allergies, most notably asthma and hay fever, it was essential to combine the expertise of the allergist and the psychiatrist in order to effect a cure.[40]

More specifically, in a chapter entitled '*Allergy con amore*,' Dunbar linked the emergence of asthma and hay fever in both children and adults to particular emotional conflicts, revolving especially around the emotional, and implicitly sexual, relationship between children and their mothers:

> There are certain specific emotions which seem to be linked especially to asthma and hay fever. A conflict about longing for mother love and mother care is one of them. There may be a feeling of frustration as a result of too little love or a fear of being smothered by too much. A second emotional conflict characteristic of the allergic is that which results from suppressed libidinal desire, often closely associated with the longing for mother. The steady repetition of this emotional history of "smother love" in the asthmatic is as marked as the contrasting history of hostility and unresolved emotional conflict in the sufferer from hypertension.[41]

Dunbar's approach, in which children were thought to be either 'in search of love' or afraid to explore their 'strong sexual curiosity,' extended to other allergic phenomena, including migraine and eczema. In eczematous patients, for example, the impact of 'smother love' was literally to smother the body in disease:

> One of the delayed-action mines of childhood explodes, appropriately enough, on the surface. The explosion takes the form of the common skin diseases, and the fuse is usually shorter than that of most other such mines. Eczema and its medical relations generally make their appearance while the victim is still young. Smother love has enveloped them so completely that, in a sense, their body is covered by it, and the skin is the part most immediately affected.[42]

By prioritising the emotional determinants of asthma, hay fever, and eczema, Dunbar did not dismiss the role of pollen or other immediate physical triggers of allergic reactions. Nor indeed did she ignore the fact that many people had a 'very keen longing for mother love' without developing allergies. Faithful to her balanced, psychosomatic vision of health and disease, she pointed out that the 'longing [for mother love] and the pollen (or dust or food) must be considered in their relation to each other and to the individual.'[43] Nevertheless, it was only through the 'acquisition of emotional stability,' mediated by effective psychotherapy, that patients with asthma were literally able to 'breathe again.'[44]

Dunbar's explicitly psychoanalytical interpretation of asthmatic children and adults, and in particular her emphasis on the mother–child relationship, found expression and support elsewhere, not only amongst colleagues in psychosomatic medicine in North America but also amongst those in Europe. In 1951, for example, Margaret Lowenfeld (1890–1973), working at the Institute of Child Psychology in London, explored the origins of childhood asthma in a presentation to the Alfred Adler Medical Society. According to Lowenfeld, 'just as there is general agreement about the phenomena and the stimuli in asthma, so there is consensus of opinion that under psychological treatment of any kind, asthmatics reveal themselves as aggressive, and that they have a smothering relationship with their mothers.'[45] A few years later, Theodora Alcock, an international expert on the Rorschach test and a member of the Tavistock Clinic of Human Relations in London,[46] similarly reviewed the personality characteristics of asthmatic children based on studies carried out in Cambridge. Citing the work of Alexander, Dunbar, Wittkower, and others, Alcock suggested that her overall conclusion, that 'the asthmatic personality appears characterized by conflicting factors, and a high degree of emotional tension without appropriate release,' was 'consistent with psychoanalytical and other findings concerning the ambivalent attitude of asthmatics based on an unresolved dependence on an omnipotent mother-imago.' Echoing Dunbar's emphasis on the interdependence of allergic constitution and emotional environment, Alcock inferred that those 'with an allergic inheritance may find an outlet in asthma, if their unconscious need is for a disorder so punishing to the patient and his parents, while also so provocative of loving attention.'[47]

While Lowenfeld, Alcock and others largely adopted Dunbar's psychoanalytical framework for understanding and treating asthma, other researchers developed a rather different version of the mind–body relationship, one in which bodily, rather than psychological, mechanisms were central. Between the 1920s and 1940s, for example, the Austrian physician Erwin Pulay (b.1899) published a series of books on allergies and other conditions in which he argued that the state of hypersensitivity was mediated predominantly by the function of the endocrine glands.[48] In *Allergic Man*, translated into English from the original German version in 1945, Pulay suggested that hypersensitivity constituted essentially a form of intolerance that became manifest in either physical or mental idiosyncrasies. Although he acknowledged the manner in which an inherited predisposition served to determine both physical and psychological characteristics, he argued nevertheless that 'the individual only achieves individuality by the guidance of his hormones,' mediated by interaction with the environment.[49] In particular, mental and physical health and disease were fashioned by the balance and functions of the sex hormones, which operated to maintain effective 'oxydisation' of the tissues. According to Pulay, the tendency to many diseases, including allergy, was particularly evident in those inhabiting what he termed an 'intersexual state,' characterized by hormonal imbalance, 'faulty oxydisation' with the build-up of toxic waste products in the body, and 'a displacement of the heterosexual tendency.'[50]

> Biological intolerance therefore always appears to be linked up with a disturbance of equilibrium among the sexual hormones themselves. Reduced to a general formula, this means that the sexual hormones intervene in allergic reactions . . . Hay-fever, like asthma and the characteristic allergic diseases, belongs to the group of diseases associated with the intersexual state.[51]

Significantly, Pulay's formulation of hypersensitivity and intolerance offered not only innovative understandings of the pathogenesis of asthma and hay fever couched in the relatively new language of hormones,[52] but also novel routes to treatment:

> The author discovered that men suffering from hay-fever, and who had not proved amenable to therapeutic treatments, could be cured if given female sexual hormone injections, while in women the attacks could be reduced in severity by the injection of anterior pituitary lobe hormone.[53]

Although Pulay's idiosyncratic approach to hypersensitivity attracted little overt support from European and North American physicians, there was clearly some clinical interest during the middle decades of the twentieth century in the relationship between allergies and endocrine function.[54] Until 1965, for example, allergic diseases were classified together with endocrine, metabolic, and nutritional disorders in the World Health Organization's influential International Classification of Diseases.[55] More broadly, Pulay's linkage between constitution and allergy and his association between the mental and physical manifestations of the allergic personality also echoed the general preoccupations of psychosomatic medicine in this period. At the same time, however, Pulay's framing of asthma and hay fever also reflected older, traditional understandings of the relationship between allergy, class, and culture. Thus, his twinned assertions that the 'allergic subject' constituted a 'representative of the highest order of the human race, in which lie rooted those principles that constitute what we recognise and value as humanity,' and that hypersensitivity was associated with 'gifts of the highest order and therefore the most brilliant accomplishments,'[56] clearly echoed the presumptions of late Victorian and Edwardian commentators such as the ear, nose, and throat surgeon Morell Mackenzie (1837–92) that hay fever and asthma were nervous diseases 'almost exclusively confined to persons of cultivation.'[57]

During the post-war years, psychosomatic formulations of asthma and other allergic conditions were not confined to the work of psychiatrists and psychologists such as Alexander, Dunbar, Lowenfeld, and Alcock. On the contrary, although clinical allergy remained largely preoccupied with perfecting the technique of desensitization or increasingly with exploiting a range of new anti-allergy preparations being developed by major pharmaceutical companies,[58] allergists were also interested in the emotional determinants of allergic diseases. In Britain, the leading allergist during these years was arguably John Freeman. Director of the allergy clinic at St. Mary's Hospital in London, Freeman devoted much of his time and energy to developing vaccines and improving the efficacy of prophylactic desensitization. However, he was also keen to identify and address the emotional triggers of asthma attacks as well as the impact of the modern home environment. Although he rejected the notion that allergy was 'all nerves,' he argued that 'emotions, moods or tensions are always part of the story,' and that from this perspective, the 'influence of the home crops up with monotonous regularity' in the case histories of allergic patients.[59]

In a substantial monograph on allergic diseases, published in 1950, Freeman explored the 'home influence' on allergies in depth. As Freeman was aware, the material domestic environment was often a trigger for exacerbations of asthma, hay fever, and eczema; plant pollen, dust mites, and pets, for example, could all be guilty of provoking attacks in sensitive individuals. However, Freeman was convinced that in many cases of intractable allergies, sometimes appearing only at home in the form of 'weekend asthma,'[60] it was not the physical contents of homes that made people sick, as his patients often assumed, but rather 'the human environment.' In particular, he argued that the homes of allergy sufferers differed 'in emotional tension from the normal homes.'[61] According to Freeman, 'asthmogenic families' or 'asthmogenic homes' were marked by 'a greater degree of emotionalism and nervous tension,' evident in 'excessive parental attention' and the corresponding 'emotional infantilism' of the children. Indeed, the correlation between the domestic emotional environment and allergies was sufficiently strong for Freeman to suggest that 'asthma or any of the toxic idiopathies thus become, so to speak, our piece of litmus paper from which we may be led to suspect an abnormally strained atmosphere in the home.'[62] Distancing himself from explicitly Freudian interpretations of asthma with characteristic panache, Freeman nevertheless, like the psychoanalysts, pointed to a disordered parent–child relationship as a major cause of asthma and other allergic conditions.

> I don't think we need invoke Oedipus complexes, though the Freudians would naturally incline towards them; indeed psychiatrists seem to detect a screw loose in both parents and children on these occasions. There

seems (to the non-psychologist at least) to be no evidence of anything more abnormal than the extreme sloppy-mindedness on the part of the parents, though of course this has led to gross and harmful mismanagement of the child.[63]

In this context, Freeman often remarked on the 'extraordinary prevalence of the Only Child in the Allergy Clinics.'[64] Although he recognized that the Second World War had dislocated family life and resulted in a decrease in family size, he did not consider that these external factors accounted for the frequency with which only children suffered from allergies and attended the allergy clinic during the post-war years. Instead, he was inclined to explain this phenomenon in terms of emotional suffocation within the home, driven by social anxieties about mothering.

> I think that all this well-meant zeal for dancing attendance on their tiny families must be due in part to the incessant propaganda to which young mothers nowadays are being subjected from books, lectures, welfare centres, clinics, the wireless, and so forth; according to some at least of these admonitory voices, the mothers cannot take too much trouble in brooding over their young: according to the evidence of the asthma clinics, they most certainly can overdo it . . . These admonitory voices of today would do better if they told the mothers to relax, to be less fussy with their children, and to interfere less; in short, they should teach the mothers to wean their children emotionally, as well as from the breast.[65]

Contemporary formulations of causative links between the home environment and asthma by British physicians in the mid-twentieth century found echoes in the work of North American allergists. Although Warren T. Vaughan (1893–1944), for example, shared many of Freeman's preoccupations with identifying and manipulating the immunological responses of allergy patients, he also regularly explored the emotional or nervous triggers of asthma and hay fever.[66] Significantly, however, in the hands of American physicians, psychosomatic theories of asthma were translated into a particular form of clinical intervention which involved removing the asthmatic child from the disordered home environment in order to effect a cure. As Carla Keirns has argued, 'parentectomy,' as it became known, was pioneered in particular by M. Murray Peshkin (1892–1980), who established the Jewish National Home for Asthmatic Children with the express purpose of treating asthmatics in a residential setting away from their parents.[67] Although he originally believed that separation reduced exposure to physical allergens, Peshkin subsequently became convinced that clinical improvement was the result of the removal of adverse emotional factors, in particular contact with the patient's mother.

> When I repeatedly observed a child in a convalescent home rendered symptom-free by his separation from his home environment and that a

> visit by his mother could precipitate a major attack of asthma, I realized more then ever before that hospitalization and removal of the child to a convalescent home was in effect the separation of the child from the asthmatogenic emotional climate which existed in the child's own home and that it was this adverse psychogenic factor which was principally responsible for pushing the asthmatic child into a state of intractable asthma.[68]

Although British allergists were generally more cautious than their North American counterparts about the value of parentectomy, since it appeared to over-simplify the factors involved in intractable asthma and lead to the 'indiscriminate separation of children from their homes,'[69] they were not entirely averse to adopting similar, although more limited, strategies that neatly removed patients from both their material and emotional domestic environments. From the 1930s through to the 1970s, for example, British asthmatic children were sent to open-air schools in rural or coastal settings or relocated for periods to residential settlements in mountainous areas in Europe, such as Font Remeu in the Pyrenees and Davos in Switzerland, where each child 'is taken away from the over-anxiety of home, visits a new country, and receives concentrated treatment in an optimistic atmosphere.'[70] While the benefits of such retreats included fresh air, a simple diet, regular exercise, and an opportunity to receive the latest pharmaceutical interventions, the popularity of such havens testified to the status and credibility of psychodynamic approaches to allergic diseases in the post-war period.

CONCLUSION

Psychosomatic interpretations of asthma and other allergic conditions did not pass unchallenged. In particular, some allergists on both sides of the Atlantic continued to emphasise the role of foods and synthetic chemicals in the environment and to resist the relentless focus on psychological factors. In 1957, for example, Ethan Allan Brown, president of the American Academy of Allergy, complained that 'in present-day journals (the editors of which should know better) there are papers (by physicians who should also know better) stating that not only asthma, but all allergy as such is "psychosomatic"'.[71]

In spite of such reservations, by the 1960s it had become a truism to suggest that asthma and other allergies could be triggered or exacerbated not only by physical irritants in the indoor and outdoor environments, but also by the emotional and psychological dynamics of the patient's home and family, especially by over-anxious parenting and a disturbed relationship between mother and child. Indeed, for many clinicians, asthma had become 'the example *par excellence* of psychosomatic illness, the clearest demonstration of that complex inter-relationship of body, intellect and emotion.'[72] More particularly, as Aaron Lask argued in a comprehensive survey of the impact on asthmatics of their 'attitude and milieu' published in 1966, the causes (and by inference the treatment) of asthma were to be located predominantly in disordered childhood experiences: 'Psycho-analytical study of asthma has revealed the complexity of the psychobiological nexus in infancy that lays down the asthmatic pathway.'[73]

Clinical adherence to psychosomatic understandings of asthma were echoed in popular accounts of the disease, evident not only in the vignettes outlined at the start of this chapter, but also in much broader media coverage of allergies in the post-war period. During the 1960s and 1970s, for example, medical reports in *The Times* regularly emphasized the emotional or psychological determinants of asthma and eczema in particular. Although readers were sometimes cautioned both about the manner in which clinicians tended to 'overstress the psychological, or psychosomatic aspect of disease' and about the dangers of treating asthmatic children as invalids, they were nevertheless reminded that emotional factors often triggered attacks, that asthma and eczema tended to occur among children who were over-protected by their parents, and that the attitudes and responses of both doctors and parents were crucial to recovery and on-going management.[74]

Significantly, asthma and eczema were not the only conditions during the middle decades of the twentieth century that were thought to be generated by emotional disturbances at home or by disordered mother-child relationships. As John Stewart and Sarah Hayes argue elsewhere in this volume, the emotional environment of the home became central to the efforts of psychiatrists, psychologists, and social workers in Child Guidance Clinics both to understand and treat 'maladjusted' children and to combat the social problems posed by juvenile delinquency. Of course, the home environment, and especially the behaviour of mothers, had for many decades been a target for public health reformers, or 'hygienists,' anxious to improve the nation's physical and mental health, to raise intelligence levels, and to reduce both infant and maternal mortality rates.[75] But in the post-Second World War period, particularly under the influence of research by John Bowlby (1907–90) in Britain and the popularizing work of Benjamin Spock (1903–1998) in North America, many social, behavioural, and physical problems were forcibly recast primarily as the products of maternal deprivation and familial disharmony.[76] Equally, during the 1970s, the German-born psychoanalyst Hilde Bruch (1904–84) suggested that anorexia nervosa and a variety of other eating disorders were largely the product of particular family expectations and dynamics.[77]

More strikingly, in 1948, the German psychoanalyst Frieda Fromm-Reichmann (1889–1957) introduced the notion of the 'schizophrenogenic mother.'[78] According to Fromm-Reichmann and her colleagues, schizophrenia, much like asthma, could be triggered by dominant, over-protective mothers. Although Fromm-Reichmann's formulation of the aetiology of schizophrenia was contested, sometimes being dismissed as a 'psychiatric myth,' it was extensively discussed amongst psychiatrists and enjoyed considerable support, particularly from proponents of existential psychiatry such as R. D. Laing (1827–1989).[79] Importantly, however, in Laing's formulation of the concept, articulated most clearly in *The Divided Self* first published in 1959, whole families, rather than just mothers, contributed to the emergence of madness. 'Not only the mother but also the total family situation may impede rather than facilitate the child's capacity to participate in a real shared world, as self-with-other.'[80]

The rising popularity of psychodynamic formulations of asthma and many other conditions as products of the emotional environment at home in the years following the Second World War depended on the ability of such theories to appeal to diverse political and professional interests and agendas. On the one hand, preoccupations with the impact of mothering on asthma echoed and reinforced conservative attempts to ensure that mothers stayed at home to rebuild families and restore domestic and social stability in the wake of the social and familial disruption wrought by global conflict. Framed by stark evidence of the impact of evacuation and homelessness on children, post-war commentators emphasized the importance of the ever-present, caring 'good mother' to ensure the healthy mental and physical development of her children.[81] The broader social and political, as well as psychological and physical, implications of women's domestic role were clear. As the *Beveridge Report on Social Insurance and Allied Services* had suggested even during the war: 'In the next thirty years housewives as mothers have vital work to do in ensuring the adequate continuance of the British race and of British ideals in the world.'[82]

On the other hand, psychosomatic theories of asthma also appealed to radical political and professional critiques of biomedical reductionism and Western forms of capitalism. Psychosomatic medicine itself emerged as a form of holisitic opposition to disease theories that prioritized the somatic over the psychological and that failed adequately to link mind and body. In this sense, psychosomatic approaches to asthma and other conditions were intended to be both humanizing and anti-reductionist. At the same time, such approaches shared much in common with social or psychosocial medicine, according to which the roots of many physical and mental conditions were located in the structures and inequalities of societies and families, not merely in individual biology. According to the Scottish playwright and doctor James Lorimer Halliday (1897–1983) writing in 1948, for example, the increased incidence of psychosomatic disorders, declining fertility, rising rates of sickness and absenteeism from work, deepening unemployment, juvenile delinquency, class war and regional nationalism, mass emigration, the decline of religious faith, and the popularity of escapist pursuits such as gambling were all attributable to progressive social disintegration and the emergence of what he termed a 'sick society.'[83] For Halliday, much like Laing and many others, the solution to such widespread psychosocial problems lay not only in effectively combining psychological with physical approaches to disease, but also in exposing and challenging the 'roots and growth of this Western civilization, including those of its typical economy, the market economy.'[84]

By the 1980s, the popularity of psychosomatic theories of asthma and other allergic conditions was beginning to wane. In some ways, psychological approaches were rendered increasingly redundant by technical developments in medicine. The identification of immunoglobulin (Ig) E in 1967 and greater clarification of the biochemical pathways involved in allergic reactions had paved the way for a new generation of anti-allergy pharmaceutical products, such as antihistamines, bronchodilators, and topical steroids, which offered immediate relief (as well as commercial profit) from disease.[85] In addition, the predominance of allergies amongst only children and small families, interpreted by Wittkower, Freeman, and others as the result of emotional suffocation, was reframed in biological terms as the product of modern hygienic lifestyles.[86] At the same time, the social and political dimensions of debates about rising trends in allergies were shifting. In particular, widespread anxieties about familial and social stability were partly displaced by concerns about the impact of modern lifestyles on the environment and, in turn, about the impact of environmental changes on health. Thus, debates about rising trends in asthma during the closing decades of the twentieth century focused more on global patterns of indoor and outdoor pollution than on psychological mechanisms or domestic harmony. While patients, families, and physicians remained alert to the impact of emotions on asthma, psychoanalytical preoccupations with the mother–child relationship and the emotional environment gradually receded.

ACKNOWLEDGEMENTS

I am particularly grateful to the Wellcome Trust for funding the research on which this chapter is based.

NOTES

1. Anon., 'Man's asthma cured by wife's death,' *The Times* (29 March 1962), 5a.
2. C. P. Taylor, *Allergy*, in Jim Haynes (ed.), *Traverse Plays* (London: Penguin, 1966), 104–39.
3. Anne Sexton, 'Man and Wife,' in Anne Sexton, *Live or Die* (London, 1966), 27–8. See also the chapter on Anne Sexton by Jo Gill in this volume.
4. See Reg Smythe's Andy Capp cartoon published in the *Daily Mirror* (11 March 1958).
5. The terms *asthmogenic home* and *asthmogenic family* appear, largely interchangeably, in John Freeman, *Hay-Fever: A Key to the Allergic Disorders*, (London: William Heinemann, 1950), 166.
6. Raphael C. Panzani, 'Seneca and his asthma: The illnesses, life, and death of a Roman stoic philosopher,' *Journal of Asthma* 25 (1988): 163–74. On the early history of asthma, see: Edmund L. Keeney, 'The history of asthma from Hippocrates to Meltzer,' *Journal of Allergy* 35 (1964): 215–26; John Gabbay, 'Asthma attacked? Tactics for the reconstruction of a diseases concept,' in

Peter Wright and Andrew Treacher (eds.), *The Problem of Medical Knowledge,* (Edinburgh, 1982), 23–48; E. Stolkind, 'The history of bronchial asthma and allergy,' *Proceedings of the Royal Society of Medicine* 26 (1932–3): 1120–6; Alex Sakula, 'A history of asthma,' *Journal of the Royal College of Physicians* 22 (1988): 36–44; Sheldon C. Siegel, 'The history of asthma deaths from antiquity,' *Journal of Allergy and Clinical Immunology* 80 (1987): 458–62; Ian Gregg, 'Some historical aspects of asthma,' *Southampton Medical Journal* (1991): 11–21.

7. Thomas Willis, *The Practice of Physick* (London, 1684), 92–6; John Floyer, *A Treatise of the Asthma* (London, 1698).
8. On the introduction and reception of these diagnostic techniques, see: Jacalyn Duffin, *History of Medicine: A Scandalously Short Introduction* (Toronto, 1999), 191–211; Jacalyn Duffin, *To See with a Better Eye: A Life of R. T. H. Laennec* (Princeton, 1998); Noel Snell, 'Inhalation devices: A brief history,' *Respiratory Disease in Practice* (Summer 1995): 13–15.
9. Walter Hayle Walshe, *A Practical Treatise of the Diseases of the Lungs* (London: James Walton, 1871), 543–56.
10. Henry Hyde Salter, *On Asthma: Its Pathology and Treatment* (London, 1860); Henry Hyde Salter, 'On the effects of local spasmodic influences on asthma,' *Edinburgh Medical Journal* 3 (1857–8): 1092–3; Henry Hyde Salter, 'On some points in the treatment and clinical history of asthma,' *Edinburgh Medical Journal* 5 (1859–60): 1109–15; Hyde Salter, 'On the treatment of asthma by belladonna,' *Lancet* i (1869): 152–3.
11. George M. Beard, *American Nervousness: Its Causes and Consequences* (New York, 1881).
12. John Gabbay, 'Asthma: A case study of the relationship between changing theoretical concepts of a disease and its treatment,' (unpublished dissertation, Cambridge, 1977), 50–1. See also: John Millar, *Observations on the Asthma, and on the Hooping Cough* (London, 1769); Sheldon G. Cohen, 'Asthma among the famous,' *Allergy and Asthma Proceedings* 17 (1996): 161–71.
13. Gregg Mitman, 'Hay fever holiday: Health, leisure, and place in gilded age America,' *Bulletin of the History of Medicine,* 77 (2003), 600–35.
14. Clemens von Pirquet, 'Allergie,' *Münchener Medizinische Wochenschrift* 30 (1906): 1457–8.
15. For further discussion, see Mark Jackson, *Allergy: The History of a Modern Malady* (London: Reaction Books, 2006).
16. Sir William Osler, *The Principles and Practice of Medicine* (New York, 8th edition, 1914), 627.
17. W. C. Hollopeter, *Hay Fever: Its Prevention and Cure* (New York: Funk and Wagnalls, 1916), 121.
18. Sir Humphry Rolleston, *Idiosyncrasies* (London: Kegan Paul, Trench, Trubner & Co., 1927), 92–102. See also the report of a paper presented by Rolleston to a British Medical Association conference in 1921 in *Lancet* ii (1921): 280–1.
19. Arthur F. Hurst, 'An address on asthma,' *Lancet* i (1921): 1113–7.
20. Rolleston, *Idiosyncrasies,* 94–5. See also references to the emotional aspects of asthma in: Alexander Francis, *The Francis Treatment of Asthma* (London: William Heinemann, 1932), 21; Alexander Gunn Auld, *The Nature and Treatment of Asthma, Hay Fever and Migraine* (London: H. K. Lewis, 1936), 10.
21. Horace S. Baldwin, 'Studies in the asthmatic state: I. The stimulus,' *Journal of Allergy* 1 (1929): 124–9.
22. Erich Wittkower, 'Studies in hay-fever patients (the allergic personality),' *Journal of Mental Science* 84 (1938): 352–69. See also Anon., 'Asthma,' *The Times* (19 November 1934), 13c–e.
23. Ibid., 358.

24. Ibid., 358–9.
25. Ibid., 360.
26. Ibid., 368.
27. For further discussion, see Jackson, *Allergy*, 56–102.
28. 'Asthma,' *The Times* (19 November 1934), 13c–e.
29. Dorothy Levenson, *Mind, Body, and Medicine: A History of the American Psychosomatic Society* (American Psychosomatic Society, 1994); Nissim Mizrach, 'From causation to correlation: the story of *Psychosomatic Medicine*,' *Culture, Medicine and Psychiatry* 25 (2001): 317–43; Jack D. Pressman, 'Human understanding: psychosomatic medicine and the mission of the Rockefeller Foundation,' in Christopher Lawrence and George Weisz (eds.), *Greater than the Parts: Holism in Biomedicine, 1920–1950* (New York: Oxford University Press, 1998); Theodore M. Brown, 'The rise and fall of American psychosomatic medicine,' available at http://human-nature.com/free-associations/riseandfall.html; Carla Christina Keirns, 'Short of breath: a social and intellectual history of asthma in the United States,' (unpublished PhD thesis, University of Pennsylvania, 2004), 169–203.
30. Cited in Mizrach, 'From causation to correlation.'
31. Levenson, *Mind, Body, and Medicine.*
32. Mizrach, 'From causation to correlation.'
33. Levenson, *Mind, Body, and Medicine*, 39.
34. Ibid.
35. Russell Viner, 'Putting stress in life: Hans Selye and the making of stress theory,' *Social Studies of Science* 29 (1999): 391–410; Mark Jackson, 'In search of stability: Hans Selye and the biology of stress,' *Wellcome History* (Summer 2006), 1–4.
36. Further biographical details are in Levenson, *Mind, Body, and Medicine.*
37. See, for example: Helen Flanders Dunbar, *Emotions and Bodily Changes* (1935); Helen Flanders Dunbar, *Psychosomatic Diagnosis* (1943).
38. Flanders Dunbar, *Mind and Body: Psychosomatic Medicine* (New York: Random House, 1947).
39. Ibid., 17–20.
40. Ibid., 175–6.
41. Ibid., 177.
42. Ibid., 190.
43. Ibid., 177.
44. Ibid., 184–90.
45. Margaret Lowenfeld, 'Asthma in childhood,' manuscript in the Wellcome Library for the History of Medicine, Special Collections, PP/LOW/C.22, p. 12.
46. Robert S. McCully, 'Miss Theodora Alcock 1888–1980,' *Journal of Personality Assessment* 45 (1981): 115.
47. Theodora Alcock, 'Some personality characteristics of asthmatic children,' *British Journal of Medical Psychology* 33 (1960): 133–41.
48. Erwin Pulay, *Ekzem and Urtikaria: Klinik, Pathogenese und Therapie* (Berlin: Urban and Schwarzenberg, 1925); Erwin Pulay, *Der Uberempfindliche Mensch* (Leipzig, 1936); Erwin Pulay, A. P. Cawadias, and P. Lansel (eds.), *Constitutional Medicine and Endocrinology* (London: Frederick Muller, 1943–7); Erwin Pulay, *Allergic Man: Susceptibility and Hypersensitivity* (London: Scientific Book Club, 1945).
49. Pulay, *Allergic Man*, 19.
50. Ibid., 53–4, 89–90.
51. Ibid., 97.
52. The term *endocrine* had been introduced in 1893 but only became popular in the early twentieth century. The term *hormone* was introduced by Ernest

Starling (1866–1927) in 1905 and was rapidly adopted. See R. B. Welbourn, 'Endocrine diseases,' in W. F. Bynum and Roy Porter (eds.), *Companion Encyclopedia of the History of Medicine,* Vol. 1 (London: Routledge, 1993), 484–511.

53. Pulay, *Allergic Man,* 97.
54. George W. Bray, 'The hereditary factor in hypersensitiveness: Anaphylaxis and allergy,' *Journal of Allergy* 2 (1931): 205–24; Albert J. Vander Veer, 'Address of the president,' *Journal of Allergy* 4 (1933): 428–9.
55. Jackson, *Allergy,* Chapter Three.
56. Pulay, *Allergic Man,* 139–40.
57. Morell Mackenzie, *Hay Fever and Paroxysmal Sneezing* (London: J. & A. Churchill, 1887), 10. For further discussion, see Jackson, *Allergy,* Chapter Three.
58. See Jackson, *Allergy,* Chapters Three and Four.
59. Freeman, *Hay-Fever,* 160.
60. Ibid., 150, 158–9.
61. Ibid., 163.
62. Ibid., 167.
63. Ibid., 169–70.
64. Ibid., 164.
65. Ibid.
66. Warren T. Vaughan, *Primer of Allergy* (St. Louis: C. V. Mosby Co., 1939), 61–2; Warren T. Vaughan, *Strange Malady: The Story of Allergy* (New York: Doubleday, Doran & Co., 1941), 219–28.
67. Keirns, 'Short of breath,' 182–203.
68. M. Murray Peshkin, 'Intractable asthma of childhood: Rehabilitation at the institutional level with a follow-up of 150 cases,' *International Archives of Allergy* 15 (1959): 91–112.
69. Philip Pinkerton and Corinna M. Weaver, 'Childhood asthma,' in Oscar W. Hill (ed), *Modern Trends in Psychosomatic Medicine 2* (London: Butterworths, 1970), 81–104.
70. Anon., 'Children saved by affection,' *The Times* (1 November 1962), 13f.
71. Ethan Allan Brown, 'American Academy of Allergy: The changing picture of allergy,' *Journal of Allergy* 28 (1957): 368. I am grateful to Matthew Smith for this reference.
72. Pinkerton and Weaver, 'Childhood asthma,' 81. See also J. J. Groen, 'Present status of the psychosomatic approach to bronchial asthma,' in Oscar W. Hill (ed.), *Modern Trends in Psychosomatic Medicine 3* (London: Butterworths, 1976), 231–59.
73. Aaron Lask, *Asthma: Attitude and Milieu* (London: Tavistock, 1966), xvi.
74. Anon, 'Implications of increase in asthma deaths,' *The Times* (13 August 1968), 7e; Anon., 'Bronchial asthma,' *The Times* (14 April 1971), 8c; Anon., 'Dermatology: eczema and emotion,' *The Times* (2 july 1971), 18e; Anon., 'Asthma: study of 400 child sufferers,' *The Times* (5 October 1973), 12c; Hugh Jolly, 'What to do about eczema,' *The Times* (18 June 1975), 7e.
75. Nikolas Rose, *The Psychological Complex: Psychology, Politics and Society in England 1869–1939* (London: Routledge and Kegan Paul, 1985).
76. John Bowlby, *Child Care and the Growth of Love* (London, 1953); Benjamin Spock, *The Common Sense Book of Baby and Child Care* (1946).
77. Hilde Bruch, *The Golden Cage: The Enigma of Anorexia Nervosa* (London: Open Books, 1978); Hilde Bruch, *Eating Disorders: Obesity, Anorexia, and the Person Within,* (London: Routledge and Kegan Paul, 1974).
78. F. Fromm-Reichman, 'Notes on the development of treatment of schizophrenics by psychoanalytical psychotherapy,' *Psychiatry* 11 (1948), 263–73.

79. Frances E. Cheek, 'The "schizophrenogenic mother" in word and deed,' *Family Process* 3 (1964), 155–77; G. Parker, 'Re-searching the schizophrenogenic mother,' *Journal of Nervous and Mental Diseases* 170 (1982), 452–62; C. E. Hartwell, 'The schizophrenogenic mother concept in American psychiatry,' *Psychiatry* 59 (1996), 274–97.
80. R. D. Laing, *The Divided Self* (London: Penguin Books, [1959] 1982), 189.
81. Angela Holdsworth, *Out of the Doll's House: The Story of Women in the Twentieth Century* (London: BBC Books, 1988), 109–30.
82. Sir William Beveridge, *Beveridge Report on Social Insurance and Allied Services* (London, 1942).
83. James L. Halliday, *Psychosocial Medicine: A Study of the Sick Society,* (London, 1948). For similar concerns expressed elsewhere at this time, see Dunbar, *Mind and Body* (New York, 1947).
84. Halliday, *Psychosocial Medicine,* 180.
85. Jackson, *Allergy,* Chapter 4.
86. Ibid., Chapter 5.

Part Two

Housing, Health, and Home

9 'Skeletons in the Medicine Closet'
Women and 'Rational Consumption' in the Inter-War American Home

Nancy Tomes

INTRODUCTION

In 1914, the home economist Christine Frederick noted the growing influence of health-related product advertising on the American home. 'Health boards may think they are responsible for the aseptic attitude of the modern housekeeper,' she wrote in the trade journal *Advertising and Selling,* 'but Platt's Chlorides, vacuum cleaners, and dustless dusters did it,' referring to three heavily advertised products whose promotional campaigns stressed the necessity for a sanitary home. Likewise, she continued: 'Pure food champions and pure food laws have told us what to avoid to keep out of an early grave, but Heinz, Beechnut, National Biscuit, and other honest manufacturers, through advertising, have told us what is pure food and how and where we can get it.'[1]

Although public health authorities would surely have objected to Frederick's dismissal of their own efforts, her point that in the United States national advertising had become a health force to be reckoned with by the 1910s was beyond dispute. Not only had manufacturers amply demonstrated their capacity to alter personal and household hygiene through extensive advertising; their successes had also inspired public health workers to adopt similar methods of persuasion. Starting in the early twentieth century, health reformers began to borrow heavily from the new 'sciences' of advertising, marketing, and public relations to promote not-for-profit health causes, from well-baby crusades to anti-fly campaigns. By the 1920s, the public health educator had begun to 'visualize his task' as that of 'a salesman selling health,' in the words of Philip Jacobs, the Publicity Director for the National Tuberculosis Association (NTA).[2]

Of course this mirroring of medical and commercial health advice was by no means a new phenomenon. As Roy Porter showed in his classic *Health for Sale,* the profitability of the so-called sick trade has long worked to blur the boundaries between science and commerce. But the rise of a mass consumer economy dependent upon aggressively marketed, brand-name goods certainly expanded the range of that confusion in the early 1900s. New forms of mass-mediated market mimicry developed, in which advertisements came increasingly to resemble public health messages, and public health messages came to resemble product advertisements. To the extent that historians have noted this convergence, they have tended to assume that the two streams of health persuasion reinforced scientific expertise in a relatively straightforward fashion. Although scholars have noted conflicts surrounding specific product lines, such as constipation remedies and infant foods, they have rarely questioned the premise that commercial advertising worked to amplify medical authority.[3]

Historical accounts of scientific motherhood and the conduct of the modern home are a case in point. In her 2006 *Perfect Motherhood,* Rima Apple argues that starting in the late 1800s, women of all classes gradually came under the influence of a reinvigorated medical authority. Expectations that doctors would be 'dominant' and mothers would be 'obsequious,' in Apple's words, emerged simultaneously in inter-war medical advice literature and advertising copy. Expert advice and commercial extortions represented a seamless web, in which advertisements reinforced the central message delivered to wives and mothers of the inter-war era: Trust your doctor, and put your faith in science.[4]

But a closer look at the inter-war period suggests that the mirroring process, whereby expert and commercial health advice came to resemble each other, eventually undermined clear-cut faith in scientific expertise. The blurring of distinctions between information and advertising raised troubling questions about the reliability and consistency of scientific 'fact.' Although advertisements appeared deferential to medical opinion, they often recommended health strategies that doctors vehemently opposed. Far from viewing commercial advertising as a beneficial ally, American doctors distrusted the advertising profession as a wily, dangerous adversary over which they had too little control. The fact that women, the traditional bulwarks of medical authority in the home, were also the prime targets for commercial persuasion made these tensions all the more significant.

To offset the influence of a market mimicry that made expert fact and advertising artifice hard to distinguish, medical leaders agreed that American consumers, in particular women, needed to be better trained to make wise choices among products, information, and advisors. They were joined by other nonmedical groups, chief among them home economists and consumer advocates, who agreed that true obedience to expert authority required learning to distinguish the 'real' truth from false claims. While the need for rational consumption applied in theory to all product choices (and to men as well), the stakes were particularly high when it came to women's shopping for health-related items. A poor choice of apparel or furnishing could be disappointing, but an ill-considered diet, drug, or cosmetic could sicken, maim, and even kill. Thus maintaining health in the modern home required new vigilance against what a 1949 article in *Hygeia* referred to as the 'skeletons in the medicine closet.'[5]

Yet as this chapter documents, the project of promoting 'rational' health consumption quickly became mired in conflict among the experts themselves.

Heated battles developed as industry groups resisted medical criticisms of their selling techniques, and lay critics questioned the medical profession's credentials as consumer advocates. Thus, women intent upon becoming 'rational consumers' increasingly encountered a host of squabbling commercial and professional groups, all claiming to be the 'true' advocate of the concerned mother and housewife.[6]

These controversies emerged early and noisily in the United States, due to the precocious development of its advertising industry and the educational emphasis of its public health movement. But the underlying tensions between simultaneously popularizing scientific expertise and encouraging a robust commercial culture were by no means unique to the United States. The problem of market mimicry, and its potential threat to scientific authority, emerged in many cultures during the same time period. Distinctive national traditions, of both medical authority and advertising regulation, ensured that those tensions played out in very different ways. But as advertising practices and consumer-centered economies expanded in the early twentieth century, concerns that modern scientific progress might be undercut by a robust, unscrupulous commercialism certainly appeared in places other than the United States.[7]

This chapter examines how these dynamics unfolded in the inter-war United States, hoping that future work will trace out how they evolved in other countries. Using the 'lady consumer' and the contents of her medicine cabinet as a focal point, I dissect the tensions generated by the simultaneous expansion of a mass consumer economy and 'democratization' of public health in the years between 1910 and 1940. In the first part of the chapter, I explore how the streams of health information generated by for-profit and non-profit health campaigns came to mingle and overlap in those years, so that in style and content, public health messages and product advertisements reinforced each other. The second part of the chapter examines the efforts by different expert groups to combat the commercialization of health advice, and to aid consumers, especially women, to distinguish advertising fiction from public health fact when making product choices. In the conclusion, I suggest some ways in which these pre-Second World War debates anticipated persistent tensions in health promotion in a modern consumer culture.

LADY CONSUMERS AND THE INTER-WAR HEALTH 'SELL'

As Rima Apple has argued, modernizing American women's roles as health consumers required replacing the traditions of domestic medicine, in which wise women handed on homemade medicines and cleaning solutions from one generation to the next, with the tasks of the modern woman shopper, carefully selecting and utilizing pre-packaged products to promote her family's health. Skilled shopping emerged as one of the key roles that women needed to master in order to function as the 'chief operating officers' of their newly rationalized homes. In the words of one inter-war mother, becoming 'modern' meant that 'you go and buy, you don't make.'[8]

Reflecting this shift from 'making' to 'buying,' personal and household care products emerged as the backbone of the inter-war mass consumer economy. While less expensive than consumer durables such as appliances and furnishings, non-durable goods such as food, cleaning products, and medicinal drugs were more quickly used up and thus more frequently purchased. Manufacturers had a huge investment in encouraging the purchase of non-durable goods, which traditionally fell to the 'lady consumer,' as the author T. Swann Harding referred to her in 1930. Women were 'the shoppers of the world,' agreed a contemporary advertising text.[9]

Women thus became the major target for a new style of health promotion that equated good health with the wise choice and use of an increasing array of product lines, from food and toothpaste to household cleaners and over-the-counter drugs. The woman consumer's responsibility for 'buying health' was made all the more challenging by the market mimicry that characterized for-profit and non-profit forms of persuasion. Commercial advertisers sought to make their promotional campaigns more scientific, while public health educators sought to make their educational crusades more effective. As a result, their styles of persuasion converged in many important ways.[10]

First, to make their products and their selling methods more respectable, leading advertising agencies began in the early 1900s to abandon the carnivalesque excess of the nineteenth-century medicine show in favour of more low-key, sophisticated appeals to buyers. Proprietary drug companies sought new respectability by making their promotional campaigns for over-the-counter drugs more science-based. Manufacturers of non-drug products, such as food, soaps, and even cigarettes, sought to exploit the burgeoning popular interest in health and beauty. The promise that the regular purchase and use of a specific product would promote good health, buttressed by elaborate appeals to modern science, became a commonplace of early twentieth-century advertising.

This aggressive use of the health sell expanded at a time when there existed relatively little regulation of advertising claims and practices. The Pure Food and Drugs Act of 1906 gave the new Food and Drug Administration (FDA) oversight only of label and packaging material; the FDA had no power to reprimand manufacturers for making false claims in their advertisements. That power rested with the Federal Trade Commission (FTC), founded in 1914, which investigated complaints about fraudulent advertisements as a form of unfair trade practice. From the late 1920s, the commission's power to compel both manufacturers and advertising agencies to appear before its special committee on fraudulent advertising helped tone down promotional claims. But until 1938, when the law was changed, the courts' requirement that the FTC prove that deceptive advertising practices hurt competitors, as opposed to consumers, limited its efficacy. Moreover, the volume of advertisements under its review meant that regulatory scrutiny focused primarily on only the most dangerous and extreme examples of proprietary medicine fraud.[11]

In addition to federal regulation, professional and trade groups promoted their own voluntary standards of what was termed 'ethical advertising.' Perhaps the best known of these was the model statute promoted by the trade journal *Printers' Ink*, which proposed to make a misdemeanor of 'any assertion, representation or statement of fact which is untrue, deceptive or misleading.' But as with the FTC, the focus of ethical advertising initiatives remained on the outer fringes of patent medicine excess. Extravagant claims for the health values of comparatively harmless products such as toothpastes or disinfectants remained acceptable so long as the advertiser stayed away from exaggerated promises to cure life-threatening diseases. '"Puffing" is one thing; lying another,' as an editorial in *Printers' Ink* put it succinctly in 1916.[12]

Between 1900 and 1920, the style of product advertisements changed in striking ways that made such puffery all the more effective. Advertisements for branded goods evolved from densely printed, text-heavy, comparatively unadorned statements of a product's virtues to a more complex visual statement combining fewer words with more images. The art of copy-writing distilled the item's appeal into a few memorable lines, while technical innovations in printing and engraving allowed advertisements to incorporate much richer visual images.[13]

Ironically, the ability of advertisers to invoke health issues in these more sophisticated messages depended heavily on the contemporaneous efforts of public health educators in these decades. From the late 1800s, health reformers had increasingly realized that public health improvements required not only strong laws and regulations, but hygienically informed and disciplined citizens. To cultivate the latter, local and state public health departments, voluntary health associations, and commercial interests such as life insurance companies began to dedicate substantial resources to popular outreach. The pioneers of the new public health publicity, as it came to be called, were often men and women with backgrounds in business, journalism, reform, and social work rather than medicine.[14]

To get their messages across, public health educators borrowed many of the same communication strategies developed by advertising professionals. The public health equivalent of copy-writing was the ubiquitous slogan, which became a hallmark of Progressive-era public health crusades. In place of the densely printed tracts distributed by nineteenth-century sanitarians, public health workers developed short, snappy phrases, such as 'Spitting spreads death' and 'Death lurks in the filth on a fly's feet.' Public health messages combined such slogans with striking symbols and social tableaux to illustrate the lessons of health.[15]

The greater scope and sophistication of popular health education only redoubled its potential for commercial appropriation. The more women shoppers came to be aware of germs, vitamins, and tooth decay, the more readily manufacturers could use that knowledge to market disinfectants, vitamin-enhanced foods, and toothpaste. By shaping selling campaigns around scientific principles of health preservation and disease prevention, manufacturers sought to reap big rewards in terms of increased sales. As an executive of the J. Walter Thompson agency explained in a 1930 staff meeting: 'The discovering of new merchandising angles and of themes for advertising campaigns which wish to be sound as well as novel, is leading more and more into territories formerly populated solely by chemists, biochemists, dieticians, doctors, specialists in all the several branches of science.'[16]

Inter-war advertisements incorporated appeals to modern science in varied ways. At a symbolic level, many surrounded their product claims with icons of the modern hospital and laboratory, such as petri dishes, microscopes, and test tubes. Representations of the white-garbed scientist/doctor and the nurse became standard characters in the repertoire of commercial art. Simultaneously, advertising copy reproduced arguments from contemporaneous public health writings, albeit in more exaggerated, dramatic fashion. A case in point was the commercial appropriation of the new public health's emphasis on 'flies, fingers, and food,' that is, the role of insect vectors, casual contact, and food contamination as sources of disease transmission. Recurrent public health warnings about death-bearing houseflies and mosquitoes were echoed in promotions for a wide range of commercial items, from Thermos bottles to insecticides. In a style strongly reminiscent of the public health slogans of the era, a 1926 Fly-Tox ad caught the reader's attention with the question, written in large type, 'What is your baby worth?,' followed by vivid descriptions of the insect 'assassins' and their innocent victims: 'With the germ of fever firing their blood, little bodies writhe in the burning torture of flaming torment. The end sometimes is tragic.' The dangers of touch and cough also furnished excellent copy for soap and disinfectant promotions, as in the 1930 Listerine appeal to the 'Careful Mother,' which equated free use of that product with a loving maternal concern.[17]

The parallels between public health message and product advertising were amplified by their placement in the mass media of the time period. As newspapers and mass-circulation magazines grew increasingly dependent on advertising revenue, the demarcations between editorial, article, and advertisement became less distinct. An editorial on vacuums might be accompanied by an article on the vacuum's hygienic virtues, which would be situated next to an advertisement for a Hoover that repeated the same arguments. Women readers could no doubt distinguish editorials from advertisements, but the convergence in their messages inevitably weakened the distinctions between the different types of information.

In addition to advertisements themselves, for-profit and non-profit enterprises also relied upon similar strategies for conducting promotional campaigns. To entice the 'lady consumer,' national corporations used attractive store displays, free samples, cents-off coupons, informational brochures, and celebrity endorsements to draw attention to new product lines. At a more local level, department stores sponsored fashion shows and developed elaborate window displays to draw in female customers, while Chambers of Commerce and Rotary Clubs sponsored fairs and other events to promote the economic health of their communities.

Public health reformers actively collaborated with these efforts, seeking to embed their work in the everyday world of the citizen-shopper. They found businesses happy to support the anti-tuberculosis campaigns and other public health initiatives as a means to improve their own public image. The spinning of public health campaigns as marketing events for the whole family is well illustrated in a 1921 article about the Rotary Club's 'Health Week' that appeared in the *American Journal of Public Health*. The author explained how local businessmen had been recruited for the event by emphasizing it as an opportunity to pitch their goods to women consumers:

> The shoe man can emphasize the merits of common sense shoes for children and grown-ups, the hardware man can bring out the value of seeking good ventilation when purchasing a furnace, the plumber the merits of sanitary plumbing, the electrical fixture man can point out the need of proper lighting. The dry goods merchant may show the hygienic features of various kinds of clothing, underwear, etc., and the grocer may bring to the fore the sanitary care with which the packages sold in his establishment are wrapped, or their nutrient values.[18]

The distribution of free booklets, a tactic thought especially well suited to women consumers, was another strategy that both non-profit and for-profit groups employed widely in the early 1900s. Between 1900 and 1940, public health departments, voluntary health societies, and agricultural extension services published and distributed millions of handouts concerning personal and household health issues, from simple 'do and don't' cards to lengthy pamphlets. Similarly, national manufacturers, following the lead of the proprietary medicine companies, began to commission attractive, often lavishly illustrated cards and booklets that combined useful health information with product promotions. Deliberately or not, the commercial booklets often resembled their non-profit counterparts, albeit in glossier form. For example, Johnson and Johnson, the manufacturer of home first aid products, produced a *Household Handbook* that bore a striking resemblance to the American Red Cross's popular home health care textbook.[19]

The commercial imitation of the child health programmes developed by the NTA and other inter-war groups offers a particularly good example of the crossover between non-profit and for-profit promotional campaigns. Originally begun in 1915 as part of the Christmas Seal campaign, the NTA's Modern Health Crusade evolved into a well-organized, widely emulated programme of child health education built around health chores such as hand washing and teeth brushing. By the early 1920s, more than

7 million American children were participating in the Modern Health Consumers' crusade through their public schools.[20]

The Modern Health Crusade's success precipitated a host of commercial imitations, which exploited the sensitivity mothers were assumed to have toward their children's requests for specific products. One of the most ambitious of these child-centered promotions was the 'HCB' club developed by the J. Walter Thompson Company in 1928 to promote Cream of Wheat. Membership entitled children to a free HCB chart and gold stars to affix to it; after four weeks of faithfully eating hot cereal every morning, participants got an HCB button and learned that the initials stood for '*H*ealth helps *C*hevaliers win *B*attles.' Like the Modern Health Consumers' Crusade, the Cream of Wheat campaign targeted public schools for participation. School districts agreeing to participate in the club got free samples of the cereal, charts to keep for each student, and health lesson plans 'emphasizing the Hot Breakfast Idea.' As the advertising executive who developed the idea explained, the school materials did not specify that children must eat any particular brand of hot cereal, but 'the psychology of this plan (as we have heard in many instances) is that the child comes running home with a sample and exclaims, "Teacher says we must eat Cream of Wheat,"' and the mother would buy that brand. Thus, he observed, 'we get the backing of the school authority without their being conscious of this questionable partiality.'[21]

These commercial 'knock-offs' of non-profit health campaigns annoyed public health educators. As voluntary health associations developed their own trademarks and promotional campaigns, they became concerned about commercial infringements upon their symbolic capital. For example, in 1919, the American Red Cross (ARC) refused to accept Johnson and Johnson advertising in its publications because the ARC felt the manufacturer unfairly invoked the red cross emblem in its promotional campaigns. Similarly, in 1920, the NTA registered its double-barred cross with the U.S. Patent Office 'to conserve the emblem so that it would not be used by unscrupulous vendors of patent medicines and organizations that were not approved by the National Tuberculosis Association,' in the words of the organization's first historian, Adolphus Knopf. The increasing prominence of commercial materials in the classroom prompted educators to develop guidelines for their use, and some states and cities passed laws prohibiting or circumscribing their presence in public schools.[22]

TEACH THE TRUTH AND THE TRUTH ONLY

The blurring of boundaries between commercial and non-commercial health promotions clearly worried medical leaders. As the noted public health authority Charles Chapin wrote in 1915, 'Clear, forceful and catchy writing is worse than useless if it fails to teach the truth and the truth only,' and sternly warned the new breed of 'publicity men' to 'stop filling your columns with tommy-rot, hot air and dope.' Likewise, editorials in medical and public health journals routinely denounced the misuse of medical authority to sell mouthwash and toilet paper. To guard against misinformation, experts needed to help American consumers, in particular the women shoppers who made the bulk of health related purchases, to acquire a more discerning sense of the difference between scientific fact and advertising fiction. Becoming more adept at resisting the health 'sell' became the mark of the responsible wife and mother.[23]

One of the most robust bids to become the woman consumer's trusted advisor came from the American Medical Association (AMA). Building on its long-standing efforts to combat medical quackery and fraud, the AMA vigorously asserted its credentials as a disinterested, reliable guide to medicines and household remedies.[24] One claim to virtue rested on the voluntary advertising codes the organization imposed on its rapidly expanding line of professional journals. In 1905, the AMA Board of Trustees decided that only preparations meeting the standards of its newly established Council on Pharmacy and Chemistry would be allowed to buy advertising space in its publications. Many of the association's constituent state medical societies, as well as other medical journals, eventually adopted the same policy. By 1930, the AMA reported that 'nearly one half the medical publications in the United States have agreed to limit advertisements for proprietary medicaments to those accepted for [the Council of Pharmacy and Chemistry's] New and Nonofficial Remedies,' thereby exercising 'a salutary influence on advertising.'[25]

The AMA's scrutiny of advertising primarily concentrated on the cancer cures and other egregious frauds that concerned the FTC and FDA in this era. Only occasionally did the association take on mainstream manufacturers for claims that the FTC had allowed to pass. A case in point was the AMA's criticism of a 1930 Listerine advertisement that touted the preparation's antiseptic action. The advertisement claimed: 'We could not make this statement unless prepared to prove it to the entire satisfaction of the U.S. Government and the medical profession.' In fact, the AMA's Chemical Laboratory tested the product and issued a report in 1931 roundly disputing its germicidal powers. While the AMA could point to this action as a sign of its vigilance, Listerine ads continued to tout its germ-fighting powers.[26]

In 1930, the AMA introduced its 'seal of approval' programme as another way to counter unscientific advertising claims. Modeled loosely on the magazine *Good Housekeeping*'s seal of approval programme (begun in 1910), the AMA's programme aimed to help women consumers distinguish between good and bad health products. As its popular health magazine *Hygeia* (later renamed *Today's Health)* explained the seal's purpose in 1944: 'One way of distinguishing between reliable statements and nonsensical advertising puffery is to look for some sign of actual consideration by a scientific group, an indication of this being the appearance on the package or in advertising matter of a 'seal' such as those of the Councils of the American Medical Association and of the American Dental Association.'[27]

The AMA's seal programmes were administered by its Councils on Pharmacy and Chemistry, Foods, and Physical Therapy. (Another committee was eventually established to screen cosmetics.) Manufacturers submitted their products and advertising material to the Councils, and if their health claims were found 'unobjectionable,' the company then got permission to use the AMA seal in its advertising. Only products bearing the seal might purchase advertising space in *Hygeia* and other AMA publications. Given the increasing size of the AMA's inter-war publishing empire, manufacturers interested in cultivating physician goodwill had considerable incentive to comply with its advertising guidelines.[28]

'CONSUMERS MUST LEARN TO READ THE LABELS'

The AMA's bid to become the trusted authority on consumer health issues faced competition in the inter-war period from a new breed of lay consumer advocates. Unlike their Progressive-era predecessors, members of this inter-war generation took a more skeptical view of physician leadership. As educated lay people, many with backgrounds in engineering, nursing, or journalism, they did not accept the argument that consumers should just follow doctors' directions. They not only felt competent to form their own judgments about health matters, but also questioned how well the medical profession was performing as the patients' advocate, especially when it came to policing health commercialism.[29]

The lay consumer advocates who emerged in the 1930s fell into two distinct and mutually hostile camps. One group, exemplified by Ruth de Forest Lamb and T. Swann Harding, emerged within the Food and Drug Administration, the federal regulatory agency set up explicitly to protect consumers' health interests. Not surprisingly, this group took a positive view of the federal government's consumer initiatives and saw stronger government regulation as the key to consumer health protection.[30] A second group emerged from the 'consumers' clubs' founded in the late 1920s; its main exemplars were Consumers' Research, a not-for-profit consumer advocacy organization founded in 1929, and its rival Consumers Union, founded in 1936, ultimately the more successful of the two groups. Compared to Lamb and Harding, the free-standing consumer groups tended to be far more critical of the federal regulatory process. So while sharing a distrust of commercial advertising and medical authority, the two factions differed in the tone and content of the strategies they recommended.[31]

For all their internal divisions, inter-war consumer advocates stressed similar themes in their advice to the modern health consumer. In articles for mass market magazines as well as popular books, they articulated the outlines of a new kind of health consumer consciousness. Consumers, especially women, had to resist the siren call of modern advertisements, and instead had to learn to read product labels, the only place where manufacturers had to conform to real 'truth in advertising.' Women needed to ignore the self-serving arguments of manufacturers and to support stronger federal regulation of advertising. Last but not least, they needed to understand that the AMA's advice about health goods reflected medicine's economic interests, and had to be approached with suitable caution.

The texture of their advice is nicely captured in an article T. Swann Harding published in the 1930 *Journal of Home Economics,* entitled 'The Consumer and the Medicine Cabinet.' As a people, he suggested, Americans were particularly prey to the influence of advertising. 'The alarm with which a comparatively empty medicine cabinet in an American bath room is habitually viewed, exemplifies admirably the power of advertising propaganda.' Not only had advertising made Americans highly 'health-conscious,' he noted, but 'we are easily cowed by pathological myths and more easily persuaded to buy what is "good" for us than any other people on earth.' Commercial interests fiercely resisted any regulation of advertising as a restraint on their rights of 'free speech,' arguing that such censorship was 'unAmerican.'[32]

In such a commercialized atmosphere, Harding noted, the 'lady consumer, who remains predominantly the home purchasing agent in this country, faces almost insuperable obstacles in the effort to get her money's worth.' To be sure, her situation was far better than her grandmother's, because the FDA now had power to regulate the safety of medicines. But the work remained incomplete, he warned, because 'human ingenuity in devising new frauds can normally outdistance the orderly processes of logic and science in authoritatively disproving the claims of old ones.' Nor could women depend on medical authorities to point them in safe directions. Physicians' advice reflected their own economic interests: Not only were doctors opposed to self-care that would rob them of a patient's fee, but also medical journals had become too dependent on advertising revenue, in spite of their advertising codes. In a slap at the latter, Harding noted: 'It is even true that the advertising pages of our best medical journals flaunt before the physician's hurried attention many drug compounds which are either impotent or have been imperfectly tested clinically and biologically.' Given the limits on current law, the modern woman consumer had to become wary in her shopping habits. 'Consumers must learn to read the labels,' Harding emphasized, because they were the only part of a product's promotional package that had to be reasonably accurate.[33]

Consumer advocates outside the ranks of government agreed with the majority of Harding's arguments, but were far less willing to make excuses for the federal regulatory process. Emphasizing instead how political pressures on the FDA and FTC rendered their judgments untrustworthy, these consumer advocates called for independent scrutiny of consumer products by groups such as their own, unbeholden to either government or industry influence. In that spirit, Consumers' Research began to compile information on consumer products and ultimately to set up its own testing facilities. In exchange for their dues payments, subscribers received regular issues of the group's *Confidential Bulletin,* which contained detailed evaluations of specific product groups. These evaluations were presented as superior to all others because Consumers' Research accepted no paid advertising or financial support from any group that might profit by its evaluations.

For the public as a whole, consumer advocates pioneered a new kind of guide to consumer products, epitomized by the 1933 best seller, *100,000,000 Guinea Pigs: Dangers in Everyday Foods, Drugs, and Cosmetics,* by Arthur Kallet and F. L. Schlink. Its success led to the publication of other 'guinea pig' books on women's hygiene, food and nutrition, and children's health. While scorned by manufacturers and the AMA alike, the idea of consumer rating of goods proved attractive enough to convince publishers to put out more 'guinea pig' books, and both Consumers' Research and Consumers Union signed up sufficient numbers of subscribers (including many physicians) to keep their work afloat even during the Great Depression.[34]

In their approach to the AMA, these groups manifested a kind of critical consumer consciousness that would become increasingly mainstream in the post-Second World War period. At the core of this consciousness was a critical awareness that physicians were not doing a very good job in their role as consumer advocates. These new-style consumer experts differed from traditional sectarian critics of the regular profession in that they espoused mainstream scientific views, and criticized organized medicine for not being scientific enough: physicians were failing to protect their patients because of economic conflicts of interest that made them soft on advertising hyperbole.

A case in point was the consumer advocates' scorn for the AMA's advertising policies, especially in its journal for lay people, *Hygeia.* Established in 1922, the magazine was intended to provide doctor-friendly advice on topics of interest to the general public, in particular wives and mothers. *Hygeia*'s early issues stressed the dangers of patent medicine, and after 1930, the magazine only accepted advertisements for products that had the AMA seal of approval.[35] Yet early in the 1930s, probably to offset the Depression's effect on its advertising revenue, *Hygeia* hired an advertising editor and began to feature a monthly column, entitled 'Among *Hygeia* advertisers,' that struck a markedly more pro-advertising tone. As Charles Mohler, the advertising editor wrote in 1934: 'True, advertising is commercial, but it is intensely human, always likely to be closely allied to one's everyday interests . . . that is why you will find it exceedingly profitable to read each and every advertisement in *Hygeia* in a careful and leisurely manner.' In another editorial, he noted: 'In this issue of HYGEIA there are examples of new and important ideas which are basically important to the industries they represent, and at the same time they mean much to the health or the comfort and happiness of people in general.' The very next sentence inquired, 'Do you know that it is now possible to have a chocolate flavored drink delivered fresh from the dairy daily?' and went on to praise Krim-Ko Chocolate Flavored Drink for allowing mothers to get their children to 'drink milk much more readily than if the plain milk were offered to them.' The editor then directed readers to the advertisement in that month's issue to find out more about the product.[36]

Consumer activists were quick to note the contradictions inherent in the AMA's advertising policies. As F. J. Schlink, one of the founders of Consumers' Research, noted in a 1932 letter, 'There are many things about the American Medical Association which are exceedingly admirable, and their technical information generally is critical and reliable to a degree which is hardly equaled by any other professional organization in America.' Yet regarding their advertising policy, 'we find much to disagree with. You need hardly go farther in coming to a judgment of their policy, than to read the page which appears in each number of HYGEIA, signed by, I believe, a Mr. Mohler, their advertising "editor"—as they term him.'[37]

From *Hygeia's* standpoint, what seemed to matter most in distinguishing the good from the bad advertisement was its portrayal of the medical profession. Many *Hygeia* advertisements couched their product's virtues in doctor-friendly terms, a trait that surely helped them pass the AMA's critical scrutiny. Extravagant or incorrect claims might be tolerated if the overall message of the advertisement supported the physician's authority and dignity. But as inter-war consumer advocates warned, this strategy let many misleading claims be passed on to the magazine's readers, and hardly entitled the medical profession to disparage consumer groups' own efforts at consumer protection. Thus they raised serious questions about the protection to be found in simply 'following the doctor's directions,' as the medical advice givers suggested.

CONCLUSION

While sharing a deep distrust of commercial advertising, physicians and lay consumer advocates arrived at different strategies for negotiating this new health information environment. The AMA developed strategies that rested on trust in medical authority, as its seal of approval programme, while lay consumer advocates emphasized a more skeptical strategy based on close label reading. Yet they remained in agreement that more strict regulation of advertisements would best serve to protect American women from these misleading claims of health puffery.

Concerns about the health risks of misleading advertisements were central to New Deal battles over strengthening federal regulatory power over advertising. Business interests wanted to preserve the widest latitude for their exercise of commercial freedom of speech; consumer advocates wanted a stricter regulation of advertising claims. After years of political manoeuvering, the U.S. Congress in 1938 finally passed the Wheeler Lea Act, which strengthened the regulatory power of both the FDA and the FTC. A major sticking point throughout the battles over the new law was the regulation of advertising. The law that resulted was a compromise: the FTC was given the power to regulate advertising as a fraud perpetuated on consumers, as well as business competitors; the FDA was given stronger powers to regulate the safety of drugs, foods, and (at last) cosmetics. But the 1938 legislation overhaul still allowed for considerable latitude in drawing the line between 'puffing' and 'lying.'[38]

In his 1940 book *Good Health, Bad Medicine,* physician Harold Aaron, the medical consultant to Consumers Union, summed up the existing situation. 'The new Food, Drug and Cosmetic Act is, in some respects, a marked improvement over the old Act, but there are still too many loopholes through which the artless consumer can be peppered by drug advertisers' dum-dum bullets.' As a consequence, health educators needed to take into account two factors fundamental to the conduct of American life: 'first, a continuous and intense advertising campaign by the proprietary food, drug and cosmetic industry; and second, a Federal Food Drug and Cosmetic law that does not adequately safeguard consumers against fraud and hazards.' In that spirit, Aaron offered his own home medical guide, which provided a more rigorous consumer-oriented division of home medical remedies into lists of approved and not approved remedies.[39]

In subsequent decades, the tensions between advertising fiction and public health fact that emerged so sharply in the 1930s would continue to intensify. The inter-war marketplace had generated an anxiety producing message: It was possible for the skillful woman consumer to 'buy' health for her family, but only by scrupulously uncovering deceptions that might transform her pantry or her medicine chest into a source of debility and death. For the modern wife and mother, becoming adept at sorting through this conflicting muddle became an increasingly important facet of running a modern home. Despite several decades of reform and regulation, the same theme would carry through into the post-Second World War period, as powerful new products such as prescription drugs came onto the market. Federal regulation would continue to block the most outrageous of drug dangers and frauds, yet leave ample room for misleading promotions aimed at 'lady consumers' and their families. Business and medical groups would continue to tout voluntary advertising codes as the best protection to combat advertising distortions while preserving commercial freedom of speech. Last but not least, consumer advocates would create an advice industry based on the simple principle that consumers should trust no one but themselves: not the manufacturers, the federal government, or the medical profession. The seeds of mistrust sown in the inter-war era would in the 1960s burst into a full-blown consumer health revolution.[40]

Over a half century later, the bitter fruits of that mistrust are now being harvested. In the post-Second World War period, a post-industrial economy highly dependent on the manufacture and sale of health-related products and services accelerated the cycle of regulation and controversy already evident by 1938. Further strengthening of the food and drug laws in 1962 would produce similar paradoxes: more stringent rules for product safety that in turn generated more fears of misuse and overuse. The growing profitability of health care has generated fierce battles over how much market forces should be allowed to operate. Business interests have played on issues of consumer choice and advertising freedom as central to allowing the market to foster scientific progress. Meanwhile, consumer advocates have become increasingly critical of how those choices are framed. The end result has been a mushrooming of consumer initiatives, from lengthy guides to the 'best and worse drugs,' to hospital score cards and databases of incompetent physicians.

But the underlying tensions evident even in the 1930s remain: American consumers face a host of confusing opinions about what it means to be an enlightened health consumer. Is the escalating use of antibiotic soap a good or bad development? Is a high-fibre, low-fat diet a preventive against breast cancer? The parties to these debates profess a common commitment to public health, yet arrive at remarkably different conclusions about the answers to such questions. Sadly, the advice first developed by consumer advocates almost sixty years ago still retains its relevance. In the words of Harold Aaron, 'Skepticism is an important requirement in all search for knowledge. In health care, next to the ability to buy competent medical care, it is perhaps the most important quality that the consumer should possess.'[41]

NOTES

1. Frederick is quoted in Andrew Heinze, *Adapting to Abundance* (New York: Columbia University Press, 1990), 164.
2. Philip Jacobs, *The Tuberculosis Worker* (Baltimore, MD: Williams & Wilkins, 1923), 17.
3. Roy Porter, *Health for Sale: Quackery in England 1660–1850* (Manchester: University of Manchester Press, 1989). On laxatives, see James Whorton, *Inner Hygiene: Constipation and the Pursuit of Health in Modern Society* (New York: Oxford University Press, 2000). On infant foods, see Rima Apple, *Mothers and Medicine: A Social History of Infant Feeding* (Madison: University of Wisconsin Press, 1987).
4. Rima Apple, *Perfect Motherhood: Science and Childrearing in America* (New Brunswick, NJ: Rutgers University Press, 2006), 56. Note that in developing her argument, Apple is well aware that many women did indeed perceive contradictions in the advice they were hearing. See especially Chapters 3 and 4.
5. Mary Helen Anderson, 'Skeletons in the medicine closet,' *Hygeia* 27 (April 1949): 250–1, 278. The drive to include cosmetics in consumer protective legislation has finally been given proper attention in Gwen Kay, *Dying to Be Beautiful* (Columbus: Ohio State University Press, 2005).
6. My understanding of the contradictions inherent in modern consumer culture is deeply indebted to two works: Lizabeth Cohen, *A Consumers' Republic* (New York: Knopf, 2003); and Charles McGovern, *Sold American:*

Consumption and Citizenship, 1890–1945 (Chapel Hill: University of North Carolina Press, 2006).

7. There is a growing literature on consumer culture, gender, and health that suggests that these issues were by no means limited to the United States: Victoria de Grazia, *Irresistible Empire: America's Advance Through 20th-Century Europe* (Cambridge, MA: Harvard University Press, 2005); Susan Strasser, Charles McGovern, and Matthias Judt (eds.), *Getting and Spending: European and American Consumer Societies in the Twentieth Century* (New York: Cambridge University Press, 1998); Victoria de Grazia and Ellen Furlough, *The Sex of Things: Gender and Consumption in Historical Perspective* (Berkeley: University of California Press, 1996); Nancy Reagin, 'Comparing apples and oranges: Housewives and the politics of consumption in interwar Germany,' in Strasser, McGovern, and Judt (eds.), *Getting and Spending*, 241–62; Anne McClintock, *Imperial Leather* (New York: Routledge, 1995); Timothy Burke, *Lifebuoy Men, Lux Women: Commodification, Consumption and Cleanliness in Modern Zimbabwe* (Durham, NC: Duke University Press, 1996); Virginia Berridge and Kelly Loughlin (eds.), *Medicine, the Market and the Mass Media: Producing Health in the Twentieth Century* (London: Routledge, 2005). To date, the majority of work on gender and advertising in relation to health has focused on tobacco and cigarettes. See, for example, Virginia Berridge, 'Constructing women and smoking as a public health problem in Britain 1950–1990s,' *Gender and History* 13 (2) (2001): 328–48.
8. Jacquelyn S. Litt, *Medicalized Motherhood: Perspectives from the Lives of African-American and Jewish Women* (New Brunswick: Rutgers University Press, 2000), 296–97. For a good overview of the "CEO" philosophy of women's roles, see Ruth Schwartz Cowan, *More Work for Mother: The Ironies of Household Technology from the Open Hearth to the Microwave* (New York: Basic Books, 1985).
9. T. Swann Harding, 'The Consumer and the Medicine Cabinet,' *Journal of Home Economics* 22 (July 1930): 558–565; quote is on p. 558; Carl A. Naether, *Advertising to Women* (New York: Prentice Hall, 1928), xiii.
10. On this dynamic illustrated in terms of germ consciousness, see Tomes, *Gospel of Germs*, esp. Chapter Seven; on vitamins, see Rima Apple, *Vitamania* (New Brunswick, NJ: Rutgers University Press, 1996). A useful survey of commercial health promotion remains James Harvey Young, *The Medical Messiahs: A Social History of Health Quackery in Twentieth-Century America* (Princeton, NJ: Princeton University Press, 1967).
11. Young, *Medical Messiahs;* Charles Jackson, *Food and Drug Legislation in the New Deal* (Princeton, NJ: Princeton University Press,1970); Blake Clark, *The Advertising Smoke Screen* (New York: Harper and Brothers, 1944); Kim B. Rotzoll and James E. Haefner, *Advertising in Contemporary Society* (Urbana: University of Illinois Press, 1996), Chapter Seven. On the often overlooked push to extend FDA authority over cosmetics, see Kay, *Dying to Be Beautiful.*
12. The *Printers' Ink* statute is reprinted in Daniel Pope, *The Making of Modern Advertisement* (New York: Basic Books, 1983), 205, at p. 219. See also Young, *Medical Messiahs*, Chapters Six and Seven. Other trade groups such as the Associated Advertising Clubs of America and the National Better Business Bureau sought to discourage irresponsible marketing practices.
13. The best overview of these changes remains Roland Marchand, *Advertising the American Dream* (Berkeley: University of California Press, 1985). An older but still useful study is Frank Presbrey, *The History and Development of American Advertising* (New York: Greenwood Press, 1968; reprint of 1929 edition).

14. Tomes, *Gospel of Germs,* esp. Chapter Four. For an excellent overview of the emergence of health education as a separate field, see Elizabeth Toon, 'Managing the Conduct of the Individual Life,' (Ph.D. dissertation, University of Pennsylvania, 1998). She discusses public health educators' perception that they had to compete more effectively with commercial messages about health.
15. Tomes, *Gospel of Germs,* Chapter Five; Nancy Tomes, 'Epidemic Entertainments: Disease and Popular Culture in Early Twentieth-Century America,' *American Literary History* 14:4 (Winter 2002): 625–52.
16. Remarks of Mr. Kimball, Minutes of Staff Meeting, 25 November, 1930, p. 2. Box 3, F 2, J. Walter Thompson Company Archives (JWT archives), Special Collections Library, Duke University.
17. The Fly-Tox ad is reproduced in Robert Atwan, Donald McQuade, and John W. Wright, *Edsels, Luckies and Frigidaires* (New York: Dell, 1979), 267. The Listerine ads are in the Competitive Files, JWT Archives. My generalizations about the increasing use of symbols associated with modern medicine are based on my survey of advertisements in the Competitive Files, JWT Archives, and in the advertising section of the *Ladies Home Journal.* See also the insightful discussion of scientific imagery in Apple, *Vitamania,* esp. pp. 102–103.
18. Donald B. Armstrong, 'National Health Council Launches Rotary Health Week,' *American Journal of Public Health,* 11 (1921): 1006–1007; quote on p. 1007. On city health campaigns, see: Judith Walzer Leavitt, *The Healthiest City: Milwaukee and the Politics of Public Health Reform* (Princeton, NJ: Princeton University Press, 1982); and Susan L. Smith, *Sick and Tired of Being Sick and Tired: Black Women's Health Activism in America, 1890–1950* (Philadelphia: University of Pennsylvania Press, 1995), esp. Chapters 2 and 3.
19. *Household Hand Book* (New Brunswick, NJ: Johnson and Johnson, 1916), Trade Catalogue Collection, Hagley Museum and Library, Wilmington, DE; Jane A. Delano and Isabel McIsaac, *American Red Cross Textbook on Elementary Hygiene and Home Care of the Sick* (Philadelphia: P. Blakiston's Son & Co., 1913).
20. Tomes, *Gospel of Germs,* 122–3.
21. The HCB campaign is described in Staff Minutes, May 1, 1929, Box 2, Folder 1, JWT archives. See also Harold Wengler, 'Transmuting and Delivering a Bowl of Cereal (Hot),' *JWT News Bulletin,* 3 (1929): 17–19. Lifebuoy Soap also developed and distributed a hand washing chart designed to encourage frequent use of their product, while dairy companies produced posters and games to promote more milk consumption. The range of commercial materials such as charts and posters is well illustrated in Saidee E. Stark, *How Schools Use Advertising Material: A Study of the Use of Advertising Material by Teachers in Schools and Colleges and by Home Economics Workers* (New York: Association of National Advertisers, Inc., 1930).
22. 'American Red Cross Bars "Red Cross" Advertising,' *Printers' Ink,* (20 March 1919): 108; Knopf, *History of the National Tuberculosis Association,* p. 154. See Stark, *How Schools Use Advertising Material,* for an overview of the debates over commercial materials in public schools.
23. Charles V. Chapin, 'Truth in Publicity,' *American Journal of Public Health,* 1915, *5:* 493–502; quotes on p. 502. On the growing ambivalence about advertising, see: Toon, 'Managing the Conduct of the Individual Life,' esp. Chapter Three; and Nancy Tomes, 'The "Great American Medicine Show" Revisited,' *Bulletin of the History of Medicine* 79:4 (Winter 2005), 627–63.

24. On the AMA's earlier battles against quackery, see James Harvey Young, *The Toadstool Millionaires* (Princeton, NJ: Princeton University Press, 1961).
25. For a good overview of the AMA's work in this period, see Young, *Medical Messiahs.* As Peter Bartrip has shown, the AMA's advertising standards were far more rigorous than its British counterparts in this period. See Peter Bartrip, 'Pushing the Weed: The Editorializing and Advertising of Tobacco in the *Lancet* and the *British Medical Journal,*' in Stephen Lock, Lois Reynolds and E. M. Tansey (eds.), *Ashes to Ashes: The History of Smoking and Health* (Atlanta, GA: Editions Rodopi B.V., 1998), 100–126.
26. For the AMA's report on Listerine, see 'The Chemical Laboratory,' *JAMA,* 96 (1931): 1303–06. Listerine continued to feature scientific themes; for example, 'The Germ Nobody Knows' (1934) presented a lengthy discussion of scientific efforts to isolate the cold virus. Both Listerine ads are in the Competitive Files, JWT Archives.
27. Austin E. Smith, 'Doctors Say . . .' *Hygeia,* 22 (1944): 658–659, 696, 698. Quote is on pp. 658–9.
28. On the AMA seal programme, see Frank D. Campion, *The AMA and U.S. Health Policy Since 1940* (Chicago: Chicago Review Press, 1984), 115–116, 469–477. The seal of approval programme continued until 1955, when it ended due to concern about potential lawsuits over injuries sustained by use of physical therapy devices carrying the official seal.
29. My generalizations here and in the next section are based on primary research in the Consumers' Research archives, Alexander Library, Rutgers University; the Consumers Union Archives, Yonkers, New York; and the T. Swann Harding papers, Library of Congress. For a more detailed discussion of these issues in relation to drug advertising, see Tomes, 'The Great American Medicine Show.'
30. Ruth de Forest Lamb, *The American Chamber of Horrors* (New York: Farrar and Rinehart, 1936); T. Swann Harding Papers, Library of Congress. See also Jackson, *Food and Drug Legislation,* for background on Lamb and Harding.
31. McGovern, *Sold American;* Lawrence Glickman, 'The Strike in the Temple of Consumption,' *Journal of American History* 88:1 (June 2001): 99–128.
32. Harding, 'The Consumer and the Medicine Chest,' 562, 565.
33. Ibid., 558, 559, 565. Lamb makes a very similar set of arguments in *The American Chamber of Horrors.*
34. Arthur Kallet and F.L. Schlink, *100,000,000 Guinea Pigs* (New York: Grosset and Dunlap, 1933). On the other guinea pig books, see Jackson, *Food and Drug Legislation,* 16–20. For the development of consumer testing, see Norman Silber, *Test and Protest: The Influence of Consumers Union* (New York: Holmes and Meier, 1983).
35. 'Report of the Board of Trustees,' Proceedings of the Annual Meeting of the AMA for 1935, 9.
36. Charles S. Mohler, 'Among *Hygeia* Advertisers,' *Hygeia,* 12 (1934): 962. The ad for Krim-Ko appears on p. 1049. The annual reports on AMA publications published in JAMA make no mention of Mohler's hiring, so I do not know when and why he was added to the *Hygeia* staff. But the annual reports do make evident that the Depression hit the magazine hard, making it plausible that he was hired to help attract and keep advertising revenue to offset its losses. Since many institutions removed the front and back matter when binding magazines, I have not yet determined exactly when the column started. 'Among *Hygeia* Advertisers' was definitely part of the magazine by 1933, and had disappeared by the early 1940s; it was replaced by a much smaller column entitled 'Adcombers' accompanied by a list of advertisers in that month's issue.

37. F. L. Schlink to L.B. Ross, Sept. 12, 1932, Box 440, Folder 21, Consumers' Research Inc., Rutgers University. In print, the lay consumer advocates tended to be much more deferential to medical authority than they were in their private correspondence.
38. Jackson, *Food and Drug Legislation.*
39. Harold Aaron, *Good Health and Bad Medicine: A Family Medical Guide* (New York: Robert McBride and Co., 1940), viii. Aaron was later instrumental in the founding of the *Medical Letter,* a guide to prescription drugs aimed at physicians, which also refused to accept any form of advertisement.
40. Tomes, 'The Great American Medicine Show.'
41. Aaron, *Good Health and Bad Medicine,* 317.

10 The Home Fires

Heat, Health, and Atmospheric Pollution in Britain, 1900–45

Stephen Mosley

INTRODUCTION

By 1900, coal smoke from Britain's home fires was widely acknowledged to be a major urban environmental problem. In providing warmth indoors, the family hearth—closely associated with the very idea of 'home'—simultaneously polluted the atmosphere outdoors.[1] Doctors, architects, anti-smoke activists, and others all drew attention to the damaging effects of domestic air pollution, which included blackened buildings, stunted vegetation, begrimed belongings, wasted fuel, diminished sunlight, and high death rates from respiratory diseases. In 1908 the *British Medical Journal* charged that house, rather than factory, chimneys were the 'greatest offenders' in polluting city air. Its report on smoke abatement concluded: 'The prevention of smoke nuisances must inevitably tend to a higher hygienic standard, to brighter cities, cleaner homes, and happier dwellers, and . . . the general improvement of the nation.'[2] Yet in spite of growing knowledge and concern, the traditional open coal fire remained unregulated and the public's preferred form of home heating throughout the first half of the twentieth century.

This chapter seeks to explain why, despite its many disadvantages, the open fire was retained in the majority of British homes during the period 1900–45. Historical studies of atmospheric pollution problems in twentieth-century Britain are currently thin on the ground. Only a few authors have attempted to unravel the political, technical, economic, and cultural complexities of smoke control after the First World War.[3] Building upon these pioneering studies, this chapter explores contemporary debates about home heating systems, indoor and outdoor air pollutants, and their interrelationships in three sections.[4] The first section surveys the main sources of urban smoke pollution, including the open fireplace, and examines its effects on human health and well-being. The next part is concerned with modernist planning for light and air, particularly inter-war housing schemes that used 'smokeless' appliances for space heating. It also looks at reformers' attempts, in the absence of any legislative restrictions, to persuade the British people to reduce domestic smoke emissions voluntarily. The third section enquires into contemporary theories about domestic air quality and thermal comfort, making the tensions between indoor and outdoor environmental conditions evident. In addition, it considers the heating choices of the British public. Paradoxically, traditional open fires—while irredeemably smoky—were highly valued for their 'hygienic advantages': for their brisk ventilation and their radiant heat. Modernist aspirations to admit more health-giving sunlight and fresh air to Britain's gloomy industrial cities were to be frustrated by a failure to tackle effectively the crucial issue of how homes were heated.

THE SMOKE NUISANCE

By the dawn of the twentieth century, most of Britain's large towns and cities had enjoyed a considerable measure of success in cleaning up environmental 'nuisances' relating to land and water. In stark contrast, a solution to the problem of reducing smoke pollution in urban areas remained elusive. In 1899 *The Builder,* the country's leading architectural periodical, reported:

> Insanitary conveniences, defective drains, foul methods of sewage disposal, polluted streams, are all being steadily improved, and so rapid has been the progress in recent years that the day does not seem far distant when they shall be known only as historical evidences of the lack of civilisation in the nineteenth century. But while other nuisances are being gradually abated, the smoke nuisance increases year by year . . . and no man can estimate the human suffering it entails by shutting out the invigorating sunshine and by poisoning the air we breathe.[5]

The sense of achievement that many contemporaries undoubtedly experienced as newly constructed water supply and waste disposal systems improved urban health and local environments was tempered by the notion that smoke pollution in Britain was going from bad to worse. In *fin-de-siècle* London, according to Bill Luckin, the city's befogged inhabitants believed that its atmospheric conditions were 'even more potentially dangerous than the water problem that had triggered catastrophic mid-century cholera.'[6] Rising levels of air pollution had gradually enveloped great cities such as Glasgow, London, and Manchester in a permanent smoke haze.

Coal smoke was hardly a new phenomenon in British cities, but by the early twentieth century the problem had reached an unprecedented scale. Between 1851 and 1911 the nation's population rose sharply from 20.8 million to 40.8 million, with almost 75 percent of Britons living in urban areas by the latter date. During the same period, coal consumption in Britain more than trebled from 60 million to some 189 million tons, substantially increasing smoke emissions in rapidly expanding cities.[7] The early and mid-Victorians, especially in the Midlands and the North, had mainly attributed large-scale smoke pollution to the forests of tall factory chimneys that dominated Britain's urban-industrial landscapes. There was a shift in focus, however, as a growing number of late-Victorian publications highlighted the various human and environmental problems caused by the less obvious emissions from private homes.[8] By 1900, it had become apparent that Britain's home fires were major polluters of city air.

During the first half of the twentieth century, anti-smoke societies—active in Britain since the 1840s—continued to build a strong case against atmospheric pollution through books, pamphlets and journal articles, press campaigns, slide shows and films, and clean air conferences and exhibitions.[9] Domestic chimneys were key targets, as Ernest Simon, Chairman of the Smoke Abatement League of Great Britain, disclosed in 1922:

> Hitherto the efforts of reformers have been directed almost entirely against factory smoke. The first step on the road to success is to realise that the house chimney is a much more dangerous enemy than the factory chimney, both because domestic smoke is far greater in quantity and far more harmful in quality than factory smoke, and because factory smoke is already rapidly decreasing, and will almost certainly be immensely reduced in the next 10 or 20 years.[10]

As emissions from industrial smokestacks gradually abated, due to tougher regulation, increased combustion efficiency, and a move from coal to gas and electricity, the nation's home fires—which were exempt from smoke control laws—came to be seen as the chief contributors to the smoke nuisance. In 1940, the consumption of coal for domestic purposes had peaked at over 50 million tons per annum: a fourfold increase on that for the 1840s.[11] And unlike industrial boiler furnaces, domestic grates had not improved much over time in terms of their efficiency.

In his 1945 Chadwick Public Lecture on 'Coal in Relation to Atmospheric Pollution,' the government scientist Albert Parker declared that: 'The domestic open fire produces more smoke per ton of coal burned than any other appliance in general use.'[12] Parker, Director of Fuel Research at the Department of Scientific and Industrial Research, supplied his London audience with estimates, reproduced in Table 1, that seemed to confirm the belief that domestic emissions constituted a more serious pollution problem than factory smoke.

While accounting for less than a quarter of the nation's annual coal consumption in the late 1930s, Parker's figures showed that the traditional open fireplace produced almost half of all urban smoke.[13] Moreover, ground-level domestic smoke emissions were considered to be more harmful than those from industrial chimneys, even though industrial coal users emitted far more acid-forming sulphur dioxide than Britain's householders.

Tall smokestacks were designed to reduce local air pollution—and placate local critics—by discharging their sulphurous emissions high into the atmosphere, to be diluted and dispersed by the prevailing winds.[14] Domestic

Table 1 Nature and Quantity of Pollution from Coal in Great Britain for 1936–38

Type and use of fuel	*Quantity of coal (millions of tons per annum)*	*Pollution produced (millions of tons per annum)*		
		Smoke	*Ash*	*Sulphur dioxide*
Coal:				
Domestic grates	42	1.1	0.1	1.0
Electricity power stations	14	small	0.1	0.4
Railways	13	0.4	0.1	0.4
Collieries and various industrial uses	68	0.8	0.2	2.4
Coke and gas:				
Coke ovens and use of coke	20	small	small	0.5
Gas industry at gas works	19	small	small	0.1
In using gas	–	nil	nil	small
In using coke	–	nil	small	0.2
Total	176	2.3	0.5	5.0

Source: *The Investigation of Atmospheric Pollution: 26th Report* (London, 1949).

fires, because of their inefficiency and the low level at which their smoke was discharged, were widely held to be the 'greater evil.' Burning coal at a lower temperature than industrial boiler-furnaces, the incomplete combustion of fuel in open grates produced more smoke particulates and 'tarry' soot in the urban environment. Household fires had a marked impact on air quality, as Thomas Horsfall, an active member of the Manchester and Salford Noxious Vapours Abatement Association, explained:

> house smoke . . . is poured into the stratum of air which supplies us with that which we breathe in the streets and in our houses, and it enters the air at so many different points that it becomes more thoroughly incorporated with the air in which we move and breathe than does mill smoke . . . sending far more soot into the lungs, the clothes, and the houses of the inhabitants.[15]

In 1920 Dr Caleb Saleeby, a noted writer, journalist and eugenist, set the tone for detractors during the inter-war years when he described Britain's home fires as 'a disgusting and deadly system of coal combustion, which neither our mines nor our national purse nor our bodies can afford.' Indeed, the same year the Newton Committee on Smoke and Noxious Vapours Abatement reported: 'We are satisfied that domestic smoke . . . causes serious danger to health and damage to property.'[16] By the early twentieth-century, evidence that linked sulphurous smoke emissions with a number of adverse health effects was mounting.

The omnipresent smoke-cloud that shrouded Britain's towns and cities was recognised as a major contributor to an upturn in mortality from common respiratory conditions. By 1901 the 'increasingly lethal' bronchitis group of respiratory diseases had, as Simon Szreter has pointed out, unobtrusively become the nation's 'most important single killer,' accounting for over 16 percent of all deaths.[17] Government concerns were voiced by Neville Chamberlain, who as Minister of Health told the House of Commons in 1923:

> I should not be surprised if, owing to the great attention which has been given to certain complaints, some Hon. Members thought that the most fatal diseases were tuberculosis and cancer. That is very far from being the case. Easily the first in their fatal effects are those diseases, which are classed as respiratory diseases—pneumonia, bronchitis, and diseases of that kind—and I am afraid that we must attribute the very high mortality which we suffer from these diseases to the congested conditions and polluted atmosphere which are to be found in our largest towns.[18]

Death rates from respiratory diseases in industrial centres stood in stark contrast to those for England and Wales as a whole, as Table 2, compiled by Dr H. Osborne, Medical Officer of Health for Salford, helps to illustrate. In his investigation into air pollution, Osborne acknowledged that the causes of bronchitis and other respiratory conditions were 'numerous and complex.' Other variables that needed to be taken into account included damp housing, cold weather, tobacco smoking and occupational exposure to harmful substances. Nonetheless, Osborne argued that these data—taken from the Registrar-General's statistical review for 1923—demonstrated a strong correlation between 'atmospheric impurity' and 'excessive mortality from respiratory disease.'[19] Anti-smoke activists consistently used high death rates from respiratory diseases to keep the issue of air pollution in the public eye.

The relationship between atmospheric pollution and respiratory illness attracted most public attention in the wake of protracted winter smog episodes, when the demand for open fires was at its peak.[20] Smog—a term neologised in 1905 by Dr Harold Des Voeux of the London-based Coal Smoke Abatement Society to describe the fusion of smoke and fog—was a recurring problem in Britain's cities. Cold and fog were thought to be relatively harmless in rural areas, but not when married together with the urban smoke cloud. It was becoming increasingly clear to contemporaries that thick sulphurous

Table 2 Death Rates from Non-tubercular Respiratory Diseases for the Year 1923

Town	*Deaths per million*
Salford	3092
Liverpool	3067
Southwark (London)	2699
St. Helens	2614
Leeds	2243
Newcastle	2199
Birmingham	2038
England and Wales (average)	1867

Source: Adapted from H. Osborne, *The Problem of Atmospheric Pollution,* (Manchester, 1924).

smog caused mortality from respiratory diseases to rise sharply, particularly among the sick and the elderly. Osborne reported that during prolonged periods of winter smog, it 'is the common experience of medical practitioners to find their bronchitic patients dying off like flies . . . Smoke-laden fog may set up respiratory disease in those previously healthy; it often kills off those already suffering from bronchitis.' In 1924 Marion Fitzgerald, an authority on domestic heating and former Sanitary Inspector for Woolwich, likened deadly smog visitations to a 'form of air raid . . . kill[ing] its hundreds of victims by acting as a sort of poison gas.' Over a decade before the infamous smog disaster of December 1952, the National Smoke Abatement Society drew attention to no fewer than eight 'fatal smoke fogs' in London, Glasgow, and Manchester, which, taken together, had claimed in excess of 5,000 lives.[21] However, concerns about the adverse effects of smoke on health were not limited to death-dealing respiratory diseases.

Smoke pollution—by absorbing and scattering light—was recognised to lower sunshine levels significantly in early twentieth-century towns and cities. It blocked out, reformers complained, as much as 50 percent of available sunlight and daylight.[22] Beneath the pall of smoke, 'sun-starved' urban populations were thought to be deteriorating physically, mentally, and morally. In 1889 a British Medical Association investigation had revealed that the incidence of rickets, a disease of childhood caused in part by sunlight deprivation, was greatest in smoky industrial towns and mining areas. The gloom and grime, which compelled families to spend more time indoors in poorly ventilated rooms, was also believed to help spread the 'White Plague,' tuberculosis. Coal smoke had long been associated with degeneration, and fears that these 'diseases of darkness' were turning Britain into a nation of 'physical inefficients' were greatly heightened after large numbers of urban recruits for both the Boer War and the First World War were rejected for active service because of their poor physiques. The smoke nuisance, Saleeby declared in 1920, was mainly responsible for the nation's cities being 'crammed with rickety, tuberculous and stunted people.'[23] But town populations were not only perceived to be undersized and unhealthy; the contaminated air and lack of light were considered to be primary factors in reducing them mentally and morally too.

Smoke meant an arduous daily battle against dirt, particularly for the nation's housewives who did most of the washing and cleaning. Maintaining high standards of domestic cleanliness—which promoted both health and respectability—in the face of 'ever-invading' soot and grime placed an unrelenting strain on women, as Salford's Robert Roberts observed:

> Women wore their lives away washing clothes in heavy, iron-hooped tubs, scrubbing wood and stone, polishing furniture and fire-irons. There were housewives who finally lost real interest in anything save dirt removing. Almost every hour of the week they devoted to cleaning and re-cleaning the same objects so that their family, drilled into slavish tidiness, could sit in state, newspaper covers removed, for a few hours each Sunday evening. On Monday purification began all over again. Two of these compulsives left us for the 'lunatic asylum,' one of them, I remember vividly, passing with a man in uniform through a group of us watching children to a van, still washing her hands like a poor Lady MacBeth.[24]

Dirty air not only entailed drudgery, it was also closely associated with mental illness and the 'degradation of the human spirit.' According to anti-smoke reformers, the murky atmospheric conditions contributed to a broad range of psychological problems and moral failings, including depression, drunkenness, gambling, criminality, and a disinclination to work. By the early decades of the twentieth century, smoke pollution was inextricably linked with death, disease, and degeneration, and restoring clean air and sunlight to Britain's 'malurbanised millions' was believed by many contemporaries to be 'the next great task of public health.'[25]

THE SMOKELESS CITY

In their 1922 book *The Smokeless City*, Ernest Simon and Marion Fitzgerald quoted an old Italian proverb: 'All diseases come in the dark and are cured in the sun.' Modern medical research, they argued, had rediscovered the importance of sunlight for public health:

> medical science has proved that sunlight is both a disinfectant and a healer . . . The germs of tuberculosis are rapidly killed by being exposed

> to the action of direct sunlight, but have been found to be virulent after two months when kept in the dark. Those towns which have their sunlight diminished through smoke are deprived to a greater extent of a powerful, natural germicide, and in such places man's bacterial enemies have every opportunity to lead prolonged and mischievous lives. That sunshine is also a healer is proved by the excellent results obtained by the sun-cures for tuberculosis and other diseases . . . It has a great stimulating effect on the skin, helps to keep the muscles well-nourished and vivifies the blood by increasing the amount of haemoglobin. If sunlight is so potent for healing it must also play an important part in maintaining the human body in health.[26]

By the inter-war years, the work of the Nobel Laureate Niels Finsen, Auguste Rollier, Sir Henry Gauvain, and others had raised public awareness of the medicinal value of the ultraviolet component of sunlight. Most domestic hygiene manuals of the day routinely proclaimed the benefits of sunshine for an individual's physical and psychological well-being. For example, in 1939 the author of *The Modern Woman's Home Doctor* wrote: 'In these times it is hardly necessary to emphasise the health-giving qualities of sunlight. Exposure to air and sunlight . . . promotes the health of the body as a whole . . . [and] creates a healthy outlook on life.' Women in particular, in their roles as homemakers and mothers, were exhorted to do everything in their power to see that children were not deprived of light.[27] It is hardly surprising, therefore, that the need to protect sunlight from pollution became a key part of anti-smoke campaigns. The propaganda of both the Sunlight League (founded in 1924) and the National Smoke Abatement Society (founded in 1929) stressed the role played by natural light in curing and preventing 'diseases of darkness,' particularly rickets and tuberculosis. In short, sunlight had re-emerged as a useful tool for rebuilding the nation's health.[28]

Anti-smoke activists shared an ambition to open up congested, 'sunless' industrial cities to light and air with Britain's first generation of town planners. Indeed, there was some overlapping membership between the two groups, with both Thomas Horsfall and George Cadbury being leading advocates of smoke abatement and town planning. Planning for sunlight, space, and fresh air, and attention to hygienic principles in design, were defining characteristics of the influential British Garden City Movement and the international Modern Movement in architecture. In 1902 Ebenezer Howard, in his *Garden Cities of Tomorrow,* had argued that workers would be healthier if 'the free gifts of Nature—fresh air, sunlight, breathing room and playing room' were maximised in urban areas, and the 'smoke fiend' banished by the development of alternative sources of heat and power, particularly electricity.[29] His ideas for the Garden City incorporated low-density housing, broad streets, open spaces, and generous gardens to facilitate air circulation and sunlight penetration. Re-interpreted by town planners such as Raymond Unwin, co-designer of Letchworth and Chief Architect at the

Ministry of Health, suburban 'garden city style' estates constructed by local authorities and private builders sprouted throughout Britain after the First World War.[30] But if aspirations to make Britain's cities brighter, cleaner, and healthier places were to be achieved, then the problem of domestic smoke still had to be addressed.

Post-World War One reconstruction—Lloyd George's government had promised to build 'Homes fit for Heroes'—offered a real opportunity to reduce urban air pollution. To ease an acute housing shortage, the Addison Act of 1919 provided state subsidies for both local authority and private housing schemes that conformed to Ministry of Health siting and design guidelines. Reformers were quick to suggest that all government subsidised housing should be equipped to utilise 'clean' fuels such as gas, coke, or electricity for cooking and heating. In 1920, the Newton Committee—whose investigations into smoke abatement had been disrupted by the war—issued an interim report recommending that the Ministry of Health should decline to approve any housing scheme that failed to use 'smokeless methods' for supplying heat and power.[31] Simon and Fitzgerald argued in *The Smokeless City* that:

> the house-building on a large scale, which is now going on, and must go on for many years to come, gives a unique opportunity for new methods, if only those responsible for housing—the Government, local authorities and private builders—will rise to the occasion and design houses from the point of view of fuel economy and smokelessness. In the past it was urged, with some reason, that it was impracticable to attempt smoke abatement by altering existing appliances . . . The situation is now changed and it is possible to construct houses provided with better methods of heating for a very small increased capital outlay, and in some cases, even for less, than on the old-fashioned method.[32]

Enterprising builders, some reformers claimed, could save between '3 to 5 percent' per house on construction costs by eliminating open coal fires and chimney stacks from future developments.[33]

During the inter-war years, a number of local authorities and private builders took up the challenge. In 1926, a survey of municipal housing schemes by the Smoke Abatement League of Great Britain highlighted several 'courageous experiments' in 'smokeless' heating. Liverpool City Council, it reported, had built 250 all-electric houses, eradicating the open hearth completely. Some local authorities, including those at Bermondsey, Gateshead, Glasgow, Hackney, Leeds, Manchester, Swansea, and Woolwich, had constructed a 'considerable number' of part-electric houses, wiring kitchens and bedrooms for electrical appliances while retaining the traditional open fireplace in the living room. In addition, councils at Acton, Dundee, and Hull had between them installed central heating systems in almost 700 new flats and houses, with the latter planning to build a further 1,100 homes along the same lines. But the survey found that gas most commonly replaced solid fuel in post-war housing schemes, especially in the kitchen. Of 362 respondents to the Smoke Abatement League's questionnaire, 172 local authorities disclosed that the smoky 'old-fashioned' kitchen range had been superseded by modern gas cookers. Answers about the provision of gas fires revealed that 26 councils had fitted them in the main room of all houses built since 1919, while some 43 councils had installed them in bedrooms.[34] However, these initiatives represented only a modest step towards the ideal of the smokeless city. The Smoke Abatement League had undertaken the survey not only to illustrate how domestic smoke emissions could be cut and to bring examples of best practice to public notice, but also in the hope of inspiring others to follow the lead of 'progressive' local authorities. This action was deemed necessary as the Ministry of Health had failed to implement extensively the Newton Committee's policy recommendation on smoke reduction in state subsidised housing. In September 1926, commenting on the construction of 'the first half million' post-war houses, Simon and Fitzgerald bemoaned a missed opportunity to clear the air, which, they argued, was mainly down to a 'lack of enthusiasm for smoke abatement on the part of the government department concerned with the health of the people.'[35]

The failure of the Ministry of Health to take sufficient action to promote smokeless heating was compounded in December 1926 when domestic coal fires were left untouched by the provisions of the new Public Health (Smoke Abatement) Act. This legislation modified the smoke clauses in the Public Health Act of 1875, tightening the regulation of industrial emissions through the introduction of stiffer fines and a broader definition of the 'smoke nuisance' (which expanded to include soot, ash, grit, and non-black smoke).[36] For many anti-smoke activists the passing of the 1926 Act was an unsatisfactory outcome to campaigning efforts, as the Sunlight League's Caleb Saleeby explained:

> this Act—the miserable triumph of a quarter of a century's agitation so far as I was concerned—may limit factory smoke, but in other respects it is reactionary, and it explicitly fails to deal with our new houses. But all new houses henceforth should be equipped, as they can be, for smokeless use. Science has shown us how to distil our coal instead of burning it like barbarians, and thus to get nothing but good out of it—fertilisers for fresh green food from the soil, artificial warmth and light for ourselves, and no obstruction to the Light of Life.[37]

Despite the lack of central government leadership on this issue, experiments in smokeless home heating continued into the 1930s, most notably with the installation of coke-burning grates on Manchester City Council's huge Wythenshawe housing estate. During the 1930s, rebuilding also took the form of apartment blocks on inner city sites as Britain's terraced slums were slowly cleared. Smokeless fuels began to be introduced in modern high-rise flats, such as the Gas, Light and Coke Company's Kensal House project, built using government subsidies in Kensington, London, in 1937. Designed as 'the last word' in working-class flat living, Kensal House comprised three five-storey blocks whose residents were warmed by a clean, efficient gas and coke fuel system. However, the vast majority of the 4 million homes built between the wars—around 1.5 million constructed with government subsidies under a series of housing acts—were still heated by smoky open fires.[38]

In the absence of any legislation that prohibited the burning of raw coal in the home, education was widely thought to be the key to abating domestic smoke emissions. Anti-smoke societies continually pushed the idea of 'good citizenship' in their publications, attempting to persuade the British people to switch to 'clean' heating technologies and cut down air pollution voluntarily. For example, in its 1913 pamphlet 'The Coal Smoke Nuisance' the Coal Smoke Abatement Society insisted that it was a 'citizen's duty' to make use of smokeless fuel in heating the home, and 'play his part in the great task of abating the smoke nuisance and of making his city a cleaner, healthier, and more sunny dwelling-place.' The crucial question was how to get people to participate and to recognise that where smoke reduction was concerned 'his or her little mite,' as the Society's treasurer Dr Harold Des Voeux put it, really did make a difference.[39] To this end, smoke abatement exhibitions were regularly staged to give householders a better understanding of their role in both causing and curing the problem, such as the 'Clear the Air' exhibit shown at Olympia, London, in 1938. Organised by the National Smoke Abatement Society, with assistance from the gas industry, its 'most arresting' feature was a diorama showing the transformation of a smoke-begrimed urban landscape into a 'clean white city bathed in vivid sunlight,' accompanied by the slogan 'We CAN work this miracle.'[40] As for the manufacturers of smokeless fuels and heating appliances, by the 1930s they were strongly emphasising health issues and good citizenship in marketing their products.

During the inter-war years, the gas and electricity industries attempted to persuade the public that their clean, convenient, and controllable heating systems were the solution to the domestic smoke problem.[41] In a hard-fought competition for customers, advertising for both the British Commercial Gas Association and the British Electrical Development Association stressed not only the labour-saving qualities of modern appliances, but also the responsibilities of householders in preventing atmospheric pollution and improving the health of their wider communities. The British Commercial Gas Association produced a remarkable range of advertisements and publicity materials addressing these themes. 'Smoke! Soot! Fogs!' exclaimed a 1931 advertisement, 'Shutting out the sun. Destroying health. Damaging property. Delaying transport. What makes our skies so filthy? Coal smoke . . . You can help to fight this evil, to clean the sky, to let in the sun. Use gas, the smokeless fuel.' Another promoting the use of

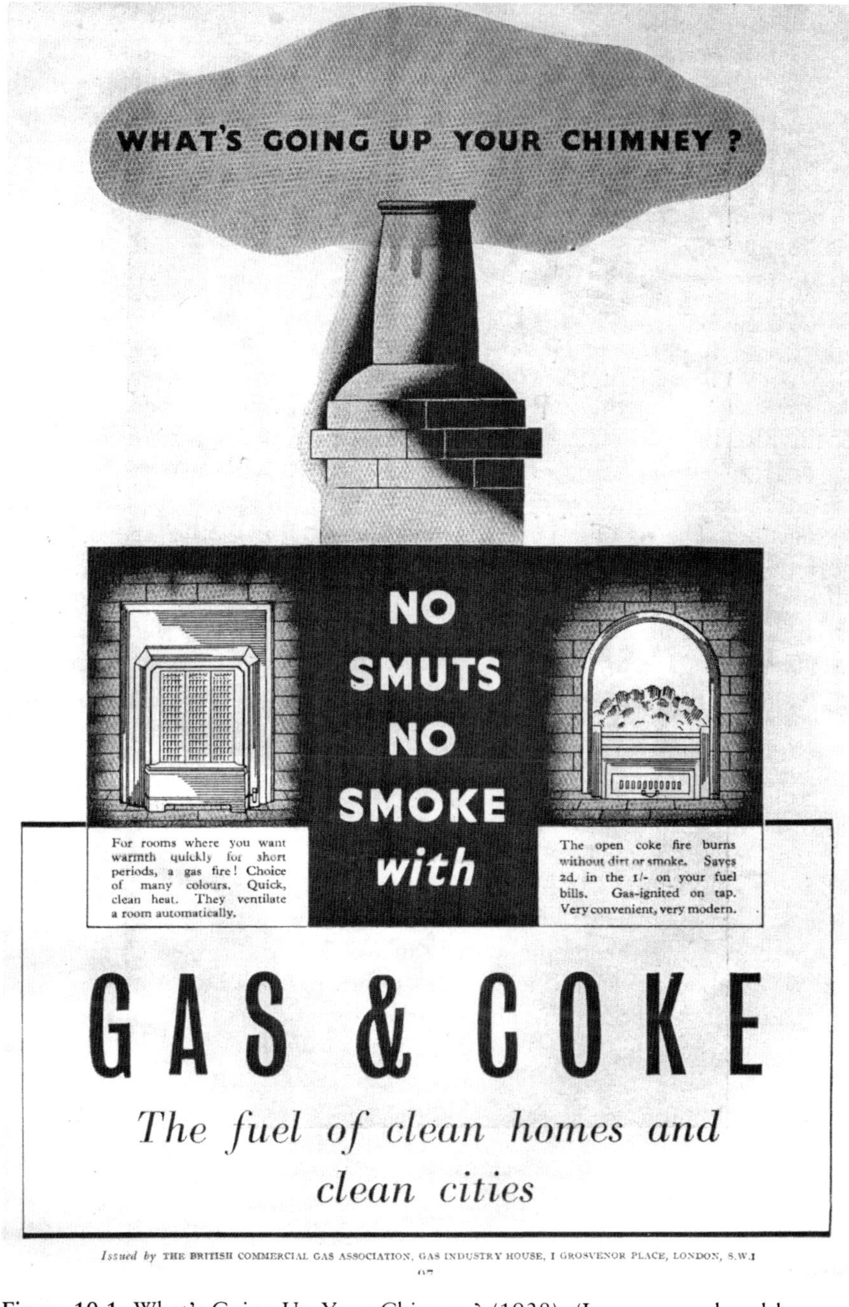
WHAT'S GOING UP YOUR CHIMNEY ?
NO SMUTS NO SMOKE *with*
For rooms where you want warmth quickly for short periods, a gas fire! Choice of many colours. Quick, clean heat. They ventilate a room automatically.
The open coke fire burns without dirt or smoke. Saves 2d. in the 1/- on your fuel bills. Gas-ignited on tap. Very convenient, very modern.
GAS & COKE
The fuel of clean homes and clean cities
Issued by THE BRITISH COMMERCIAL GAS ASSOCIATION, GAS INDUSTRY HOUSE, 1 GROSVENOR PLACE, LONDON, S.W.1

Figure 10.1. What's Going Up Your Chimney? (1938). (Image reproduced by permission of the National Gas Archive, Warrington.)

gas and coke fires (Figure 10.1) inquired: 'What's going up your chimney? No smuts, no smoke with gas and coke, the fuel of clean homes and clean cities.' In an intensive campaign, the gas industry also sponsored a documentary film *The Smoke Menace* (1937) and distributed a lavishly illustrated anti-smoke booklet *Britain's Burning Shame* (1938) in which Kensal House—rechristened as 'Cleanliness House'—featured prominently. In the 1940s Mr Therm, one of the best known contemporary advertising characters, even taught the nation's children that a 'magic smokeless city' could be brought into being if coal was properly converted into gas.[42]

The electricity industry was 'significantly under-advertised' in comparison with its rival, but British Electrical Development Association propaganda (Figure 10.2) similarly promised 'Cleaner cities, healthier cities, and happier people' if householders substituted electric fires and cookers for their coal-fuelled counterparts. In 1934 Caroline Haslett, Director of the Electrical Association for Women, argued that as this new energy source reached more and more homes it was 'no vain dream to visualize brighter cities, clear of smoke'—liberating women from 'soul-destroying drudgery.'[43] The manufacturers of solid smokeless fuels also harnessed both public spiritedness and health concerns in their advertising. According to Lt-Col. W. A. Bristow, Managing Director of Low Temperature Carbonisation, air pollution was 'sapping the vitality of the race,' and the company's advertisements reminded readers: 'Be a Good Neighbour by burning Coalite smokeless coal.' But such appeals, and related educational activities, met with only limited success in reducing domestic smoke emissions.[44]

While there are few comprehensive statistics regarding the installation and use of heating appliances in inter-war Britain, a number of reports and surveys conducted by organisations such as Political and Economic Planning (PEP), Mass Observation, and the National Union of Townswomen's Guilds provide valuable data on the types of heating employed in the home and the public's preferences. Reports on fuel supply and the demand for household appliances published by PEP, an independent non-party organisation committed to furthering national reconstruction, showed that right up to the end of the Second World War over 90 percent of working-class dwellings depended on the traditional coal fire or range to heat the main living room. Although smokeless heating appliances were beginning to become common in new suburban housing (mainly in bedrooms) and multi-storey blocks of flats (where the delivery and storage of coal presented difficulties), PEP's investigations revealed that the majority of low-income, inner-city households rarely used gas or electric fires. However, PEP estimated that in 1939 there were 10.1 million gas and electric cookers in use, shrinking the smoke clouds over cities, with most British housewives choosing to cook with gas. But it pointed out that 'the gas or electric cooker is mainly or exclusively used in summer,' with over half of all households reverting to the smoky coal-fired range

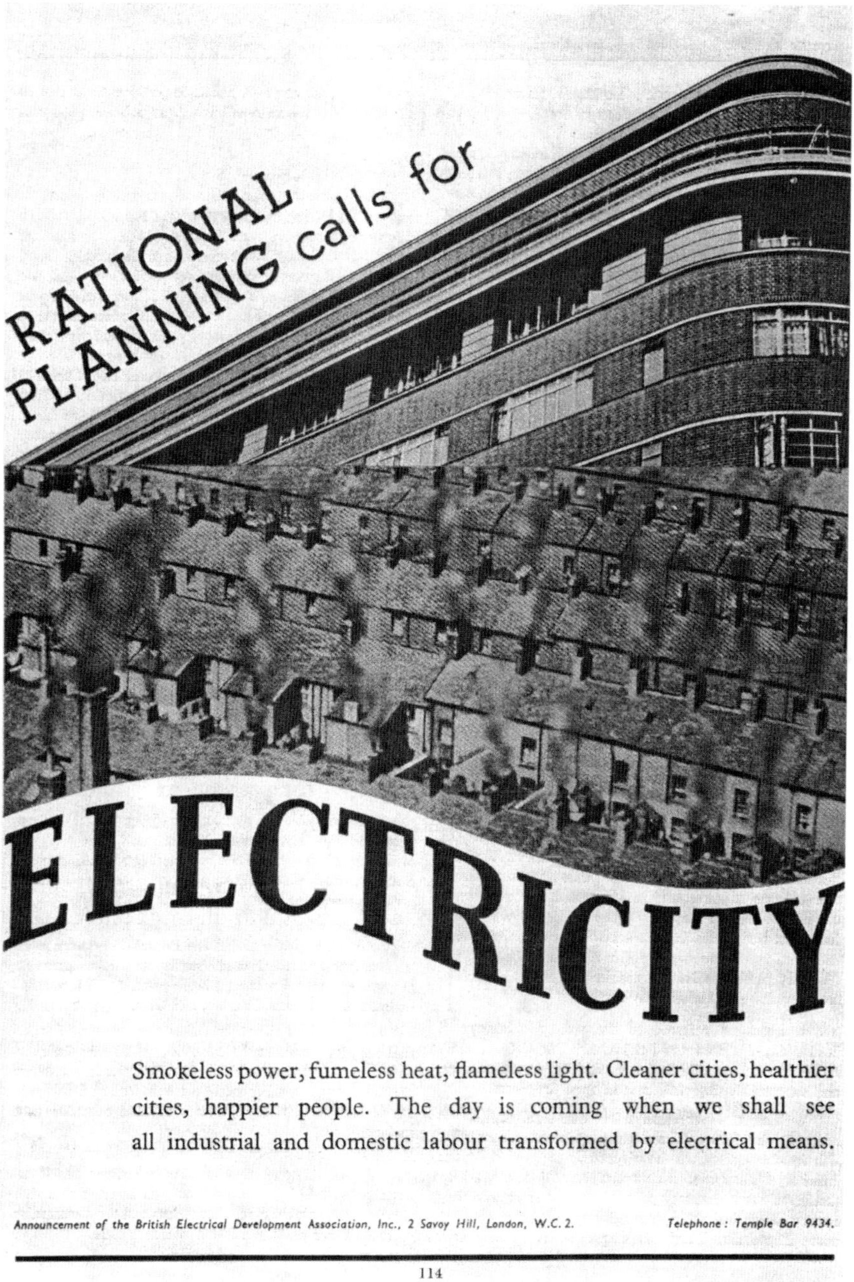

Figure 10.2. Rational Planning Calls for Electricity (1938). (Image reproduced by permission of the Senior Archivist, Museum of Science and Industry in Manchester).

during the winter months as it combined heating with cooking.[45] Social survey data also helped to highlight the public's continuing attachment to the open coal fire. During the summer of 1939 Mass Observation, as part of an enquiry into people's homes, asked the question: 'What type of heating would you like if you could choose?' Some 73 percent of respondents opted for an open coal fire or range, 11 percent for an open coke fire, with the remaining 16 percent split between gas, electric and other forms of domestic heating.[46] An extensive wartime housing survey by the National Union of Townswomen's Guilds found 88 percent of English respondents in favour of coal fires, with the figure rising to 91 percent in Scotland, while a 1943 report on the design of dwellings by the Society of Women Housing Managers concluded: 'Evidence from all parts of the country showed an overwhelming demand for an open coal fire in the living room.'[47] Thus, a different question now arises: 'Why did the British insist on a traditional open hearth for home heating?'

THE HOME FIRES

During the first half of the twentieth century, despite concerted anti-smoke propaganda and advertising campaigns, the majority of British homes—old and new—were still heated by open fires. National figures for domestic fuel consumption show that in 1938 bituminous coal (with minimal assistance from anthracite) provided heat in 80 percent of all households, gas and coke 10 percent and 6 percent respectively, with electricity warming just 4 percent of British homes.[48] As late as 1952, a survey for the Coal Utilisation Council found that the 'great mass' of city-dwellers were still 'one room families,' living and eating around the open coal fire. Contemporary reports and surveys clearly indicate that smokeless fuels and appliances played only a 'subsidiary role' in domestic heating systems, with modern gas and electric fires generally being used 'intermittently' by the better-paid to warm bedrooms for short periods. Furthermore, they demonstrate that most Britons definitely preferred coal fires to any other means of warming living rooms, even though a switch to the 'instant heat' of gas and electricity would do away with the dirty and time-consuming daily chores of lighting, refuelling, and ash removal. This reluctance to adopt new technologies undoubtedly frustrated reformers and power companies alike, and according to Arnold Marsh, General Secretary of the National Smoke Abatement Society, it presented 'perhaps the most formidable obstacle on the road to a smokeless Britain.'[49] At a time when expectations of cleanliness, comfort, and convenience were rising, the 'old-fashioned' open hearth continued to hold its own against all competitors.

The British favoured open coal fires for a number of interconnected reasons. Coal maintained its popularity for home heating partly because it was relatively cheap, and partly because householders were unwilling to bear the costs of installing and running smokeless appliances. The running costs of gas and electricity, particularly in the early decades of the twentieth century, were often 'prohibitive for cottage tenants,' while space heating appliances were usually 'landlord's fixtures': it was therefore 'prudent' for tenant-occupiers—most housing was rented before 1945—to continue to use existing solid-fuel systems. In 1946 a government committee on domestic fuel policy, chaired by the indefatigable Ernest Simon, reported: 'Coal has been so cheap in the past that, in spite of its very low efficiency, the cost of heating by the open coal fire has not been regarded as excessive.' Unsurprisingly, smoke abatement and higher fuel efficiency standards were key objectives of the Simon Report, which also recommended the establishment of 'experimental' smokeless zones in urban areas. Nonetheless, it noted that for the 'continuous heating of rooms' coal-fuelled appliances still cost the consumer only 'about half as much as gas or electricity.' In addition, the Simon Report recognised that supplies of affordable proprietary solid smokeless fuels, such as Coalite and Suncole, were extremely limited between the wars. Coke, though more plentiful, was hard to sell: it was difficult to ignite and often made a poor blaze in the hearth.[50] There were, then, compelling economic and practical reasons for the open coal fire to remain the householder's first choice.

However, cost, practicality, and availability were not the only factors that delayed the adoption of cleaner fuels and smokeless appliances. Overcoming misgivings about technological change, as Sydney Bushell and Catherine Gordon observed in 1926, was also an obstacle to reform. 'Any woman,' they wrote, 'will naturally feel somewhat daunted when she begins to inquire about smokeless methods of warming rooms, heating water and cooking. She may have little or no experience of the alternatives which are offered to her.'[51] To those who were accustomed to using a coal fire for all purposes, the prospect of abandoning a tried and tested technology and familiar work practices could be genuinely alarming.

Sentiment as well as habit bound the British people to the domestic hearth. It not only performed vital household functions, providing heat, light, hot meals, and boiling water, but was also the hub around which home life revolved. In 1904 Hermann Muthesius, architect and cultural attaché to the German embassy in London, pithily encapsulated its socio-cultural significance when he declared:

> To an Englishman the idea of a room without a fire-place is quite simply unthinkable. All ideas of domestic comfort, of family happiness, of inward-looking personal life, of spiritual well-being centre around the fire-place. The fire as the symbol of home is to the Englishman the central idea both of the living room and of the whole house; the fire-place is the domestic altar before which, daily and hourly, he sacrifices to the household gods. This is why the English have never thought, and will never think, of relinquishing the fire-place, however irrational it

> is, however much trouble it causes and however doubtful its practical value. To the English, to remove the fire-place from the home would be like removing the soul from the body. Out of love for the fire-place they overlook all its faults . . . In England the fire-place remains and will always remain.[52]

At roughly the same time, the *British Medical Journal* anticipated a 'very long and arduous conflict in weaning the Englishman from the essentially national pleasure of a bright coal fire.' And over three decades later, the Mass Observation report on housing conditions listed 'homeliness' and 'cheerfulness' as two of the main reasons the public gave for preferring the traditional open fireplace. 'Non-coal heating,' Mass Observation concluded, 'fail[ed] to satisfy some deep-seated aesthetic demand that is satisfied by the old-fashioned, dirty, smoky, coal-fire.'[53]

Widely appreciated by contemporaries for its uplifting 'homely' attributes, the open hearth was also considered to be a more hygienic choice for domestic heating than many of its smokeless rivals. More than any other domestic appliance of the day, the open fireplace was deemed to be an 'essential feature of British comfort and British health.' Unlike gas and electric fires, a blazing coal fire could be used to incinerate most household refuse, both improving home hygiene and reducing the volume of municipal waste for collection and disposal. In addition, Britain's home fires were highly prized as ventilators of interior spaces. As the chief Ministry of Health architects Raymond Unwin and S. Pointon Taylor emphasised in 1926, 'the value of the smoke flue for ventilation is one of the reasons why people cling to the coal fire.'[54] During the first three decades of the twentieth century, long-standing concerns over 'vitiated' indoor atmospheres often eclipsed anxieties about smoke pollution outdoors. The sanitarian Alfred T. Schofield put the problem simply in his popular book *The Directory of Domestic Hygiene* (1927): 'the foulest outdoor air is purer than the best indoor; and the evils of cities is not the air of their streets, but the indoor lives of their inhabitants.'[55] Hygiene writers regularly warned that the 'stagnant' air of overcrowded and ill-ventilated housing was just as pernicious a health hazard as contaminated food and water. When too many people were crammed into too little domestic space, they stressed, oxygen levels fell, carbon dioxide levels rose, and concentrations of dangerous bacteria increased (including tubercle bacilli), as did accumulations of 'organic effluvia' produced by human respiration. It was assumed that air exhaled from the lungs contained an 'anthropotoxin' (a small proportion of the 'waste poisons' of the human system), and the authors of domestic advice manuals from *Mrs Beeton's Book of Household Management* (1906) to *The Property Owners' Handbook* (1922) routinely cautioned readers against the inhalation of 're-breathed air.' Indeed, Agnes Baden Powell's *Handbook for Girl Guides* (1912) warned Britain's future homemakers: 'People's breath is poisonous; do not breathe the air which other people have used already.' The harmful effects of continually breathing the 'vitiated' air of confined spaces were thought to include headaches, dizziness, nausea, and, ultimately—as numerous experiments on laboratory animals had appeared to show conclusively—death.[56] Paradoxically, the open fireplace, although smoky and inefficient, had crucial work to perform in safeguarding the home against these potentially deadly pollutants.

The traditional open hearth was recognised to be the primary ventilating agent in most early twentieth-century homes. In 1927, for example, Schofield wrote in *The Directory of Domestic Hygiene:*

> There is no doubt that the great safety valve of most rooms is the open chimney, which is of far more importance as an air shaft than as an outlet for the smoke. Were it not for the English love for an open fireplace, and hence an open chimney, it is hard to say what would become of large numbers of the population. No chimney ought, therefore, to be stopped up; and under ordinary circumstances, no room should be without one.[57]

In 1936, a Building Research Station study showed that an apartment heated by an open fire provided 4.5 air changes per hour: a ventilation rate more than sufficient to keep the indoor atmosphere in a 'wholesome' condition. As the *Encyclopædia Britannica* explained, 'when a bright fire is burning in an open grate, it rarely happens that any other outlet for foul air from a room need be provided.' The Model Byelaws for buildings issued in 1937 only insisted on the provision of special means of ventilation in the rooms of new houses if they did not contain an open fireplace.[58] The British public long remained unenthusiastic about gas and electric fires, and the closed stoves that were popular in the United States and continental Europe, not only because they were considered unattractive, but also because they were believed to be of negligible value for ventilation purposes. Furthermore, as early gas heaters were often badly designed and constructed, it was regularly pointed out that they posed an ever-present threat to home health, as the dangerous carbon monoxide gas they produced during combustion often leaked into rooms, causing headaches, lethargy, and sometimes even death. In 1926, R. Storry Deans MP informed the House of Commons that 'although I may be told that the smoke from my coal fire assists in poisoning the people outside, I prefer that very much to being poisoned myself by a gas fire within my own house.'[59] The notion that gas fires were insalubrious and inadequate ventilators in comparison with open fires took a long time to die away.

There was another health-related explanation for the householder's reluctance to use closed stoves and modern heating appliances—overheated air. Worries that stove-heated rooms undermined health by excessively drying the air had a long lineage. In 1843, for instance, Dr Andrew Ure remarked upon the 'sallow and withered complexions' of foreigners subjected to the malign influence of closed stoves, contrasting their hot, stuffy apartments unfavourably with the 'fresh invigorating atmosphere of an English parlour, as heated by the open cheerful grate.'[60] By the early twentieth century, ideas about overheating had assumed national importance as climatological theories about human progress gained ground. The influential American geographer Ellsworth Huntington's *Civilization and Climate* (1915), for example, explicitly linked cool, changeable climates and Euro-American superiority, dynamism, and productivity. Monotonous heat both outdoors and indoors, Huntington argued, played a major role in impairing a population's health, vigour, and efficiency. As the belief that national destinies were shaped by climate spread during the inter-war years, public health experts on both sides of the Atlantic sought to answer the thorny question: 'What should the ideal indoor environment be like?'[61]

Leonard Hill, Director of Applied Physiology at the National Institute of Medical Research, perhaps did most to define what constituted 'ideal' atmospheric conditions in the British home environment. By the mid-1920s, his research had begun to overturn the erroneous idea that 're-breathed air' was a prolific source of ill-health in overcrowded dwellings. Rather, Hill insisted that it was 'the mischief of coddling indoors in overheated and draughtless rooms' that caused listlessness and increased susceptibility to illness, particularly colds, tuberculosis, and 'nervous troubles.'[62] As early as 1913, he complained that 'heat stagnation' often accompanied the installation of modern heating systems:

> Central heating, gas-radiators, and other contrivances are now displacing the old open fire and chimney. This change greatly improves the economical consumption of coal and the light and cleanliness of the atmosphere. But in so far as it promotes monotonous, windless, warm atmospheres, it is wholly against the health and vigor of the nation. The open fire and wide chimney ensure ventilation, the indrawing of cold outside air, streaky air—restless currents at different temperatures, which strike the sensory nerves in the skin and prevent monotony and weariness of spirit. By the old open fires we were heated with radiant heat. The air in rooms was drawn in cool and variable of temperature. The radiator and the hot air system give us a deadly uniform heat—the very conditions we find unsupportable on a close summer's day.[63]

Central heating, seldom encountered outside of public buildings and blocks of flats or offices before the 1950s, was roundly condemned as 'hygienic decadence' by one inter-war commentator, as its uniform warmth was physically unchallenging to the hardy British race. To ensure a healthy home, according to Hill, atmospheric conditions indoors needed instead to closely resemble those of a sunny and stimulating spring day outdoors. In choosing a space heating appliance, he advised his readers that the 'essential principle' was to 'avoid heating the air and secure a sufficient movement of cool fresh air . . . while warming the body by radiant heat.'[64] The human body was believed to be 'better adapted' to radiant heating technologies, particularly the blazing coal fire, which replicated the way in which the sun warmed the earth. During the inter-war years Hill, who was also the vice-president of the Sunlight League, continually pressed for the adoption of improved gas fires (with adequate flues and a brighter radiant output) as a measure to prevent smoke pollution. But he nonetheless maintained: 'We must see to it that the method of house warming is contrived on the same lines as the open fire, otherwise we may lose in health . . . more than we gain from light.'[65]

At a time when the importance of sunlight to health was unquestioned, defenders of the traditional open fire were quick to stress the purported 'beneficial properties' of its radiant heat. In 1926 Marie Stopes, an expert on the composition of coal as well as family planning, argued that:

> A glowing coal fire gives out something subtle, yet intensely 'nourishing' to the system, 'nourishing' in a way that vitamins and ultra-violet rays are 'nourishing.' Whatever this stimulating influence may be, it is either absent or very weak in radiation from anthracite stoves or gas and electric fires. Hence, for health, a brightly glowing coal fire should be present in every nursery, and in the chief living room of every house . . . in the interests of the race, of the health and happiness of the individual, as well as in the name of science, may I stress the immense importance of not flouting the natural instinct of the British people to use bright *coal fires*.[66]

The Coal Utilisation Council, founded in 1932 to promote the better use of coal (and to better compete against gas and electricity), quoted Stopes's views on the value of Britain's home fires to health in an early sales brochure entitled *No. 1 Paradise Street: The House of Your Dreams:*

> "I say emphatically that any woman who can afford it and yet rears her children without exposing them daily in winter to the beneficial radiation of a bright coal fire, is doing them a deliberate injury." These are strong words, but they represent the considered opinion of a famous woman scientist, who adds that such a fire gives out something subtle yet intensely nourishing to the system . . . Nowadays we all appreciate the benefits to be derived from allowing the rays of the sun to play upon the bare skin. The rays from a coal fire have a similar effect and, apart from the comfort of having their ordinary bath in front of the nursery fire, the children will derive real benefit from having a "bath" in the rays of the fire itself.[67]

Overheating also featured prominently. The brochure advised against installing other types of fire on the grounds that they scorched the air, dried the skin, and made children 'fretful and feverish.' While few health experts and household manuals of the day made such forceful and extravagant claims, many recommended the use of radiant heat in the living room—and radiant heat remained synonymous with the open coal fire.[68]

Although the alleged benefits of radiant heat received scant attention in the 1946 Simon Report, a lengthy appendix summarised the latest research on thermal comfort requirements in the home. It concluded that overheating and incorrect humidity—and not 'vitiated air'—were the main causes of discomfort and ill-health (although the harmful effects of draughts and underheating were not neglected). It also specified the conditions that made for 'a pleasant and invigorating' indoor atmosphere, which included: air free from 'objectionable odours' ('anthropotoxins' no longer merited discussion as a threat to health); adequate and variable air movement, 'for the body is stimulated by ceaseless changes of environment'; and room temperatures 'as cool as is compatible with comfort.' While it was 'notoriously difficult' to define a 'comfort zone' that suited all people, the Simon Report suggested that an air temperature between 62 and 70 degrees Fahrenheit, with a relative humidity between 30 and 60 percent, constituted its lower and upper limits in winter. A moderate 65 degrees Fahrenheit was the generally accepted 'ideal' indoor temperature, adjudged to be the most compatible with health and comfort.[69] The Simon Report, which played a major role in setting heating standards in Britain's post-Second World War homes, recommended that all new dwellings should be provided with 'a flue suitable for a solid fuel appliance' in the living room, supplemented by the means to heat one bedroom by gas or electricity. Such a combination of heating and ventilation would avoid the thermal monotony thought so harmful to health and native vitality and, Simon and his colleagues hoped, help to open up the British home ('In cold weather . . . the smallest in the civilised world') by allowing families to make better use of previously 'wasted space' upstairs.[70] The inefficient open coal fire, however, was to be gradually replaced by improved heating appliances capable of burning solid smokeless fuels, preferably slow-combustion stoves that could be opened when the living room was occupied to reveal a homely, 'cheerful' glow. But echoing the words of the Newton Committee's 1920 interim report on domestic smoke that there was 'still a strong prejudice' in favour of the open hearth, the Simon Report cautioned that the traditional method of heating rooms 'has been and still is very popular . . . Indeed, the open coal fire is a national institution.'[71] Despite being marketed as a 'cosy' form of open fire, efficient, labour-saving 'openable' stoves were to be found in only a small proportion of British homes by 1950.[72]

CONCLUSION

During the first half of the twentieth century, a growing body of evidence linked the nation's home fires to a wide range of health and environmental problems. Yet, as Lord Newton noted, any move to outlaw the traditional open hearth was commonly viewed 'in the nature of high treason.'[73]

Without public support, politicians of all parties were reluctant to interfere with the rights of millions of Britons to enjoy an open coal fire in their own homes. Despite growing awareness of its damaging effects, the open fire had retained its place in the public's affections for three main reasons: firstly, the 'homely hearth' was still central to everyday British family life; secondly, the lack of an acceptable and economic alternative technology; and thirdly, the popular notion that the traditional open fireplace was a 'healthier' choice for domestic heating and ventilating than many of its 'modern' rivals. While the socio-cultural, economic, and technical obstacles to smoke abatement have thus far attracted most historical interest, this chapter has shown that the important health dimensions of the question should not be neglected.

By 1945, most of Britain's newer homes had mixed heating systems. In general, open fires took pride of place in the living room, supplemented by gas and electricity in the kitchen and bedrooms. The increased use of gas and electricity for cooking did help to reduce levels of urban air pollution, particularly during the summer months. However, during the inter-war years these 'modern' fuels made only a modest contribution to smoke abatement.[74] That the coal fire was still fitted as standard in both local authority and private housing developments—sanctioned by the Ministry of Health—was a major concern for those working towards the modernist ideal of the sunlit, smokeless city. Responses to wartime investigations into home heating were equally worrying for anti-smoke activists and utility companies, as householders indicated overwhelmingly that they were willing to sacrifice the cleanliness and convenience of gas and electricity for a cheerful blaze in the hearth. At a time when ideas about making a family comfortably warm in winter were being redefined, the notion that Britain's heating systems should resemble its changeable climate—providing robust ventilation and variable, 'invigorating' radiant heat—added another positive aspect to the open fire's attractions. Its use to maintain a healthy atmosphere indoors undoubtedly obstructed efforts to improve air quality outdoors.

'Homes for All' was the slogan after the Second World War, with the newly-elected Labour Party committed to 'building a better Britain.' The 1943 pamphlet 'Your Home Planned by Labour' stated that:

> The men and women who have fought and toiled to make victory possible must not live out their lives in cramped and ugly streets. Children shall not be denied sunlight—or opportunity. Women must be released from the endless drudgery of tenement or slum. Labour means to get new homes for the British people. Modern. Sunlit. Labour-saving. Labour plans to end the long era of mean streets and stunted lives.[75]

But despite the promise of a brighter future, the smoky open fire continued to be the main source of heat in Britain's homes. It took the catastrophic

'Great Smog' of December 1952, which claimed the lives of some 4,000 Londoners, to persuade the British people to give up their open coal fires.[76]

NOTES

1. Stephen Mosley, *The Chimney of the World: A History of Smoke Pollution in Victorian and Edwardian Manchester* (Cambridge: White Horse Press, 2001), 75–8. See also: Paul Langford, *Englishness Identified: Manners and Character, 1650–1850* (Oxford: Oxford University Press, 2001), 108–21.
2. Mosley, *Chimney of the World;* Bill Luckin, '"The Heart and Home of Horror": The Great London Fogs of the Late Nineteenth Century,' *Social History* 28 (2003): 31–48; Peter Brimblecombe, *The Big Smoke: A History of Air Pollution in London since Medieval Times* (London: Routledge, 1988); 'Smoke Abatement,' *British Medical Journal* (August 29, 1908): 615.
3. John Sheail, *An Environmental History of Twentieth-Century Britain* (Basingstoke: Palgrave, 2002), chapter 8; Bill Luckin, 'Pollution in the City,' in Martin Daunton (ed.), *The Cambridge Urban History of Britain, Volume III 1840–1950* (Cambridge: Cambridge University Press, 2000), 207–28; Brian W. Clapp, *An Environmental History of Britain since the Industrial Revolution* (Harlow: Longman, 1994), chapters 2 and 3; Tim Boon, '"The Smoke Menace": Cinema, Sponsorship and the Social Relations of Science in 1937,' in Michael Shortland (ed.), *Science and Nature: Essays in the History of the Environmental Sciences* (Oxford: Alden Press, 1993), 57–88; Brimblecombe, *Big Smoke;* Eric Ashby and Mary Anderson, *The Politics of Clean Air* (Oxford: Oxford University Press, 1981); *idem,* 'Studies in the Politics of Environmental Protection: The Historical Roots of the Clean Air Act, 1956: III. The Ripening of Public Opinion, 1898–1952,' *Interdisciplinary Science Reviews* 2 (1977): 190–206.
4. For an earlier discussion of indoor air pollution, see: Stephen Mosley, 'Fresh Air and Foul: The Role of the Open Fireplace in Ventilating the British Home, 1837–1910,' *Planning Perspectives* 18 (2003): 1–21.
5. 'The Smoke Nuisance,' *The Builder* 77 (1899): 143–4.
6. Luckin, 'Heart and Home,' 33.
7. Richard Lawton and Colin G. Pooley, *Britain 1740–1950: An Historical Geography* (London: Edward Arnold, 1992), Table 6, 91; Clapp, *Environmental History,* Table 2.2, 16.
8. For instance, see: F. A. R. Russell, *London Fogs* (London: Edward Stanford, 1880); Thomas C. Horsfall, *The Nuisance of Smoke from Domestic Fires, and Methods of Abating It* (Manchester: John Heywood, 1893).
9. Boon, 'Smoke Menace,' 80–84.
10. Ernest D. Simon and Marion Fitzgerald, *The Smokeless City* (London: Longmans, Green & Co, 1922), 3–4.
11. Clapp, *Environmental History,* 16; Roy Church, *The History of the British Coal Industry, Volume 3, 1830–1913: Victorian Pre-eminence* (Oxford: Oxford University Press, 1986), Tables 1.3, 19.
12. Albert Parker, 'Coal in Relation to Atmospheric Pollution,' *The Investigation of Atmospheric Pollution: 26th Report* (London: HMSO, 1949), 116–125, at p. 124.
13. Figures were uncertain and disputed. For example, in 1931 the National Smoke Abatement Society estimated the amount of domestic smoke produced at over 3 million tons per annum. National Smoke Abatement Society, *The Smoke Abatement Handbook* (Manchester: Service Guild, 1931), 11.
14. However, this strategy led to an increase in the production of acid rain and extensive damage to regional ecologies. See: Mosley, *Chimney of the World,* 35–45;

Matthew Osborn, 'Uplands Downwind: Acidity and Ecological Change in the Southeast Lancashire Moorlands,' in E. Melanie Dupuis (ed.), *Smoke and Mirrors: The Politics and Culture of Air Pollution* (New York: New York University Press, 2004), 77–99; Harold Platt, '"The Invisible Evil": Noxious Vapor and Public Health during the Age of Industry,' in ibid., 27–50.

15. Horsfall, *Nuisance of Smoke*, 3.
16. Caleb W. Saleeby, *National Health and the Smoke Nuisance* (London, 1920), 8; Ministry of Health, *Committee on Smoke and Noxious Vapours Abatement: Interim Report*, Cmd. 755 (1920), reprinted in Ministry of Health, *Committee on Smoke and Noxious Vapours Abatement: Final Report* (London: HMSO, 1921), 37.
17. Simon Szreter, 'The Importance of Social Intervention in Britain's Mortality Decline c.1850–1914: A Re-interpretation of the Role of Public Health,' *Social History of Medicine* 1 (1988): 1–37, p. 16.
18. *Parliamentary Debates* 165 (1923), col. 2575.
19. H. Osborne, *The Problem of Atmospheric Pollution*, (Manchester: John Heywood, 1924), 16 and 29.
20. Mosley, 'Fresh Air and Foul,' 1–2; Luckin, 'Heart and Home,' 32–3.
21. Osborne, *Problem of Atmospheric Pollution*, 7; Marion Fitzgerald, *Cleansing the Sky: The Case for Smoke Abatement* (Warrington: John Walker & Co., 1924), 3; National Smoke Abatement Society, *The Case Against Smoke: The Evidence of the Authorities* (Manchester: National Smoke Abatement Society, 1936), 6.
22. For example, see: Simon and Fitzgerald, *Smokeless City*, 15; Caleb W. Saleeby, *Sunlight and Health* (London: Nisbet & Co., 1929), 105; National Smoke Abatement Society, *The Importance of Smoke Abatement* (Manchester: National Smoke Abatement Society, c.1934), 2.
23. Isambard Owen, 'Reports of the Collective Investigation Committee of the British Medical Association: Geographical Distribution of Rickets, Acute and Subacute Rheumatism, Chorea, Cancer, and Urinary Calculus in the British Islands,' *British Medical Journal* (January 19, 1889): 113–16; Mosley, *Chimney of the World*, 63–4, 102–07; Saleeby, *National Health*, 5–7.
24. Robert Roberts, *The Classic Slum: Salford Life in the First Quarter of the Century*, (Harmondsworth: Penguin, 1990), 37. See also: Arnold Marsh, *Smoke: The Problem of Coal and the Atmosphere* (London: Faber & Faber, 1947), 114–15.
25. Millicent Jast, *How the Citizen Takes the Air: The Personal Significance of the Smoke Problem* (Manchester: Pontefract Bros., 1933), 8; J. E. W. Wallin, *Psychological Aspects of the Problem of Atmospheric Smoke Pollution*, (Pittsburgh: University of Pittsburgh, 1913); National Smoke Abatement Society, *Case Against Smoke*, 8–9; Caleb W. Saleeby, 'Sunlight and Disease,' *Nature* 111 (1923): 574–76, at p. 576.
26. Simon and Fitzgerald, *Smokeless City*, 15.
27. Richard Hobday, 'Sunlight Therapy and Solar Architecture,' *Medical History* 42 (1997): 455–72; W. Arbuthnot Lane (ed.), *The Modern Woman's Home Doctor* (London: Odhams Press, 1939), 343–44; Elizabeth S. Chesser, 'Sunlight, Health and Happiness,' *New Health* (April, 1927): 60–1.
28. Saleeby, *Sunlight and Health;* Edward J. Deck, *The Sun and How to Use It* (London: The Sunlight League, 1926); National Smoke Abatement Society, *Smoke Abatement Handbook*, 13–15; National Smoke Abatement Society, *Case Against Smoke*, 8–10. See also: John Hassan, *The Seaside, Health and Environment in England and Wales since 1800* (Aldershot: Ashgate, 2003), chapter 4; Ken Worpole, *Here Comes the Sun: Architecture and Public Space in Twentieth-Century European Culture* (London: Reaktion, 2000); Joanna

Bourke, *Dismembering the Male: Men's Bodies, Britain and the Great War* (London: Reaktion, 1999), 203–09.

29. Worpole, *Here Comes the Sun;* Pyrs Gruffudd, '"Science and the Stuff of Life": Modernist Health Centres in 1930s London,' *Journal of Historical Geography* 27 (2001): 395–416; Ebenezer Howard, *Garden Cities of To-morrow* (Cambridge, MA: MIT Press, 1965), 55 and 127.
30. Mervyn Miller, *Raymond Unwin, Garden Cities and Town Planning* (Leicester: Leicester University Press, 1992); Dennis Hardy, *From Garden Cities to New Towns: Campaigning for Town and Country Planning, 1899–1946* (London: E. & F. N. Spon, 1991).
31. Richard Rodger, 'Slums and Suburbs: The Persistence of Residential Apartheid,' in Philip Waller (ed.), *The English Urban Landscape* (Oxford: Oxford University Press, 2000), 233–68, p. 250; Ministry of Health, *Interim Report,* 46.
32. Simon and Fitzgerald, *Smokeless City,* 27.
33. J. W. Beauchamp, *The Influence of Electricity on the Domestic Smoke Problem* (Manchester: J. F. Tangye, 1924), 8; Saleeby, *National Health,* 8.
34. Ernest D. Simon and Marion Fitzgerald, 'Municipal Housing Schemes and Smoke Abatement,' in Smoke Abatement League of Great Britain, *Report of the Smoke Abatement Conference held at Bingley Hall, Birmingham, September 7th, 8th and 9th—1926* (Manchester: Smoke Abatement League of Great Britain, 1926), 29–37, pp. 30–32.
35. Ibid., 29–30. See also: Saleeby, *National Health,* 8; 'The Minister of Health on Smoke,' *Journal of the National Smoke Abatement Society* 9 (1938): 111–13.
36. Ashby and Anderson, *Politics of Clean Air,* 95–96.
37. Caleb W. Saleeby, 'The Benefits of Sunlight,' in W. Arbuthnot Lane, (ed.), *Blazing the Health Trail* (London: Faber & Faber, 1929), 62–71, p. 71.
38. C.V. Malcolm, 'Smokeless Zones—The History of Their Development,' *Clean Air* (Spring, 1977), 4–10, p. 8; Compton Mackenzie, *The Vital Flame* (London: British Gas Council, 1947), 36–37; Elizabeth Darling, 'What the Tenants Think of Kensal House: Experts' Assumptions versus Inhabitants' Realities in the Modern Home,' *Journal of Architectural Education* 53 (2000): 167–77, at p. 167; Lawton and Pooley, *Britain,* Table 16.3, 313; Eric Hopkins, *The Rise and Decline of the English Working Class* (London: Weidenfield & Nicolson, 1991), 23.
39. Coal Smoke Abatement Society, *The Coal Smoke Nuisance: Why It Should Be Abated* (London: Coal Smoke Abatement Society, 1913), 3–4; 'Conference on Smoke Abatement,' *The Builder* 83 (1905): 643–44, at p. 644. See also: Boon, 'Smoke Menace,' especially 72, 74, 78–80.
40. 'Britain's Burning Shame and the Gas Campaign,' *Journal of the National Smoke Abatement Society* 9 (1938): 101–03, at p. 101.
41. These utilities were, however, major polluters in their own right. See: Peter Thorsheim, 'The Paradox of Smokeless Fuels: Gas; Coke and the Environment in Britain, 1813–1949,' *Environment and History* 8 (2002): 381–401; Stephen Murray, 'Bankside Power Station: Planning, Politics and Pollution,' *The Local Historian,* 33 (2003): 99–111; John Sheail, *Power in Trust: The Environmental History of the Central Electricity Generating Board* (Oxford: Oxford University Press, 1991).
42. National Smoke Abatement Society, *Smoke Abatement Handbook,* facing cover; Boon, 'Smoke Menace,' 85; Hugh Gee and Sally Gee, *Pictures in the Fire* (London: British Gas Council, 1947), 32.
43. Bill Luckin, *Questions of Power: Electricity and Environment in Inter-war Britain* (Manchester: Manchester University Press, 1990), 26; Caroline Haslett, 'The New Adventure,' in Peggy Scott, *An Electrical Adventure* (London: Jas. Truscott & Son, 1934), 108–09, p. 109. The issue of drudgery and women's household

work is explored earlier in this volume in chapters by Rhodri Hayward, Jo Gill, and Ali Haggett.

44. Anon., *Smoke Pollution is Sapping the Vitality of the Race* (Leicester: Reader Printing Co., c.1929), 1; *Journal of the National Smoke Abatement Society* 9 (1938): 120.
45. Political and Economic Planning (PEP), *Report on the Gas Industry in Great Britain* (London: Stanhope Press, 1939), 79; *idem, The Market for Household Appliances* (London: Stanhope Press, 1945), 70 and 92–128. See also: Alison Ravetz, *The Place of Home: English Domestic Environments, 1914–2000* (London: E. & F. N. Spon, 1995).
46. Mass Observation, *An Enquiry into People's Homes* (London: John Murray, 1943), 136.
47. PEP, *Household Appliances,* 125; Association for Planning and Regional Reconstruction, *Housing Digest: An Analysis of Housing Reports 1941–1945* (London & Glasgow: Art & Educational Publishers, 1946), 51.
48. Ministry of Fuel and Power, *Domestic Fuel Policy: Report by the Fuel and Power Advisory Council,* Cmd. 6762 (London: HMSO, 1946), Table III, 38. See also: Ministry of Works, Post-War Building Studies No. 19, *Heating and Ventilating of Dwellings* (London: HMSO, 1945), Appendix 1, Heating of Dwellings Inquiry.
49. Coal Utilisation Council, *A Survey into the Domestic Use of Solid Fuel and Solid Fuel Appliances in Great Britain* (London: Coal Utilisation Council, 1953), 14; Mass Observation, *People's Homes,* xvi and 135–41; PEP, *Gas Industry,* 86–87; Marsh, *Smoke,* 216.
50. Margaret Fishenden, 'Solid Fuels and Smoke Prevention,' in Cyril Elliott and Marion Fitzgerald, (eds.), *Homes Fires Without Smoke: A Handbook on the Prevention of Domestic Smoke* (London: Ernest Benn, 1926), 1–16, at p. 4; Raymond Unwin and S. Pointon Taylor, 'Clean Air and Clean Houses,' in Smoke Abatement League of Great Britain, *Smoke Abatement Conference,* 38–44, at p. 43; PEP, *Household Appliances,* Table 12, 116; Women's Advisory Committee on Solid Fuel, *Heating, Cooking and Hot Water Supplies for the Post War House* (London: Unwin Bros., 1944), 9; Ministry of Fuel and Power, *Domestic Fuel Policy,* 13 and 17–19; Robert Roberts, *A Ragged Schooling: Growing Up in the Classic Slum* (Manchester: Manchester University Press, 1976), 73; Ravetz, *Place of Home,* 126–27. Economic and fuel supply issues are examined after 1945 by Catherine Mills in the following chapter.
51. Sydney Bushell and Catherine Gordon, 'The Housewife and Smoke Prevention,' in Elliott and Fitzgerald, *Homes Fires,* 46–58, p. 46.
52. Hermann Muthesius, *The English House* (Oxford: Blackwell Scientific Publications, [1904] 1987), 181.
53. 'Smoke Abatement,' *British Medical Journal* (August 29, 1908): 615; Mass Observation, *People's Homes,* 136–7.
54. 'Domestic Lighting and Heating,' *Nature* 117 (1926): 198; L. C. Parkes and H. A. Des Voeux, 'Discussion on the Smoke Problem in Large Towns,' *Journal of the Royal Sanitary Institute* 28 (1907): 485–506, at p. 505; Ministry of Works, *Heating and Ventilating,* 81; Unwin and Taylor, 'Clean Air,' 44.
55. Alfred T. Schofield, *Directory of Domestic Hygiene, With Hints as to Health, Life, Food, and All Matters Relating to the Person and the Home* (London: Pickering & Inglis, 1927), 131.
56. *Mrs Beeton's Book of Household Management* (London: Ward, Lock & Co., 1906 edn.), 1821–22; M. Cheverton-Brown, *The Property Owners' Handbook* (London: A. Brown & Sons, 1922), 213; Agnes Baden-Powell and Robert Baden-Powell, *The Handbook for Girl Guides: Or How Girls Can Help Build the Empire* (London: Thomas Nelson & Sons, 1912), 345; Leonard Hill,

'Ventilation, Sunshine and Clothing,' in *The Preventive Aspects of Medicine: A Series of Lectures Delivered at King's College Hospital Medical School* (London: The Lancet, 1934), 10–11; C.E.A. Winslow, *Fresh Air and Ventilation* (New York: E. P. Dutton, 1926), 33–50.
57. Schofield, *Directory of Domestic Hygiene*, 136.
58. Thomas Bedford, *Basic Principles of Ventilation and Heating* (London: H. K. Lewis, 1948), 176 and 269; Ministry of Works, *Heating and Ventilating*, Table 3.2, 27; *The Encyclopaedia Britannica, Volume 27*, (Cambridge: Cambridge University Press, 1911), 1009; Lane, *Modern Woman's Home Doctor*, 10; Stewart Swift, *Housing Administration: A Practical Handbook for the Use of Public Health Officials, Students and Others Interested in Housing* (London: Butterworth & Co., 1938), 41.
59. *Parliamentary Debates*, 200 (1926), col. 1837.
60. *Parliamentary Papers* (House of Commons), 1843 (583) VII, q.2062.
61. Ellsworth Huntington, *Civilization and Climate*, 3rd ed. (New Haven, CT: Yale University Press, 1939), esp. 165–73. See also: S. F. Markham, *Climate and the Energy of Nations* (New York: Oxford University Press, 1944); C. E. A. Winslow and L. P. Herrington, *Temperature and Human Life* (Princeton, NJ: Princeton University Press, 1949); Marsha E. Ackerman, *Cool Comfort: America's Romance with Air-Conditioning* (Washington, DC: Smithsonian Institution Press, 2002); Elizabeth Shove, *Cleanliness, Comfort and Convenience: The Social Organization of Normality* (Oxford: Berg, 2003), chapter 2.
62. Leonard Hill, 'Ventilation and Heating,' in Smoke Abatement League of Great Britain, *Smoke Abatement Conference*, 54–58, at p. 55; *idem, Report on Ventilation and the Effect of Open Air and Wind on the Respiratory Mechanism* (London: Jas. Truscott & Son, 1914); *idem, Sunshine and Open Air* (London: Edward Arnold, 1925), 36–44; Leonard Hill and Mark Clement, *Common Colds: Causes and Preventive Measures* (London: William Heinemann, 1929), 25–30 and 86–90.
63. Leonard Hill, Martin Flack, James McIntosh, R. A. Rowlands, and H. B. Walker, *The Influence of the Atmosphere on Our Health and Comfort in Confined and Crowded Places* (Washington, DC: Smithsonian Institution, 1913), 8–9.
64. Harry Roberts, *The Practical Way to Keep Fit* (London: Odhams Press, 1939), 90–91; Hill, 'Ventilation and Heating,' 55; *idem, Sunshine and Open Air*, 37.
65. P. L. Garbutt, 'Healthy Forms of Heating,' in W. Arbuthnot Lane (ed.), *The Golden Health Library*, Volume 5, (London: British Books, 1929–30), 1507–11; Hill, Flack, et al., *Influence of the Atmosphere*, 44.
66. Marie Stopes, 'Domestic Heating,' *Nature* 117 (1926): 343.
67. Coal Utilisation Council, *No.1 Paradise Street: The House of Your Dreams* (London: Coal Utilisation Council, n.d.), 4 and 32.
68. Ibid. 7–8, and 30. For example: Garbutt, 'Healthy Forms of Heating'; and M. Mackenzie, (ed.), *The Family Physician*, Volume 1, 2nd ed. (London: Caxton, 1953), 292–6; PEP, *Gas Industry*, 79.
69. Ministry of Fuel and Power, *Domestic Fuel Policy*, 46–9; Ministry of Works, *Heating and Ventilating*, 16.
70. Ministry of Fuel and Power, *Domestic Fuel Policy*, 34 and 50.
71. Ibid. 5; Ministry of Health, *Interim Report*, 45.
72. Joya Doyle, 'To be Cosy at Home,' in M. Sherman, (ed.), *Daily Mail Ideal Home Book, 1951–52* (London: Associated Newspapers, 1952), 162–71, at p.169; Coal Utilisation Council, *Domestic Use of Solid Fuel*, 14.
73. Simon and Fitzgerald, *Smokeless City*, vii.
74. Ministry of Fuel and Power, *Domestic Fuel Policy*, 45.
75. Helen Meller, *Towns, Plans and Society in Modern Britain* (Cambridge: Cambridge University Press, 1997), 68; Patricia Garside, '"Unhealthy Areas":

Town Planning, Eugenics and the Slums, 1890–1945,' *Planning Perspectives* 3 (1988): 24–46, at p. 42; The Labour Party, *Your Home Planned by Labour* (London: Labour Party, 1943), 14.

76. However, new research suggests that around 7,000 more people lost their lives. See: Devra Davis, *When Smoke Ran Like Water: Tales of Environmental Deception and the Battle Against Pollution* (Oxford: Perseus Press, 2002), 42–54. The influence of London's Great Smog on the smoke abatement movement is discussed in more depth by Catherine Mills in the following chapter.

11 Coal, Clean Air, and the Regulation of the Domestic Hearth in Post-War Britain

Catherine Mills

INTRODUCTION

In July 1956, Anthony Eden's Conservative Government successfully steered a bill for clean air through parliament and on to the Statute book.[1] The Clean Air Act substantially strengthened the regulatory controls in place at the end of the Second World War. It predetermined a national standard of air quality, created a tariff of financial penalties, established a Clean Air Council to monitor pollution levels and co-ordinate research, and removed the necessity for the plaintiff to demonstrate in court that smoke created a nuisance. The main thrust of legislation was the regulation of domestic smoke emissions. The Act encouraged local authorities to introduce and enforce smoke pollution controls: the burning of bituminous coal would be prohibited or heavily restricted in a zone by zone progression across towns and cities, particularly those identified as 'black' by the House of Commons Committee on Air Pollution in 1953, namely urban and industrial areas that were prone to high levels of atmospheric pollution and frequent natural fogs.[2]

The introduction of alternative cleaner fuels for domestic space and water heating posed economic and logistical problems for local authorities, placed an additional financial burden on individual households, and demanded sweeping technological and cultural changes. Moreover, as Stephen Mosley has suggested in the preceding chapter, there was strong and persistent popular resistance to any restriction of domestic coal burning throughout the 1940s and into the 1950s.[3] The traditional open coal fire was regarded by many as a birthright; it provided a cheap source of domestic heat and hot water, a means of hygienic rubbish disposal, and healthy ventilation. The roaring flames symbolised warmth, comfort, and prosperity, and represented the very heart of the home around which family life revolved.[4] A recent study by Peter Thorsheim has also revealed that the nation's coal miners perceived smoke control as a potential threat both to their future employment and to their fiercely guarded concessionary coal allowances.[5]

Yet by 1970, the British love affair with the open coal fire appeared to be in decline. Ninety percent of the 324 'black' authorities had either planned or implemented smoke control programmes.[6] Domestic coal consumption had fallen from 37.5 million tons in 1956 to 19 million tons in 1970.[7] In contrast, sales of electricity for the same period had risen from 23,755 gigawatt-hours to 78,989, and gas from 2,591 million therms to 6,133.[8] This shift in energy sources was reflected in improvements in air quality. Nationally, domestic smoke emissions had fallen from 1.32 million tons in 1956 to 0.64 millions tons in 1970 and sulphur dioxide from 0.88 to 0.5.[9]

Historical accounts of urban air pollution in post-war Britain have largely provided a broad political survey of the background to the 1956 Act.[10] Scholars such as Parker, Brimblecombe, and Ashby and Anderson have argued that the occurrence of the London smog in December 1952, which is now thought to have claimed as many as 12,000 lives, operated as a catalyst for government intervention.[11] Subsequent implementation of policy at local level has attracted very little study. Scarrow has suggested that variables such as a local authority's geographical proximity to established smoke control areas, their status and financial resources, their perception of need, and the nature of their local industry all influenced the speed and success of implementation.[12] This chapter seeks to explain what strategies local authorities employed and exploited to overcome resistance and implement successful smoke control programmes, and how local and national factors shaped these policies.

The opening section of this study draws upon the previous chapter and sets out contemporary tensions at play, which in the post-war period revolved more specifically around the 1956 Act. This is followed by two contrasting local authority case histories of Sheffield, including the small neighbouring Urban District Council of Rawmarsh dominated by coal mining, and Coventry.[13] Sheffield had a reputation for high quality steel products, and for low environmental quality. This contrasts with Coventry's image as a centre of light industry and modern housing. Both authorities were declared 'black' by the Beaver Committee, and subsequently introduced successful smoke control programmes. These two studies highlight the extent to which the home became a focus of government intervention, and expose class and gender dimensions explicit in local initiatives. Local government officials targeted prosperous homes and housewives, partly through the rhetoric of health, but primarily by exposing economic and environmental aspects of pollution in order to convince local populations of the importance of compliance.

CONFLICTING TENSIONS

Although gas and electricity were permitted fuels under the 1956 Act, these were relatively expensive options and it was proposed that coke and manufactured solid smokeless briquettes, such as Coalite and Rexco, would largely replace coal as a domestic energy source.[14] Efficient combustion of solid smokeless fuels required either the adaptation of the traditional open fireplace or the installation of new appliances, together with a gas poker for clean ignition.[15] Slum clearances were underway, and fire grates capable of burning smokeless fuels had been incorporated into Harold Macmillan's ambitious social housing programmes. Nevertheless, the *Committee on Air Pollution* (hereafter the Beaver Committee, named after the chairman Sir Hugh Beaver) estimated that roughly 12 million fireplaces in England and Wales still required conversion in 1953.[16] The average cost per household for the owner-occupier and private tenant was estimated at £10.[17] The local authority was responsible for up to 70 percent of the total costs, but the remaining expense fell to the householder, and only in cases of extreme hardship would a total grant be made available.

Although solid smokeless fuels were of a similar calorific value to coal, they were more expensive, difficult to light, and glowed rather than producing flames. Coke was roughly 50 percent cheaper than the branded smokeless fuels, but supply was dependent on the production of town gas and was often erratic.[18] Domestic supplies of coke had the 'last call' on production, which amounted to roughly 15 to 25 percent of the total.[19] At the end of 1953, carbonisation was only up to pre-war production levels, and a recommendation to increase output had fallen on 'stony ground.'[20] Fireplaces in London County Council Flats in Peckham had been converted to burn coke, but local coal merchants had insufficient supplies to meet their needs.[21] Coke was also bulky, and it was not profitable for fuel merchants to sell small quantities, yet many householders did not have sufficient storage space for an economically viable order. As an anonymous contributor rather flippantly pointed out in the *Medical Officer*, you 'can't lay in stock . . . if you live in a tower block.'[22]

Moreover, coke was often associated with poverty; it was commonly known as 'cinders' particularly amongst the elderly, and often described as 'second hand coal' or 'coal with the goodness burnt out.'[23] Many erroneously believed coke combustion produced toxic fumes that would both poison the occupants of the room,[24] and cause severe damage to the lining of the chimney.[25] In contrast, as Mosley has already suggested, a coal fire was often defended as a healthy heating option.[26] As one Sheffield resident suggested: 'Give me a good coal fire any day. I have to keep warm, I have bronchitis.'[27] Soot and smoke were imbued with antibacterial properties that cleansed the atmosphere, the open grate provided a constant source of ventilation that removed the build up of stale air in the home, and the radiant heat of coal allegedly produced the British complexion and 'nourished' the human body.[28]

Although the Beaver Committee made it abundantly clear that air pollution 'fosters disease and can cause death' and confirmed an association between pollution and 'the incidence of bronchitis and other respiratory disease,' the scientific evidence was equivocal.[29] The specific role of coal smoke in the pathogenesis of respiratory disease was poorly understood. Exposure to polluted air had a non-specific effect, typically but not exclusively on persons already suffering from cardio-respiratory illnesses, particularly the elderly. Establishing a causal relationship between respiratory diseases and air pollution relied on epidemiological studies. Editorial comment in the *Medical Officer* claimed that pioneers in the field had been ridiculed as 'cranks,' and their methodology had been 'thrown back in their teeth by those who like a nice coal fire.'[30] The main criticism was that there was no means of separating out the specific effects of exposure to smoke, which in itself was a chemical cocktail, from environmental factors, such as temperature and background infections.[31] It was also suggested that the introduction of the National Health Service had increased the number of elderly sufferers being kept alive, and dirty air simply advanced their death and artificially inflated rates of mortality.[32] Amongst the industrial working classes, unremitting dirty air and chronic bronchitis had largely become accepted as part of everyday life.[33] As suggested in the preceding chapter, appeals and educational activities had met with only limited success, and abatement activists predicted apathy and resistance to change amongst the urban population, particularly in relation to their health.[34]

Sir Hugh Beaver had identified the 'pressure of public opinion' as a critical factor in securing government interest in domestic smoke control. Demand for reform stemmed from concerned politicians such as Norman Dodds, Member for Dartford, and Anthony Greenwood, Member for Rossenthwaite, public figures such as Caroline Haslett, the president of the Women's Electrical Association, and the National Smoke Abatement Society (NSAS).[35] Dodds had consistently warned of a potential repeat of the London smog disaster as the winter months of 1953 approached, and Greenwood pressured for greater regulation and control.[36] Haslett promoted the use of electricity in the home environment.[37] The NSAS, in contrast, had lobbied parliament for the regulation of domestic emissions since the late nineteenth century, and had funded Gerald Nabarro's Private Members Bill in 1955 in response to the government's apparent indifference to the recommendations of the Beaver Committee.[38]

These individuals and groups of individuals, who were convinced of the environmental and health benefits of smoke control, were a select minority and were far from representative of the industrial working classes. The NSAS was described as a 'voice crying in the wilderness,' whose meetings were 'attended by a few enthusiasts who believed in the cause.'[39] Their membership primarily consisted of local authorities and interested organisations such as the Solid Smokeless Fuels Association (SSFA), and the National Coal Board (NCB). By their own admission, the NSAS had aimed its propaganda at the 'better informed sections of the community.'[40] There had been no substantial grass-roots activism for regulation and control of the domestic hearth since either the London smog disaster in 1952 or the subsequent publication of the Beaver Committee reports, and nothing to indicate that there had been any substantial change in thinking amongst either the mining communities or the majority of urban dwellers burning bituminous coal in the terraces, back-to-backs, and pre-war developments in Britain's industrial cities and towns. Moreover, the claims in West Bromwich that regulation violated 'the right of a householder to manage his own affairs according to his circumstances and inclinations,' following the County Borough's attempts to be the first authority to obtain orders under the 1956 Act, did not bode well for other local authority initiatives.[41]

SHEFFIELD

Set amongst the foothills of the southern Pennines, Sheffield was often described as 'a dirty picture in a beautiful frame.'[42] Residents who were born after 1920 had never seen the cream stone of the civic buildings, buses were withdrawn on roughly fifty days per year, the horizon was never visible, to hang out washing to dry was fruitless, and in 1956 the rate of mortality from bronchitis for the County Borough was roughly 17 percent above the national average.[43]

Two key features contributed to Sheffield's pollution problem: its topography and an economy based on steel. River valleys converge from the south and the west and drain into the main river Don, producing a rough radial pattern. Spurs and bold ridges separate the valleys, and the range of relief extends from 45 metres above sea level in the northeast to 450 metres in the southwest. The city originated at the convergence with the Don and developed out along the valley bottoms. Heavy industry and associated housing largely concentrated in the Don basin to the northeast of the city and the later more prosperous residential developments on high ground to the south and west.[44]

A substantial amount of fuel was required to process steel, and it was estimated that more coal was burned in a 10 square mile area of Sheffield than in any other European city.[45] The close proximity of roughly 15,000 domestic dwellings each with at least one open hearth burning bituminous coal significantly increased the amount of smoke discharged to the atmosphere, and it was claimed that more 'dirt' fell on the industrial east end than anywhere else in the world (Figure 11.1).[46] During the winter months, temperature inversions locked polluted air into the valley bottoms, whilst the surrounding higher ground would often be bathed in sunlight.[47] The landscape produced marked variations in both measured pollutants and individual experiences of dirty air, and highlighted the role of the natural setting of a city in shaping its environmental problems.

In the early 1950s, Llywelyn Roberts, the Medical Officer of Health (MOH) for Sheffield, drew attention both to the significant rise in nuisance complaints from the public and to an improvement in the cooperation shown by industry towards the Corporation's smoke inspectors.[48] The City Authorities, in conjunction with their neighbours, had begun seeking greater controls over both industrial and domestic smoke.[49] In 1955, the Sheffield Citizens' Committee for Clean Air was launched under the direction of the Socialist Medical Association,[50] and in July 1956, the Bishop of Sheffield

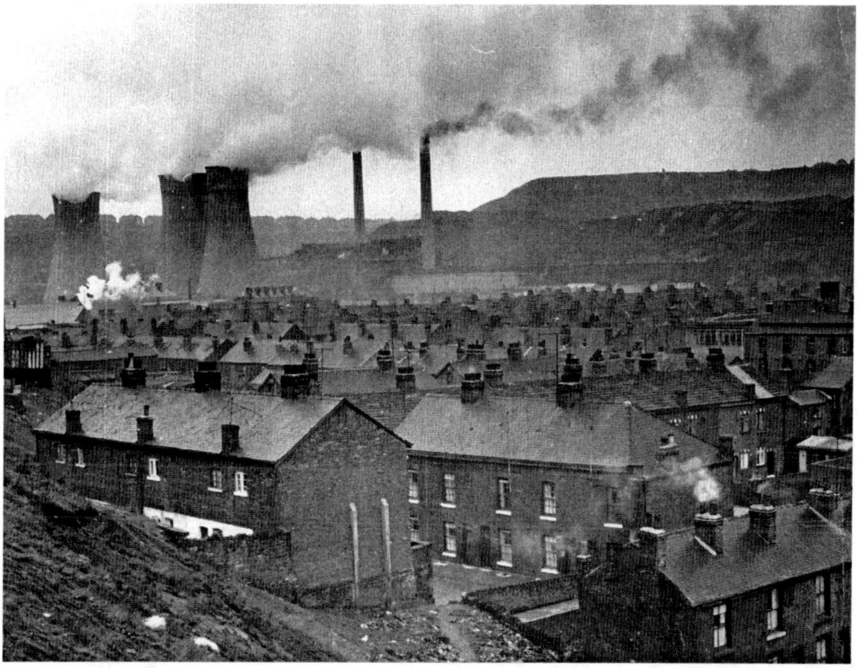

Figure 11.1. Neepsend Power Station in the Don Valley, illustrating the close proximity of housing to industry. Local Studies, Sheffield Libraries.

presided over a 'Brains Trust,' a panel of experts responding to questions on the 'probable effects' of regulation of the city's pollution problem.[51] Roberts suggested that increased support for smoke abatement was a result of post-war coal shortages that had fostered an appreciation for new efficient appliances, and a developing awareness of the effects on health of breathing dirty air highlighted by the London smog deaths of 1952.[52]

However, when regulation of domestic smoke was made possible under the new legislation, public support for clean air appeared to have dwindled. An estimated 90 percent of the city's urban dwellers were identified as either having no interest in, or being openly hostile towards, conversion to smokeless fuels, largely upon the grounds of cost.[53] Local press coverage had probably exacerbated resistance. The *Sheffield Star* reported that legislation would add six pence on to the cost of the rates, and the *Sheffield Telegraph* claimed that the quality of 'coke was in doubt.'[54] To combat any potential public misunderstanding and resistance, the Corporation embarked on an intensive programme of public education largely carried out under the auspices of the Superintendent Smoke Inspector, Joe Batey, known locally as 'Smokey Joe,' together with the Health Education Service.[55] The City Authority had first appointed smoke inspectors in 1854 and, with the exception of a brief period in 1875, the position remained a specialist technological appointment in Sheffield.[56]

Nationally, campaigns to combat resistance and misunderstanding had a long continuity in smoke abatement reaching back to the 1880s.[57] In terms of intervention, Sheffield also had a wealth of experience and support to draw upon. The Corporation had pursued an active smoke abatement policy throughout the nineteenth and early twentieth centuries.[58] The early focus was industrial emissions, and offenders had often been prosecuted with vigour.[59] The Sheffield and Rotherham Clean Air Committee, originally established in 1927, had in its various guises accumulated some 30 years of experience, and was the first of its kind to possess statutory powers of abatement. The intention behind a regional framework was to address the problem of smoke drifting across authority boundaries. Richard Winterbottom, the Labour Member for Sheffield Brightside, had played a prominent role in the drive for national policy initiatives. He maintained active communication between central Government and local industrialists, and had at one time supported the use of nuclear power to alleviate Sheffield's pollution problem.[60] Roberts, Batey and Alderman Patience Sheard, Chair of both Health and Clean Air Committees, were also all active and enthusiastic supporters of the proposed smoke control programme.

The city became the focus of much research, and by the time the first smoke control order became operational in 1959, this provided a readily accessible body of knowledge. In 1949, the University of Sheffield's Fuel Research Department had resumed a programme of research under the direction of Professor R. J. Sergeant. This study was primarily aimed at preventing industrial pollution. Towards the end of 1956, the Medical Research Council had selected the University's Department of Social and Industrial Medicine to study the medical effects of air pollution. Later in 1962, a further research unit was established in the Department of Geography, jointly funded by the Ministry of Technology, the Centre for Environmental Studies, and the Gas Council, to explore pollution problems in relation to the physical environment.[61]

The clean air campaign was intensive. Those living within the proposed smoke control area were visited in their homes, information leaflets were distributed to all ratepayers, the media were provided with data sheets containing 'facts and figures' relating to Sheffield's pollution problem, and a press conference was held.[62] Local women's organisations and youth clubs were targeted. Posters were displayed on the side of all public vehicles. There were competitions, and the library service showed promotional and educational films and handed out free bookmarks and car stickers. The Director of Education sent a circular and teaching material to all school heads suggesting ways in which the clean air campaign could be incorporated into lessons.[63] The promotion culminated in a civic luncheon presided over by Edith Summerskill, Member of Parliament for Warrington and a vocal supporter of clean air, and a public exhibition. According to the local press, Summerskill was deliberately chosen by the Corporation to appeal to women. She carried with her a jar of air, 'Sheffield's muck,' which represented 'dirty curtains, covers and paintwork, doorsteps that turn black, nylon slips that turn grey the minute you put them on, the ceaseless toil in an atmosphere where you hesitate to put your washing out, the backbreaking, heart breaking job of keeping your home clean in an industrial area.' [64]

The notion that the home environment could be harmful in this way resonates with broader themes developed in this volume. As with health educational campaigns directed at women, attempts to ally women in the battle against urban air pollution had a long history, linked to Victorian notions that cleanliness was central to respectability.[65] During the middle decades of the twentieth century, William Beveridge reinforced the role of women as protectors of family health and the home environment.[66] In the post-war years, the idea that the use of an open coal fire 'blackened' a woman's reputation as an effective homemaker, originally asserted by Caroline Haslett in a letter to the *Times,* was a theme that the NSAS fully exploited. [67] Although women had often been featured taking an active part in the more technological aspects of pollution control in the Society's journal, *Smokeless Air,* a conference was organised specifically for women designed to both highlight and promote their potential role in domestic smoke abatement.[68] In 1949, 'Smokeless Homes' was introduced as a regular journal feature, and provided comment on domestic aspects of smoke abatement. The Society reinforced its perception of female responsibilities under the 1956 Act at its annual conference with an afternoon session entitled 'Clean Air and the Housewife,' chaired by Mrs. D. Charlton of the Women's Advisory Council on Solid Fuel.[69] The conversion to cleaner burning fuels also became a theme featured in women's journals, such as an article in *She,* which offered advice on 'Hiding the Fireplace';[70] and in education, clean air became the remit of domestic science rather than of science education.[71] The women of Sheffield and Coventry, where propaganda was less focused and intense (see later discussion), appeared neither to rally to the cause nor to resist reform. Similarly, in West Bromwich, plans to invite a group of housewives to join the County Borough's Clean Air Committee failed to come to fruition.[72] This apparent indifference to smoke control may simply have reflected a continued acceptance of restriction and public control that persisted in the aftermath of war.[73]

Sheffield's public exhibition was declared open by six-year-old Susan Ward, a 'citizen of the future,' who was dressed in white to contrast with the black smoke.[74] The display stands were deliberately placed so that visitors had to move round the exhibition in a clockwise direction designed to show the problem of air pollution, the solutions, and the end result: a clean and modern environment both inside and outside the home.[75] Smoke-damaged lungs were displayed, and the education package for local schools was themed 'Smoke Spells Danger' and contained data relating to respiratory diseases and urban air pollution.[76] Nonetheless, in comparison to civic pride, the potential health benefits of smoke control were minimised.[77] The focus on a clean and attractive urban space was linked into a wider publicity campaign, 'Sheffield on the Move,' which was designed to promote a refashioned image of the city.[78]

A 'low intensity campaign' continued until the first smoke control area became operational on the 1 December 1959 in a small mixed area in the southwest of the city. This was immediately followed by an area containing relatively prosperous suburban housing on the pollution free southern and western fringes of the city. This measure was to serve as a warning to the industrial valleys in the northeast that the Corporation intended to pursue smoke control in an area-by-area extension over the next five years, whilst offering industry, in particular, time to prepare. It also offered the Corporation an administrative and economic advantage. The houses were described as 'of a better class,' built after 1951, and most would already be equipped with closed grates capable of burning smokeless fuel demanded under local by-laws as part of Sheffield's earlier smoke abatement measures.[79] The occupiers were also more likely to be able to afford both the cost of smokeless fuels and the 30 percent charge towards conversion of fire grates if required, and consequently less likely to resist regulation.

From commencement of the first order in 1959 through to 1974, there were only six objections to smoke control, two of which reached the inquiry stage and were subsequently rejected.[80] Public responses to smoke control largely mirrored the Corporation's policy of implementation; householders in the more prosperous residential suburbs that had experienced the benefits of clean air ranked damage to property and contents over health concerns, and openly supported smoke control.[81] Batey had recognised this notion of experience as a positive motivator of change early in the campaign, when he noted that 'the contribution that the domestic chimney makes to the pollution of the city air, is only appreciated when people can see for themselves the improvement in the clarity and cleanliness of the atmosphere.'[82] Although he did not refer to the journal, this concept had been originally advocated in the *Medical Officer* in 1951.[83] In contrast, the residents of Carbrook, a less prosperous area of dense industrial terracing in the Don Valley earmarked for slum clearance, were anxious about their health, but lacked enthusiasm for smoke control despite living in a visibly polluted environment.[84] Nationally most domestic violations involved low-income households.[85] Although in cases of hardship householders could claim the full cost of a modern closed fire grate, there was no similar subsidy for fuel. Only a 'small percentage' of residents initially defied the new regulations,[86] and throughout the period under scrutiny, there was only one prosecution.[87] This may reflect the Corporation's adoption of a policy of persuasion and advice that followed the recommendations of the NSAS, which believed that manpower would be better employed in the extension of smoke control rather than in its enforcement.[88]

By the end of the 1960s, Sheffield was in a position to promote a new image, 'the clean air city,' vigorously supported by the local press, which devoted considerable space to smoke control and the benefits it brought to the city.[89] 'The buildings had lost their soot and grime . . . the horizon was visible on a winter's day . . . housewives could take clean washing from the line and relief was brought to sufferers of bronchitis.'[90] When the final smoke control area became operational in 1972, Sheffield claimed to be the cleanest industrial city in Europe,[91] and in a position to compete in tourism and conference markets. Reflecting the national trend, levels of smoke pollution had fallen from an average 255 micrograms of smoke per cubic meter in 1959 to 47.5 micrograms in 1972, the number of 'smoggy days' had reduced by 80 percent, and the rate of bronchial mortality had fallen in line with the national average.[92] Capitalising on this success, attention was subsequently shifted towards 'invisible pollutants,' particularly from vehicle exhausts.[93]

The picture was different in Rawmarsh. A small urban district council dominated by coal mining, and located fourteen miles northeast of Sheffield, Rawmarsh had remained a member of the Sheffield and District Smoke Abatement Committee despite the withdrawal of neighbouring Rotherham in 1955. Whilst Sheffield celebrated success, Rawmarsh was named and shamed as 'a polluter' in the national press. The Council's civic head Ernest Payne claimed that 'there is nothing like a coal fire . . . smokeless fuels took hours to make a good fire and then had poor heating quality . . . I just do not believe that domestic coal causes damage to health.' He attributed high levels of respiratory disease amongst the urban population to labour in heavy industries.[94]

Rawmarsh was a coal mining community and Payne was an ex-miner, as were a majority of its councillors. Their persistent rejection of government requests to implement smoke control supports assumptions that urban district councils were too small, and the houses of insufficient rateable value, to raise adequate funds to bear the cost implications of smoke control,[95] and that coal mining communities were unwilling to implement changes that would challenge the dominance of the industry or devalue miners' concessionary coal allowance.[96] The high coal consumption per capita in Sheffield, Scarrow suggested, made the progress of the city 'especially impressive.'[97]

COVENTRY

Coventry had been an important engineering centre with a history of car production since the 1890s. During the Second World War, engineering expertise was turned over to the construction of aircraft parts, tanks and armaments. As a consequence the city was heavily bombed. During Operation Moonlight Sonata on 14 November 1942, roughly 4,300 homes and three quarters of the city's factories were destroyed in a single night,[98] and post-war reconstruction removed many of the structural problems experienced in Sheffield.

Plans for redevelopment were ambitious,[99] and Coventry emerged as 'an exemplar of a new type of city, in tune with the demands of a modern, more democratic and equitable age.'[100] As part of the redevelopment programme, the Corporation embarked on the cumbersome process of establishing the authority to both introduce a smokeless zone in 35 acres of the civic and commercial centre of the city, and to demand 'prior approval' of industrial fuel burning installations under a Local Act of Parliament which was granted in 1948.[101] The 1936 *Public Health Act* defined the emissions of smoke, soot, ash, grit and gritty particles as a nuisance, and local authorities were empowered to serve abatement notices and instigate court proceedings for non-compliance. The 1936 Act, however, contained no provision for the declaration of a smokeless zone or 'prior approval'; these measures could only be achieved with the enactment of separate orders.

The Corporation had agreed that failure to protect their new symbols of civic pride and consciousness from the 'blackening and corrosive effects of urban pollution' would be 'a short sighted policy,' without a conscious effort to ensure clean air.[102] When the smokeless zone became operational in March 1951, the city was established as 'the leading authority in the field' of smoke abatement,[103] and claimed an atmosphere that was 'remarkably free of smoke pollution of a serious nature.'[104] It was much to the chagrin of the Chief Public Health Officer (CPHO) Ronald Williams that the city was designated 'black' by the Beaver Committee in 1953.[105]

Implementation of smoke control orders under the 1956 Act began with a process of education and propaganda similar to events in Sheffield. An exhibition entitled 'Down with Smoke' was opened by Sir Hugh Beaver in 1957. It consisted of lectures, demonstrations, displays and a competition to win a modern gas appliance.[106] Posters were displayed in public areas, and a small mobile exhibition stand was created (Figure 11.2).[107] The early emphasis on civic pride continued, since the lower than average national rate of bronchial mortality (0.46 per 1000) in the County Borough offered little health incentive to cleanse the air.[108] Officers of the public health department visited all homes in the proposed smoke control areas to answer questions, assess attitudes, offer advice and information, and preempt any hostility. To combat potential storage difficulties resulting from conversion to smokeless fuels, the Corporation entered into an agreement with the West Midlands Gas Board (WMGB) that deliveries of coke would be made fortnightly.[109]

Although the women of Coventry, as in Sheffield, were targets of clean air propaganda, in contrast the Public Health Department opted to focus on the 'citizens of the future' in the struggle against urban air pollution. Under the auspices of the Warwickshire Clean Air Council, city and county

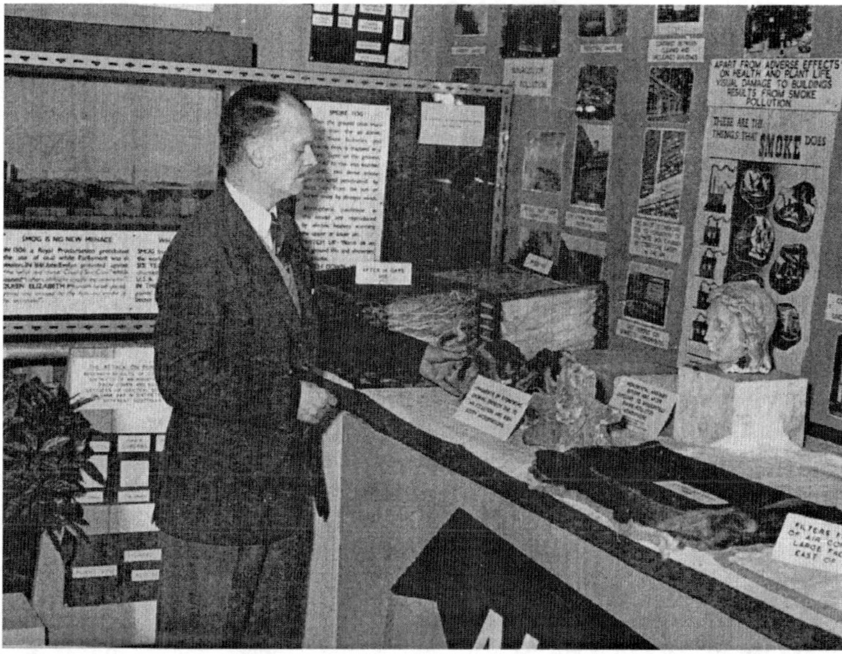
APART FROM ADVERSE EFFECTS ON HEALTH AND PLANT LIFE VISUAL DAMAGE TO BUILDINGS RESULTS FROM SMOKE POLLUTION
THESE ARE THE THINGS THAT SMOKE DOES

Figure 11.2. 'Public Health Inspectors Department Stand, Coventry Clean Air Exhibition 5th–8th February 1957'. Coventry Libraries and Information Service.

schools were provided with pollution monitoring equipment, and senior pupils took daily measurements under the supervision of teaching staff.[110] The instruments were part of Warwickshire's monitoring network and the data was sent to the Corporation analyst.[111] In 1960, a special conference for schoolchildren was held.[112] This became an annual event and involved pupils in demonstrations, lectures, exhibitions, films, and organised visits. In 1963 a tour of the local gas works was arranged for senior pupils to observe the production of smokeless fuels,[113] and a poster competition was devised for junior pupils, both activities designed to 'foster interest in the young minds.'[114]

The first two smoke control orders under the 1956 Act, Tile Hill and Allesley in the west of the city, became operational on 1 September 1961. As in Sheffield, these areas offered the Corporation similar geographical and administrative advantages. Their location ensured the city benefited from the prevailing westerly winds. Tile Hill constituted two large corporation estates already fitted with approved appliances capable of burning smokeless fuels, and Allesley Park comprised a new private development of owner-occupied homes.[115]

In December 1961, Coventry experienced a dense and persistent smog with an attendant rise in mortality from respiratory and cardiac diseases, particularly in the over sixty-fives.[116] A proactive broader based education programme with a much stronger emphasis on health, entitled 'Smoke Kills and Blights,' began the following year. Invitations were sent to ratepayers associations, local societies, women's organisations, and local schools to attend a public exhibition and a discussion.[117] Demonstration vehicles from the WMGB, SSFA, and NCB toured both the operational and proposed smoke control areas.[118] The NCB also opened a Housewarming Centre in the City to supplement the work of the Public Health Department by offering advice, demonstrations, and the opportunity for local authority tenants to view and select replacement appliances before installation.[119]

In 1962 conversion grants were revised in response to impending shortages of coke. This was a result of experiments by the gas industry to produce town gas from oil.[120] The revision offered the householder a wider choice in domestic fuel. It also facilitated the city's Medical Officer of Health, Dr. Thomas Morrison Clayton, in his vigorous encouragement of what was a growing trend towards gas and electrical heating in the city, and initiated a further shift in the focus of the campaign focus towards the promotion of the modern home: '[H]eating one room in our houses and leaving the rest as ice boxes is more appropriate to the stone age and not the space age,' he commented, whilst noting that an unnamed assurance company suggested from their records that elderly people live on average five years longer in a centrally heated home.[121]

Although many residents had pre-empted smoke control orders and voluntarily adopted cleaner burning fuels, there were small pockets of resistance to the early orders.[122] Local coal merchants exploited a loophole in the 1956 Act that was not closed until its amendment in 1968, and continued to sell bituminous coal in smoke control areas.[123] Householders who contravened orders at Tile Hill received letters and were visited by public health officers. A number of tenants experienced difficulty in lighting coke fires. In these instances, the gas board provided individual demonstrations on the use of coke.[124] Allesley Park was a development of predominately young people who were struggling to buy their first home and could ill afford the cost of conversion.[125] Many of these householders initially responded to proposed smoke control 'as a splendid idea,' but enthusiasm had waned when it was understood additional costs were involved, estimated at roughly £6.00 per residence.[126] Although ample warning was given, roughly two thirds of the residents had failed to carry out conversions by the agreed date, and 400 cases were referred to the Health Committee for authority to serve statutory notices. The Chief Public Health Officer, however, believed that the failure to adapt fireplaces was a result of delay during the summer followed by a sudden demand on local builders, rather than a demonstration of strong objections.[127]

The Corporation was vigilant in its enforcement. Fuel merchants who were suspected of supplying or encouraging the use of coal in a smoke control area were reported to their governing body. To prevent a small minority who persistently burnt bituminous coal under the cover of darkness and the weekends, public health staff were drafted onto night and weekend duties. These offences, Morrison Clayton believed, were motivated by a desire to 'get one up on the Corporation.' Like Joe Batey in Sheffield, he too similarly observed that once the benefits of clean air had been experienced individual resistance dissipated.[128]

Local economic difficulties in the late 1960s resulted in a temporary suspension of smoke control orders until the early 1970s.[129] Fortunately for the Corporation, emissions of smoke had peaked in 1963 at 130 micrograms per cubic meter and from then onwards had declined steadily. By 1966, only 30 percent of homes still used smokeless fuel as their primary source of heat; the remaining 70 percent used piped fuels, of which 15 percent had whole house or central heating.[130]

CONCLUSION

For both Sheffield and Coventry Corporations, the potential obstacles that cleansing the air posed in 1956 were either self-limiting or readily resolved. The financial provisions contained within the Clean Air Act eased some of the economic burden of conversion to modern and efficient fire grates for individual households. Local government officials addressed the technological and cultural challenges posed by smoke control through the medium of public education campaigns, designed to dispel residual ignorance and misconceptions surrounding both solid smokeless fuels and the 'cosy coal fire.'

Scarrow has argued that there was an emerging trend in the use of cleaner burning fuels, and it is difficult to evaluate the success of the local authority campaigns. [131] On the eve of Sheffield's first order in 1959, a large majority of the city's population still believed that smoke control would entirely prohibit an open fire in the home.[132] As pointed out in the late 1970s in relation to smoke control in Manchester, 'an absolute standard made offenders so obvious they were quickly reported by the public or neighbours.'[133] However, once householders had been regularly supplied with coke of a consistent quality and practice had led to satisfactory methods of combustion, there was minimal resistance to the prohibition of the coal fire in the two local authorities. With the exception of the coal mining districts, particularly in Yorkshire, this was generally the position for England as a whole.[134] Inadequate supplies of coke often resulted in a suspension of orders specific to individual localities.[135] Although it is unclear whether the programme in Sheffield was impeded, in Coventry scarcity of coke led to the promotion of piped fuels.

The promotion of clean and efficient heating systems in the domestic environment by city authorities paralleled and fed into wider campaigns to refashion and modernise the urban space. Although it is possible to suggest that the technological background of Joe Batey explains the stronger emphasis on civic pride as opposed to health imperatives in Sheffield's clean air campaign, Batey worked in close liaison with Roberts, the city's Medical Officer of Health. Roberts, however, had already adopted an environmental focus in the city's slum clearances, and stressed the need to stimulate an appreciation not only of improved housing but also of their immediate surroundings.[136] Similarly, Beaver, in a paper presented before the NSAS's annual conference at Scarborough in 1954, had also asked 'that people turn their minds' to the 'oasis in the centre of Manchester,' the 'clean white' of Nottingham's suburbs, and 'other civic efforts.'[137]

Pollution problems varied greatly between the two cities, and explanation for the variance in emphasis placed on health imperatives between the two campaigns may lie in differing perceptions of risk. Sheffield's dirty air was unremitting but familiar, and attendant health risks had become an accepted part of everyday life. Coventry, in contrast, experienced episodic smog against a backdrop of relatively clean air and the early introduction of smoke control. It was the unfamiliarity of the increase in morbidity and mortality from cardio-respiratory diseases that provoked the health initiatives behind Coventry's campaign, and the arousal of health anxieties expressed by residents of the Don Valley, who had the misfortune to witness both episodic and chronic high levels of smoke pollution.[138]

The ambiguity of health imperatives in the local histories of smoke control parallels the preliminary analysis of the relationship between respiratory health and the politics of clean air within the national context. This suggests that health anxieties were often obscured by competing tensions in the political, socio-economic, and medical arenas, and were visibly influential only at the time of the London smog disaster in 1952. In the immediate post-war period there was grumbling unease surrounding the incidence of disease in urban rather than rural settings. The medical evidence was equivocal and what little debate there was on air pollution focused upon fuel efficiency. The publication of Doll and Hill's cohort study in 1957, establishing a close correlation between cigarette smoking and respiratory diseases, largely displaced the anxieties surrounding urban air pollution.[139]

It is unlikely that a campaign promoting health would have been any more successful in achieving local smoke control. It was only when the polluted atmosphere was cleansed and the benefits became tangible, in terms of both health and the material environment, that an interested response, albeit still rather muted, was observed. However, if popular enthusiasm for smoke control was dependent on personal experience of clean air, the method of implementation adopted by local authorities disadvantaged those who were most likely to benefit from reform. The zone-by-zone expansion that focused upon new corporation housing and the prosperous residential suburbs denied the occupants of the urban industrial terraces the advantages of early progress, and the experience of a smoke-free environment, that would in turn promote a greater desire for change.

ACKNOWLEDGEMENTS

This chapter forms part of an ongoing and more extensive postdoctoral project exploring the relationship between respiratory health and the politics of clean air in post-war Britain 194–1975 generously funded by the Wellcome Trust. Thanks are also due to Donald Hindmarsh and the staff at Local Studies, Sheffield Libraries, Sheffield Archives, and Andrew Mealey, Coventry Libraries and Information Service, for their assistance.

NOTES

1. 4 & 5 Eliz.2, Clean Air Act, 1956 Ch. 52.
2. *Committee on Air Pollution, Interim Report,* Cmd. 9011 (hereafter *Beaver-Interim*), British Parliamentary Papers, 1953, Appendix 1 Map; Air Pollution.
3. See Stephen Mosley's chapter in this volume.
4. S. Mosley, *The Chimney of the World: A History of Smoke Pollution in Victorian and Edwardian Manchester (*Cambridge: White Horse Press, 2001), 69–78.
5. P. Thorsheim, *Inventing Pollution: Coal, Smoke and Culture in Britain since 1800,* 'Smokeless Zones' (Ohio: Ohio University Press 2006), Chapter 11, 173–192; also see R. Parker, 'The Struggle for Clean Air,' in P. Hall, H. Land, R. Parker, and A. Webb (eds.) *Change Choice and Conflict in Social Policy* (London, 1975), 371–409 at p. 381.
6. H. A. Scarrow, 'The Impact of British Domestic Air Pollution Legislation,' *British Journal of Political Science,* 2:2 (1972): 262–82, Tables 1 and 2, at p. 265.
7. B. L. Mitchell, *British Historical Statistics* (1988), 258–9.
8. Mitchell, *Statistics,* 264 and 269.
9. *National Survey of Air Pollution 1961–71,* Volume 1, Warren Spring Laboratory (HMSO, 1972), Table 2:1, 11.
10. E. Ashby and M. Anderson, *The Politics of Clean Air* (Oxford, 1981); P. Brimblecombe, *The Big Smoke: A History of Air Pollution in London since Medieval Times* (London, 1987); M. Jackson, 'Cleansing the air and promoting health,' in V. Berridge and K. Loughlin (eds.), *Medicine, the Market and the Mass Media: Producing Health in the Twentieth Century* (London: Routledge, 2005), 221–43; and Parker, 'Clean Air,' 371–409. For discussion on number of deaths see M. L. Bell, D. L. Davis, and T. Fletcher, 'A Retrospective Assessment of Mortality from the London Smog Episode of 1952: The Role of Influenza and Pollution,' *Environmental Health Perspectives,* 112, 1 (2004): 6–8.
11. Ashby and Anderson, *The Politics of Clean Air;* Brimblecombe, *The Big Smoke;* Parker, 'Clean Air.'
12. Scarrow, 'Air Pollution Legislation,' 262–82
13. The selection of Sheffield and Coventry for study was largely determined by the survival of extensive documentary evidence.
14. *Committee on Air Pollution, Report,* Cmd. 9322 (hereafter *Beaver-Report*), British Parliamentary Papers, 1954, paragraph 72.
15. The question of gas poker was raised by Edith Summerskill, Member for Warrington, see *Hansard,* Vol. 545, House of Commons, 3 November, 1955, col. 1246.
16. *Beaver-Interim,* para. 59.
17. *Beaver-Report*, para. 86.

18. See *Hansard,* House of Lords, 18th November, 1953, col. 389, Earl of Selkirk.
19. *Medical Officer* (6 October 1951): 141.
20. *Medical Officer* (12 December 1953): 280.
21. Comment by Freda Corbet, Peckham, *Hansard,* Vol. 563, House of Commons, 4 February, 1955, col. 1465.
22. 'Chapter on Fog,' *Medical Officer* (12 December 1953): 280.
23. *Beaver-Report,* para. 79.
24. *Beaver-Report,* para. 81.
25. See debate, *Hansard,* House of Lords, 24 April 1956, col. 1168, Lord Amulree.
26. See Mosley's chapter in this volume.
27. Comments of an elderly resident of Mushroom Lane, Sheffield to a journalist and subsequently reported in the *Sheffield Star,* 1 December 1959, cited in C. Binfield, R. Childs, R. Harper, D. Hey, D. Martin, and G. Tweedale (eds.), *The History of Sheffield 1843–1993,* Vol. I, 'Politics,' 'Optimism and Growth 1951–1973,' 119–205 at p. 131.
28. Mosley, *Chimney of the World,* 78–84; S. Mosley, 'Fresh Air and Foul: The Role of the Open Fire Place in Ventilating the British Home 1837–1910, *Planning Perspectives,* 18 (2003): 1–21; and Jackson, 'Cleansing the Air,' 225.
29. *Beaver-Report,* paras. 12–23.
30. *Medical Officer* (19 July 1952): 25.
31. Ibid.
32. Parker, 'Clean Air,' 377–8.
33. Ibid. 377.
34. See Mosley's chapter in this volume; A. Marsh, *Smoke: The Problem of Coal and the Atmosphere* (London 1947) 265.
35. For reference to Women's Electrical Association, see B. Luckin, *Questions of Power: Electricity and the Environment in Interwar Britain* (Manchester 1990), Chapter 3, 'Targeting Women,' 39–51.
36. For examples see Greenwood's speech on smoke pollution, *Hansard,* Vol. 484, House of Commons, 27 February 1951, cols. 2056–2069, and for Dodd, see *Hansard,* Vol. 515, House of Commons, 8 May 1953, cols. 845–856.
37. *The Times,* 'Letters to the Editor' (12 December 1952): 9e.
38. See B. Sanderson, 'The National Smoke Abatement Society and the Clean Air Act,' *Political Studies,* 9 (1961): 236–56.
39. *Medical Officer* (17 October 1953), Notes and Comments, 'Smoke Abatement Winning the Battle,' 186.
40. Sanderson, 'The National Smoke Abatement Society,' 238.
41. *The Times* (15 April 1957), 7a; *Midland Chronicle and Free Press,* 26 October 1956, p. 8, and 12 April 1957. Smoke control began in West Bromwich in 1958.
42. G. Wall, 'A Preliminary Report on the Perception of Air Pollution in Sheffield, Paper presented at a seminar on the social dimensions of air pollution,' University of Edinburgh, 2–4 January, 1972, Local Studies, Sheffield Libraries, 6.
43. Data sourced from *The Registrar-General's Statistical Review of England and Wales* (London: HMSO, 1956).
44. For description of the topography see A. Garnett, 'Sheffield Emerges from Smoke and Grime,' *Geographical Magazine* (November 1970): 123–8 at p. 123.
45. D. Peschek, 'Sheffield—The Clean Air City,' *Town Hall Talk,* Vol. 18, No. 110 (October 1971): 28–9.
46. *Medical Officer of Health for Sheffield, Annual Report* (hereafter *MOH-Sheffield) (*1949), 86.
47. A. Garnett, 'Climate, Relief, and Atmospheric Pollution in the Sheffield Region,' *Advancement of Science,* 13 (1957): 331–41 at p. 331.

48. During the period 1952 to 1953 complaints had risen from 87 to 167: *MOH-Sheffield,* 1953, 127.
49. Binfield et al. (eds.), *Sheffield,* 130.
50. Ibid.
51. 'Clean Air,' *Quality of Sheffield* (July 1956), 32.
52. *MOH-Sheffield,* 1952, 142.
53. 'Clean Air,' *Quality of Sheffield* (July 1956), 32; also see 'Sheffield Clean Air Report 1959/60' (hereafter Sheffield Clean Air Report), which is a scrapbook of mementos and newspaper cuttings collected for the MOH by his Health Education Officer, SY 11/21/1, Sheffield Archive Service, 8.
54. 'Sheffield Clean Air Report,' 65 and 81.
55. 'Sheffield Clean Air Report,' 1 and 3.
56. J. W. Batey, 'Cleaner Air and Smoke Abatement,' 216–8 at p. 217 in *MOH-Sheffield,* 1956.
57. Thorsheim, *Inventing Pollution,* 94–9.
58. Batey, 'Cleaner Air,' 216–8.
59. Ibid.
60. Binfield et al. (eds.), *Sheffield,* 130. Also see bundle of correspondence, reference CA 151/1 Sheffield Archive Service.
61. Garnett, 'Sheffield,' 123–8 at p. 126.
62. 'Sheffield Clean Air Report,' 2.
63. Ibid.
64. Cited in unreferenced news cutting in 'Sheffield Clean Air Report,' 54.
65. See Thorsheim, *Inventing Pollution,* 81; also see ibid. pp. 80–109.
66. W. Beveridge, *Special Insurance and Allied Services,* 1942 (Cmd. 64040) (London: HMSO, reprint 1968), and *Voluntary Action, A Report on Social Advance* (London 1948), 264. Also see: N. Tomes, 'The Private Side of Public Health: Sanitary Science, Domestic Hygiene, and Germ Theory 1870–1900,' *Bulletin of the History of Medicine,* 64 (1990): 509–39; A. Gugliotta, 'Class, Gender and Coal Smoke: Gender Ideology and Environmental Justice in Pittsburgh, 1868–1914,' *Environmental History,* 5, 2 (2000): 165–93; H. L. Platt, *Shock Cities: The Environmental Transformation and Reform of Manchester and Chicago* (Chicago, 2005), 468–91; and S. M. Hoy, 'Municipal Housekeeping: The Role of Women in Improving Urban Sanitation Practices, 1880–1917,' in M. V. Melosi (ed.), *Pollution and Reform in American Cities 1870–1930* (Texas 1980), 173–98.
67. *The Times* (12 December 1952), 9e.
68. 'Women of the Future,' *Smokeless Air,* 8 (1941): 34; and 'The Homes of Tomorrow,' *Smokeless Air,* 9 (1941): 64–9.
69. 'Smoke Abatement Conference,' *Medical Officer* (12 October 1956): 230.
70. *She* (July 1956): 54.
71. For example see E. F. Stephen, *Solid Fuel Housecraft* (London, 1950), and A. M. Kaye 'Teaching Clean Air,' *Smokeless Air,* 1, 2 (1939): 55.
72. Public protest succeeded in obtaining a postponement of orders until 1 November 1958. See note 36 above and *The Times* (27 November 1957), 7a.
73. I am grateful to Professor Virginia Berridge for this interesting suggestion.
74. *MOH-Sheffield,* 1959, 193.
75. 'Sheffield Clean Air Report,' 7.
76. Ibid., 1.
77. Ibid.
78. Wall, 'Preliminary Report,' 10.
79. Wall, 'Preliminary Report,' 3.
80. 'A History of the Campaign Against Pollution in Sheffield and District,' paper presented by A. Maule, Senior Advisor, Sheffield and District Clean Air

Committee, at the Clean Air Spring Seminar 26th to 28th March, National Society for Clean Air, Brighton, p. 5 (Miscellaneous Papers MP5081M), Sheffield Local Studies Library.
81. Wall, 'Preliminary Report,' 14.
82. *MOH-Sheffield,* 1958, 20.
83. *Medical Officer* (6 October 1951), Notes and Comments, 'Coke as a Smoke Reducer,' 141.
84. Wall, 'Preliminary Report,' 13.
85. Scarrow, 'Pollution Legislation,' 282
86. G. Tomlin, 'Civic Warning to Clean Air Abusers,' *Sheffield Telegraph* (3 December 1959), 7.
87. Scarrow, 'Pollution Legislation,' 282.
88. Ibid.
89. Wall, 'Preliminary Report,' 9–10.
90. Peschek, 'Sheffield,' 28.
91. Boundary shuffles actually thwarted this claim, and Sheffield was finally declared 'smokeless' in 1985. See data taken from *The Ambient Air Quality Monitoring Strategy for Sheffield,* Health and Consumer Services (no publication details, typed report received by Sheffield Local Studies 7th July 1992), paragraph 2.4, p. 8.
92. Peschek, 'Sheffield,' 29. The national rate of bronchial mortality was 0.6 per 1000, data sourced from *The Registrar-General's Statistical Review of England and Wales* (London: HMSO, 1972).
93. See 'Cleaner Air for Sheffield—The Air Quality Action Plan' and 'Promoting Clean Air in Sheffield-What We Can All Do!,' Sheffield City Council, Local Studies, Sheffield Libraries, Miscellaneous Papers 5627M.
94. *The Times* (25 March 1970), 12.
95. Scarrow, 'Pollution Legislation,' 267–70.
96. See Thorsheim, *Inventing Pollution;* Scarrow, 'Pollution Legislation,' 269–70.
97. Scarrow, 'Pollution Legislation,' 270.
98. See D. McGrory, 'The Coventry Blitz' at http://www.CWN.org.UK/heritage/blitz.
99. See P. Hubbard, L. Fare and K. Lilley, 'Remembering Post-war Reconstruction: Modernism and City Planning in Coventry 1940–1962' at http://www-staff.lboro.ac.uk/~gypjh/history.html, and J. Hasegawa, *Replanning the Blitzed City Centre* (Oxford: Oxford University Press, 1992), 4. 'Replanning the City Centre—Coventry 1940–45,' 30–46.
100. N. Tiratso, *Reconstruction, Affluence and Labour Politics, Coventry 1945–1960* (London, 1990), 1.
101. 11 & 12 Geo. 6, xxxvi, *Coventry Corporation Act,* 1948.
102. *Annual Report of Chief Public Health Officer for Coventry* (hereafter *CPHO-Coventry*), 1957, 22.
103. *Medical Officer of Health for Coventry, Annual Reports* (hereafter *MOH-Coventry*), 1957, 8.
104. *Coventry Evening Telegraph* (hereafter *CET*) (28 February 1951), p. 5, cols. 2–3.
105. *CPHO-Coventry,* 1958, 30.
106. *CET,* 22nd January, 1957, p. 8, cols. 5–6.
107. *CPHO-Coventry,* 1957, 24.
108. Data sourced from *The Registrar-General's Statistical Review of England and Wales* (London: HMSO, 1956).
109. *CET,* 14th November, 1957, p. 6, cols.3–6.
110. *CPHO-Coventry,* 1957, 14; also see *The Times* (8 December 1959), 17g.
111. *CET,* 29th December 1959, p. 12 col. 2.
112. *CPHO-Coventry,* 1960, 30.

113. *CPHO-Coventry,* 1962, 43.
114. *CPHO-Coventry,* 1961, 35.
115. *CET,* 5th November, 1957, p. 11, cols. 1–2.
116. *CPHO-Coventry,* 1961, 37.
117. *CPHO-Coventry,* 1962, 40.
118. *CPHO-Coventry,* 1962, 26.
119. *CPHO-Coventry,* 1963, 39.
120. *CPHO-Coventry,* 1963, 26.
121. *MOH-Coventry*, 1963, 12–3.
122. *CPHO-Coventry,* 1961, 29.
123. *CPHO-Coventry,* 1968, 46.
124. *CPHO-Coventry,* 1961, 29.
125. *CET,* 4th December, 1957, p. 3, col. 5.
126. *CET,* 14th November, 1957, p. 6, cols. 3–6.
127. *CPHO-Coventry,* 1961, 28.
128. *MOH-Coventry*, 1963, 13.
129. *CPHO-Coventry,* 1960, 26.
130. *CPHO-Coventry,* 1966, 46.
131. Scarrow, 'Pollution Legislation,' 276–7.
132. *MOH-Sheffield*, 1959, 194.
133. C. Malcolm, 'Smokeless Zones-The History of Their Development, Part 2, The Development of Smokeless Zones 1934–1958,' *Clean Air* (Spring 1977): 4–10 at p. 8.
134. 'The Clean Air Conference,' *Medical Officer* (10 October 1958): 231.
135. Parker, 'Clean Air,' 404.
136. L. Roberts, 'Post War Slum Clearances,' *The Medical Officer* (8 March 1952): 191
137. See 'Beaver Archives,' London School of Economics, 40/4/76 D23. Beaver's address was also reported in *Medical Officer* (1 October 1954): 179.
138. Broad parallels can be drawn here with 'fright factors' in current theories of risk perception. P. Bennett and K. Calman (eds.), *Risk, Communication and Public Health* (Oxford: Oxford University Press, 1999), 6.
139. See R. Doll, 'The First Reports on Smoking and Lung Cancer,' in S. Lock, L. A. Reynolds, and E. Tansey (eds.), *Ashes to Ashes: The History of Smoking and Health* (Amsterdam: Rodopi, 1998), 130–42.

12 Cockroaches, Housing, and Race

A History of Asthma and Urban Ecology in America*

Gregg Mitman

INTRODUCTION

On July 7, 1961, a 46-pound, 12-year-old, malnourished boy from a Rio de Janeiro *favela*—or slum—stepped off a plane in Denver hoping to escape the shackles of poverty and longing for a life free from the struggle to breathe. It was just one week after photojournalist Gordon Parks's exposé of life among Latin America's urban poor appeared in *Life* magazine. Flavio da Silva had been living with his family in Catacumba, one of the many squatter settlements of Rio. The family had fled the rural poverty of northeastern Brazil in search of a better life, but had found instead—like many of the *favelados,* or slum dwellers, that made up roughly 10 percent of the city's population—an equally harsh existence in the urban environment. Illness, exacerbated by poverty, had taken its toll on the eldest da Silva son. At night, or when the smoke of the open cooking fire filled the da Silvas's six-by-ten-foot home, Flavio would succumb to violent coughing. With heaving chest, blue-tinged skin, and throbbing veins, his whole body would be consumed in the fight to breathe. This fight with bronchial asthma had left a visible mark on the boy; when doctors at the Children's Asthma Research Institute and Hospital (CARIH) in Denver saw Flavio in *Life,* they recognized his expanded chest and knew its cause. Convinced that the boy, in their institution, could be saved from the death that would soon meet him in his Rio slum, CARIH doctors wrote to the magazine's editors and offered free treatment. Other concerned and inspired Americans also reached out, sending hundreds of letters and donations to *Life* to help rescue Flavio from a life without hope.[1]

Gordon Parks, *Life*'s first African-American photographer, had been sent to Brazil in March of 1961 to capture in pictures and words the tragedy of poverty in Latin America. His article focused on the life of Jose da Silva, his wife, and their eight children. It was the second of a five-part series titled 'Crisis in Latin America' that *Life*'s editorial board had planned for that spring. Fearful that poverty, widespread illiteracy, and social injustice offered a fertile ground for Communist revolution, President John F. Kennedy announced early in his administration a $500-million plan—the Alliance for

Progress—to end hunger, disease, and illiteracy in Latin America. While Kennedy's advisors struggled with how to implement their Cold War plans for universal education and economic development in the Western Hemisphere, Americans took comfort that summer in knowing that the compassion of a nation had rescued Flavio, a 'symbol of impoverished millions,' from the grip of want, disease, and despair.[2]

But while the nation seemed fixated on this Brazilian child, the weak cries of American children, suffocating under the weight of economic, environmental, and racial injustice, remained largely unheard. When a *Life en Español* version of Parks's article appeared, the Brazilian magazine *O Cruziero* was outraged by the hypocrisy in America's neglect of its own urban poor and sent reporters to document the harsh conditions of New York City's slums. Unfamiliar with the city's geography, the *O Cruziero* reporters searched the Wall Street district and chose a Puerto Rican family as their subject. Several staged shots later—a sleeping child covered in cockroaches, another crying in anguish from hunger—their work was done.[3] The *O Cruzeiro* reporters need not have gone to such lengths if they had only known where to look. In New York City, Chicago, New Orleans, and other American cities, conditions of despair approximating those of Catacumba were commonplace, even if a veil of inattention kept them hidden. As the Spanish Harlem writer and activist Piri Thomas observed, in America 'there ain't no bright sunlight to reveal the stark naked truth of garbage-lepered streets.'[4]

The truth of America's urban ghettoes—overcrowded conditions and decaying housing, high infant mortality, crime, poverty, and disease—began to well up in the early 1960s. So, too, did asthma, a disease that had mysteriously begun disproportionately to afflict African-Americans and Puerto Ricans living in poor urban neighbourhoods. Some 40 years later, public health experts, physicians, and community activists have expressed dismay at the alarming increase of childhood asthma morbidity and mortality at the turn of the millennium, particularly among people of colour living in impoverished inner city communities. Among Blacks and Latinos in New York City, for example, hospitalization and death rates are 3 to 5 times those of Whites. In East Harlem, where hospitalization rates for asthma are 10 times the national average, an estimated 23 percent of children suffer from the disease.[5] To date, a host of factors, including genetic differences based on ethnicity, socioeconomic status, exposure to dust mite and cockroach allergens, air pollution, and inadequate access to health care, have been cited to account for asthma's rise. But the roots of this urban public health crisis extend deep into our past, at least as far back as when Flavio first came to the United States to be cured. Under what conditions asthma became visible in urban America, and how those conditions of visibility and invisibility have shaped divergent explanations and strategies for action, is the subject of this chapter. America's urban asthma epidemic, long in the making, is a product of the ecology of injustice that structures urban space and life.

ASTHMA, GEOGRAPHY, AND RACE

In the fall of 1962, Dr. Leonard Greenburg noticed something peculiar about the pattern of emergency clinic admissions for asthma reported by New York City hospitals. Greenburg had spent the past decade looking for convincing evidence of a link between air pollution and higher rates of illness and death in New York City. As the first commissioner of New York City's Department of Air Pollution Control, he had been relatively ineffective in containing the city's growing air pollution menace. Even when a six-day siege of smoke, haze, and smog paralyzed the city in November of 1953—shutting down LaGuardia Airport, crippling commuter traffic, and halting bus service—Greenburg was unable to mobilize city officials to take action.[6] Despite sulphur dioxide concentrations that far surpassed those of London's 1952 killer fog and regardless of increased hospital admissions, Greenburg could offer little proof that air pollution jeopardized the health of New York City's residents. Without sufficient funds, staff, political will, or conclusive scientific data, Greenburg could do little but watch as major polluters, such as the electric company Consolidated Edison, and numerous apartment-house incinerators added to the thousands of tons of particulate matter, sulphur dioxide, and other air pollutants each year. When he resigned as air pollution commissioner in 1960 to take up a position as professor and chairman of the department of preventive and environmental medicine at Yeshiva University, Greenburg devoted his career to finding the smoking gun that he lacked as chief watchdog and regulator of New York City's air quality.[7] Many physicians assumed that a relationship existed between air pollution and asthma, suspecting that air pollution contributed to increased sickness and death. To test this assumption, Greenburg combed the records of New York City hospitals during periods of high levels of air pollution looking for a corresponding increase in asthma patient admissions. But Greenburg found no such correlation. What he did find was far more puzzling and surprising.[8]

Increasing numbers of asthma patients had been inundating emergency rooms in New York City over the previous decade with no obvious correlation to days of poor air quality. Among four New York City hospitals, Greenburg and his colleagues found a two-and-one-half- to eightfold increase in the number of asthma visits to emergency clinics from 1952 to 1962. No one knew the cause. But two hospitals stood out, both located in upper Manhattan and serving poor, minority communities. At Harlem Hospital, located on Lenox Avenue between 136th Street and 137th Street, one out of every four visits to the emergency room, excluding trauma and obstetric visits, was for asthma. At Metropolitan Hospital, located on East 97th Street and Second Avenue, one out of every seven visits was for asthma.[9]

Similar patterns were occurring in other major U.S. cities. Beginning in August 1958, officials from the United States Public Health Service and their affiliated Robert H. Taft Sanitary Engineering Laboratory in Cincinnati,

Ohio, worked closely with Tulane University researchers to investigate a recurring asthma epidemic in New Orleans. Since the mid 1950s, an unusual annual pattern of spikes in asthma admissions to Charity Hospital, which catered to the city's urban poor, appeared each summer and fall. The New Orleans asthma zone—the communities that radiated outward from Clairborne Avenue, the thriving main street of New Orleans' Black community and main thoroughfare of the city's largest African-American Mardi Gras parade—was surrounded by three of the largest city landfills, one of which was known to local residents as Dante's Inferno because of the spontaneous ignition of toxic chemicals that occurred during the drier months of the year. October and November were the worst months. On some days, more than 200 patients, many of them under the age of 30, streamed into the emergency room for the first time, struggling to breathe. On normal days, the average number of asthma admissions was 25.[10] By the early 1960s, the fall outbreaks of asthma among poor, African-American communities in New Orleans had become so common that local New Orleanians referred to the annual event as the fifth season.[11] An emerging epidemic appeared tied to the urban ecology of America's inner cities and was symptomatic of the disparate spaces in which Americans lived and breathed.

The environmental conditions endured by the African-American community that Harlem Hospital served were as bad as those faced by the asthma patients of New Orleans. The great migration of Blacks from the rural South to northern industrial centers after the First World War had turned Harlem into a vibrant centre of Black literary and artistic life during the 1920s and continued apace after the Second World War. Fleeing Jim Crow and a depressed agricultural economy, 1.5 million African-Americans left during the 1950s what Kenneth Clark described as the 'miasma of the South, where poverty and oppression kept the Negro in an inferior caste.'[12] Seeking educational and economic opportunities in the North, Blacks encountered instead the harsh realities of an urban environment isolated spatially, socially, and economically from the goods, services, and employment that sustained the health of the city and the majority of its White residents.

Of the 240,000 residents who lived in 1960 in Central Harlem (a three-and-one- half square mile area lying between 110th Street to the south and the Harlem River to the northeast) 94 percent were African-American. Limited largely to low-paying, unskilled or semi-skilled service jobs, Harlem residents earned one-third less than the average New Yorker. A severe housing shortage coupled with inflated rents resulted in overcrowded and dilapidated housing conditions that were unparalleled elsewhere in the city. Decaying tenement buildings built before 1929 provided the bulk of available housing. Slum landlords showed up when high rents were due but were absent when renters pressed for repairs. More than half of the housing units in Harlem were classified in the 1960 Census as unsafe, inadequate, or in need of major repair. Many units lacked heat or plumbing; often apartment dwellers relied upon gas ovens as their only source of warmth in cold winter months. 'Rats and roaches,' one resident living on West 117 Street complained, 'were literally moving the tenants out of the building.' More often than not, the Department of Health failed to prosecute landlords for housing code violations.[13]

Such conditions, exacerbated by the discriminatory policies of the city's social and health agencies, led to significant health disparities. The infant mortality rate in Central Harlem was nearly double that of New York City as a whole in 1961. Tuberculosis afflicted twice as many Harlem residents as it did those living in the rest of the city. Poverty, poor housing, and inadequate access to medical care were just a few of the factors that contributed to a population vulnerable to diseases that were less threatening under other economic and ecological circumstances. In the 1960s, few middle-class suburban Whites were likely to view asthma as a deadly illness. But nearly half of New York City's poor, Black welfare mothers surveyed in 1966 considered asthma to be a very serious disease.[14]

Similar conditions of poverty, degraded housing, and poor quality health care prevailed in the neighbourhood served by Metropolitan Hospital, where Greenburg's team found the second highest rate of hospital asthma admissions in New York City. Located on the southern edge of Spanish Harlem, heart of New York City's Puerto Rican community, Metropolitan became the primary health-care provider for the city's poor, Hispanic population. In the prosperous post-war economy of the United States, many Puerto Ricans saw migration as a path to upward social mobility. Of the roughly 800,000 Puerto Ricans who came north for low-paying jobs in the blue-collar trades and manufacturing industries between 1940 and 1960, almost 80 percent flew from San Juan to New York City.[15] Many expected to return to their beloved *isla verde* once their economic future was secure. But '*los Estados Unidos*,' observed Dolores Montanez, could be a 'cold place to live—not because of the winter and the landlord not giving heat but because of the snow in the hearts of people.'[16] In Spanish Harlem, the median income was roughly equivalent to that of Central Harlem and far below that of other New York neighbourhoods. 'Old-law' tenement buildings dating back to the nineteenth century were common in East Harlem. In these five- or six-story buildings, families lived in crowded quarters; three or more people often occupied a single room that lacked adequate ventilation and sunlight. Rates of respiratory infections and tuberculosis were high in these crowded conditions. A survey of 80 Puerto Rican families living in East Harlem, undertaken in the 1950s, showed 14 percent had a member of the household with chronic bronchial asthma. In the majority of cases, the family member was a child whose symptoms developed after immigration.[17]

In the early 1960s, the hot zones of urban asthma in New York City were geographic areas with high concentrations of African-American or Puerto Rican families, many of whom had come north after the Second World War. Both epicentres of these concentrations—Central Harlem and Spanish Harlem—also had the greatest concentration of poverty in New York City and some of the highest population densities per square mile in the world. Epidemiologists puzzled over whether population or environment could account for the unprecedented rise in hospital admissions for asthma. Events that transpired in Harlem and throughout the nation, however, quickly transfixed attention upon race as the determining factor.

On a hot summer evening in July, just two weeks after President Lyndon B. Johnson signed the Civil Rights Act of 1964 into law, thousands of Blacks in Harlem, many of them teenagers, took to the streets in anger and protest. It was neither the beginning nor the end of a series of long hot summers that saw riots and devastation in the cities of Chicago, Cleveland, Detroit, Newark, and Los Angeles. Frustration and anger that set ghettoes burning would be later channelled into calls for Black Power; out of the ferment of youth came the energy that tore down and built a new image of the Black ghetto, one founded upon self-help, community action, and racial pride.[18]

While the Black community transformed anger and rage into a positive force of social change, White psychiatrists and clinical allergists looked upon such emotions as the pathological seat of the nation's rising asthma epidemic. In late July of 1965, irate Watts residents and a prickly Los Angeles police force and National Guard clashed in a firestorm that left 34 people dead and hundreds injured on the West coast. The events prompted *New York Times* reporter John Osmundsen to popularize the first of several explanations for the sharp rise in asthma among New York City's African-American and Puerto Rican populations. 'An emotional epidemic that has probably never been paralleled in the annals of medicine' was sweeping the urban ghetto, Osmundsen wrote. Medical authorities suspected, he reported, that 'tensions arising from the civil rights movement' were its likely cause.[19]

The impulse to invoke race to explain the increase in urban asthma first witnessed in the early sixties speaks both to the popularity of psychosomatic explanations of asthma during the period and to the medical profession's deep and ongoing history of looking to racial difference to account for observed health disparities. Osmundsen acknowledged that other factors, including air pollution, housing, socioeconomic status, and geography, might be involved in inner-city asthma. But he noted that whatever role such factors played, they were 'doing so against a background of emotional conflicts which have been reported widely in medical literature to be associated with asthma attacks.'[20]

Many psychiatrists regarded asthma as based upon deep-seated emotional insecurities coupled with an intense dependent need. Nevertheless, the mechanisms by which emotional process interacted with the respiratory, immunological, and central nervous systems remained obscure. According to psychosomatic theories of asthma, anger, which a child might repress for fear of losing his mother's affection, could provoke an asthma attack. Another provocation might be the conflict between a wish for independence and a felt dependent need. In the case of White children, psychiatrists ascribed such emotional tensions to such factors as an overprotective mother, which factored into Murray Peshkin's parentectomy treatment at CARIH.[21] As asthma rates among African-Americans and violence in American ghettos soared, some psychiatrists and clinical allergists working in the field of asthma seized upon the 'Black personality' as a likely cause of the disease in African-American children and the increasing preponderance of asthma within the Black ghetto.

The associations of asthma with the psychology of race owed much to social science research in the post-war era that painted a portrait of a Black psyche damaged by centuries of racial prejudice and discrimination. In their highly influential 1951 book *The Mark of Oppression,* Columbia University psychiatrists Abram Kardiner and Lionel Ovesey argued that self-hatred was a common trait of the Black personality. Black children, seeing their parents as members of a 'despised and discriminated-against group,' aspired to be White. 'Accepting the White ideal,' these physicians argued, was a 'recipe for perpetual self-hatred, frustration, and for tying one's life to unattainable goals.' Hatred of White society was another mark of oppression that the psychiatry community saw manifested in the Black psyche as uncontrolled rage. To liberal social scientists, the violence and aggression witnessed in the urban race riots of the 1960s were unhealthy. Not only did they lead, as Helen V. Mclean at the Institute for Psychoanalysis in Chicago argued, to a greater number of health problems in the Black community, they also threatened liberal hopes for an integrated society by propelling the civil rights movement toward Black nationalism.[22]

To epidemiologists and physicians, the epidemic wave of asthma among poor African-Americans was symptomatic of the damaged Black psyche and the pathology of racial prejudice in America. In his *New York Times* article, Osmundsen suggested that it was not 'hard to see how' asthma, 'precipitated by conflicts between hostile feelings and dependent needs,' could 'arise among members of racial minority groups on whom civil rights activities focus.'[23] Signs that psychiatrists used to evaluate the Black personality also became a part of the clinical diagnosis of the Black asthmatic child. Records of medical evaluation conferences at the Children's Asthma Research Institute and Hospital in Denver, for example, reveal that the psychology of race figured prominently in the evaluation of Black children admitted to the home. When Mary, an eight-and-a-half-year-old African-American child from a poor neighbourhood in Kansas City, entered CARIH in 1959, part of the discussion for treatment centered on her alleged 'feelings of racial inadequacy.' 'She believes that her color is bad and is obsessed with being different and inferior in color,' wrote one attending physician. 'She's struggling with this inside herself, but she hasn't really resolved this at all.' Two years later, physicians regarded Mary's resolution of these racial conflicts, achieved through the help of play therapy, as one indication of her successful rehabilitation.[24]

COCKROACHES, HOUSING, AND ASTHMA

To presume that asthma emerged from the psychological blight of a segregated society ignored the environmental inequities of the urban ghetto visible to African-American and Latino residents. The ecology of injustice was evident everywhere in the deteriorating conditions of the inner city where poor people of colour lived. The distribution of allergens and pollutants was not equal in the economically and racially segregated spaces of the city. Neither was medical care. But the inability of epidemiologists and physicians to perceive such environmental inequities only points to how White privilege blinded medical authorities and prevented them from recognizing that the urban ecology of asthma was different from other breathing spaces where predominately White middle- and upper-class Americans lived.[25]

In the early 1960s, the ghetto was among the places least familiar to those in the clinical field of allergy. Consequently, they had few clues in their doctor's bag of skin tests and allergenic extracts to help identify important environmental factors that might be responsible for the increase of asthma observed within the city's poor African-American and Latino communities. Allergists neither knew nor worked with nature in the urban ghetto. And when they did turn to nature as an explanation for the rise in urban asthma, they were quick to give it agency through the voice of racial privilege.

Racial assumptions and prejudices about the sanitary habits of ethnic minorities focused attention on the cockroach as the next likely suspect in the seemingly unending search for the cause that could account for the marked increase in urban asthma. To call someone a cockroach was to invoke the vile behaviours of this most despised insect. It was a common racial slur levelled against New York City's immigrant Puerto Rican population.[26] And it led, along with the growing reports of occupational asthma in the pest control trade, two Washington, DC, physicians, Dr. Harry Bernton and Dr. Halla Brown, to the first of numerous studies on asthma, cockroach infestation, and exposure in the urban ghetto.

Working with allergy clinics in seven hospitals in New York City, the physicians tested 589 patients for sensitivity to an extract derived from the body parts of the German cockroach, *Blattella germanica,* the most common urban pest. The two physicians classified patients and their responses according to four ethnic groupings—Puerto Rican, 'Negro', Italian, and Jewish. Bernton and Brown based the design of their study on an unpublished survey of cockroach infestations in New York City slums that allegedly found the dwellings of Puerto Rican and 'Negro' families to have the severest infestation rates, while the homes of Italian and Jewish residents had fewer cockroaches. In the entomological survey, ethnicity rather than class served as the primary category of analysis; differences in median income or housing conditions were left unexamined. Among the patients screened in public clinics, Bernton and Brown found that 59 percent of Puerto Ricans and 47 percent of African-Americans were sensitive to cockroach allergen. In contrast, only 17 percent of Italians and 5 percent of Jews reacted positively. The order of cockroach sensitivity by ethnic group corresponded almost identically to the severity of cockroach infestations found by the cockroach survey. Furthermore, 63 percent of the patients involved in the study were reported to be asthmatic. These findings, Bernton and Brown argued, emphasized the need for urban allergy clinics to make screening for cockroach sensitivity a standard part of clinical diagnosis and, they suggested, offered a plausible explanation for the city's growing asthma epidemic.[27]

Although Bernton and Brown acknowledged class to be a confounding factor in the differential exposure of ethnic groups to cockroaches, such subtleties were easily lost in the popular press. Furthermore, in drawing attention to the heritability of asthma, their paper made it easy to infer that differential asthma rates might be explained according to biological racial differences. Just weeks after Bernton and Brown published their findings in the *Southern Medical Journal,* the *New York Times* announced in early September 1967 that allergy to cockroaches had been identified as a possible cause of the 'startling rise in recent years in the incidence of asthma among New York Negroes and Puerto Ricans.'[28]

Cultural attitudes toward the cockroach played heavily into epidemiological assumptions that highlighted race rather than class as the primary determinant in understanding the New York City outbreaks of asthma. But to downtrodden African-Americans and Latinos, cockroaches had nothing to do with their cleanliness or behaviour. Rather, cockroaches spoke to the despicable ways of slumlords that turned the ghetto into a colony of White America. To the residents of Harlem and Spanish Harlem, the life of the cockroach was linked, not to race, but to the inhumanity of beings toward one another. In their eyes, the cockroach spoke, not through the voice of privilege, but through the protest cries against economic, racial, and social injustice.

Contrary to popular opinion, cockroaches possess few filthy habits. They are in fact the felines of the insect world, constantly grooming their antennae, which they use to detect precious water and food resources. In the tropics, where the majority of the estimated 4,000 cockroach species abound, the relatively constant warm temperatures and high humidity are paradise to this water-loving, heat-craving insect. But cockroaches have been on this planet a long time—Thomas Henry Huxley believed them to be the archetypal insect—and throughout their evolutionary history they have managed to adapt to virtually every ecosystem on Earth. Less than 1 percent of the known species have come into close contact with humans. Of these, the German, American, and Oriental cockroach are the most common domestic species. None of them are endemic to North America; they came from tropical Africa and east Asia, successfully colonizing the temperate urban landscape.[29] In torrid climates, exposure to these allergenic species is directly related to social status. In the Dominican Republic, for example, scientists have found that among poor children inhabiting drafty wood-frame homes, where moisture sources such as toilets and sinks are generally located outside the living quarters, the incidence of cockroach sensitivity is low. In these shanties, the ideal abode for cockroaches—high humidity and limited air movement—is lacking. In contrast, the tight masonry construction characteristic of better built homes eliminates rapid air exchange and creates pockets of dead air with higher humidity, a virtually five-star hotel for the ubiquitous urban cockroach. The incidence of cockroach allergy among the human residents of Dominican homes of better quality construction is significantly greater than among those who live in drafty wood-frame homes.[30]

In northern American cities, however, a different set of environmental factors—human and natural—conspired to create a quite different ecology of human–cockroach interactions. Old tenement apartment buildings that made up the majority of housing stock in Harlem in the 1960s were fertile breeding grounds for *Blattella germanica* and its domestic cousins. Cockroaches were a nightmare, not only for the residents of urban, low-income apartments, but also for pest control experts hired to exterminate them. In buildings with falling plaster, cracks in the ceilings and walls, leaky faucets and toilets—all the result of years of neglect by landlords who skirted around the New York City's Board of Health and ignored the pleas of tenants—cockroaches found a welcome home. Leaky pipes offered a source for the cockroach's most valued natural resource: water. Their antennae are like dowsing rods that can search through the subterranean caverns of wood, brick, and mortar to find a prized moisture source. Garbage left by landlords to accumulate under the stairways of tenement buildings also served as a magnet for these highly gregarious creatures that congregate in kitchens and other food outlets, coming together, like humans, for conversation and a meal. The German cockroach is also highly mobile. Plumbing connections, heating and venting systems, and electrical conduits all serve as express highways for the frequent migration of cockroaches from one apartment to another to escape the application of pesticides or to find better food and water supplies. The much higher cockroach populations found by urban entomologists and pest control experts in lower socio-economic communities were a function not of race but of deteriorating housing conditions that provided a perfect ecological niche for this pre-eminent evolutionary survivor of the insect world.[31]

When Gordon Parks turned his camera on the American ghetto in 1968, he found conditions of poverty that equaled those of any Rio de Janeiro slum. In his *Life* essay on the Fontenelles, a Black family struggling to survive in Harlem, Parks confronted White middle-class readers with another America of their own making. The Fontenelles lived in a 'building ain't fit for dogs' and owned a cat 'to keep the roaches and rats in check.'[32] While the Brazilian magazine *O Cruzeiro* had pasted cockroaches on the face of a Puerto Rican child in its fabricated story of New York City poverty, such scenes of cockroaches crawling on the faces of sleeping infants were a common part of life in New York City slums. The *New York Amsterdam News*, the Black newspaper of Central Harlem, regularly featured advertisements for rat and roach pesticides like 'Kill Jo Paste' next to Primatene tablets, an over-the-counter asthma medication. In *The Cool World*, Warren Miller's gritty 1961 novel of life in Harlem, only 'E Z Kill roach powder' and 'Kill Kwik rat pellets' lined the shelves of the local hardware store. By the 1960s, epidemiological evidence and everyday experience confirmed that asthma and roaches had become part of the urban ecology of America's choking cities.[33] But to isolate cockroaches as the cause of the first epidemic wave of urban asthma would be to miss the larger environmental inequities at work in the ghetto that combined to make conditions ripe for the spread of an emerging disease and an opportunistic insect.

THE URBAN ECOLOGY OF ASTHMA

Race riots, not asthma, were what finally brought national attention to the conditions of poverty, poor housing, and lack of quality medical care that prevailed in the ghetto and contributed to the urban ecology of a disease. The passage of the Economic Opportunity Act by Congress in August 1964, just weeks after the country looked with trepidation upon the summer firestorm in Harlem, formed the backbone of President Johnson's 'War on Poverty.' An infusion of funds over the next eight years into existing and newly established federal programmes including Aid to Families with Dependent Children, Food Stamps, Head Start, and Medicare and Medicaid helped to lessen the toll of poverty—hunger, poor health, economic insecurity, and lack of opportunity—that faced an estimated 10 million poor Americans living in urban areas in 1964. When the Kennedy administration first turned its attention to poverty in America, rural Appalachia, not the inner city, was the place foremost in its mind. But the incendiary racial violence that erupted and spread across America's urban landscape in the summers of the mid-1960s fixed the eyes of the White House on another America in their midst. The need to secure the Black vote for the Democratic Party in the upcoming 1964 re-election campaign likely played a part as well. In looking to the root cause of racial disorder, Washington officials found themselves confronting deep structural economic and social inequalities. When the Economic Opportunity Act passed, just two months after the Civil Rights Act became law, the federal government put poverty and race at the centre of efforts to address the problems that plagued America's cities and stirred social unrest.[34]

New York City proved an important testing ground for the future direction of federal anti-poverty programmes. In the early 1960s, Richard Cloward, professor at the Columbia School of Social Work, helped to create Mobilization for Youth (MFY) on Manhattan's Lower East Side. A pilot experiment in combating poverty, MFY was built upon principles of opportunity and empowerment. Lack of access to education and employment and the absence of political power had locked inner-city youth into a cycle of poverty and despair. This was the argument Cloward and his Columbia colleague Lloyd Ohlin advanced in their highly influential book *Delinquency and Opportunity*, which captured the interest of Kennedy's circle of advisors. With funds from the President's Committee on Juvenile Delinquency,

Cloward and others put theory into practice and built MFY into an organization that relied upon community residents, rather than professional social workers from outside, to teach and train one another. MFY also invested resources into community action programmes. Through its legal services unit and its community action workers, MFY counselled residents on issues of direct relevance to their lives. Staff members also advised on the recourse citizens had in affecting change. Lawyers, for example, informed tenants of their rights regarding landlords, including the provision to strike and refuse to pay rent when a landlord did not provide the minimum services required by law. 'Inclusion of the poor,' Cloward insisted, 'will help to overcome a long-standing colonialism in the social welfare field.'[35] The federal War on Poverty embraced this grass-roots community activist approach, mandating that federal anti-poverty funds be distributed to agencies in which the poor had an active voice and local control. Tensions mounted between local community action groups and established social service agencies. The agencies feared that federal dollars were being used to harass city agencies and redistribute power within municipal government and society at large. Shortly after the Harlem riot, City Council President Paul Screvane accused MFY of instigating racial unrest through subversive tactics, including rent strikes, civil rights protests, and the printing of inflammatory literature.[36]

Community empowerment was an issue not of 'administrative efficiency and experience, but of justice.'[37] As the community members gained a voice and power in controlling the places in which they lived, worked, and played, the political economy of inequality shaped protest and action. Health became a political watchword and rallying cry. Harlem Area Youth Opportunities Unlimited (HARYOU) was an MFY analogue created in 1962 with the aid of the Harlem Neighbourhoods Association and the President's Committee on Juvenile Delinquency. It saw the 'problems of the Central Harlem community' as 'but symptoms of a wider social pathology.' 'Social action' and 'social protest' offered the means by which the community could 'move from disorganization and pathology to health.' High rates of infant mortality, tuberculosis, venereal disease, suicide, and asthma were but indicators of larger forces at work that suffocated the life of a community and its residents. 'Nothing short of a concerted and massive attack upon the social, political, economic, and cultural roots of this pathology is required,' argued HARYOU board members, 'if anything more than daubing or a displacement of the symptoms is to be achieved.'[38]

Housing offered a politically potent issue around which citizens and activists organized to address the integrated problems of economic, environmental, and social injustice. To Harlem residents, housing was the most visible environmental problem they confronted on a daily basis. Housing starkly revealed the system of economic dependency and exploitation that characterized the socioeconomic conditions in Harlem. It also highlighted the costs of a degraded environment on physical, psychological, and social well-being. Through HARYOU, Harlem youth, who might have otherwise been immersed in the politics of street gangs, got a taste of the power of protest and social action in affecting environmental change when they worked as aides to the Community Council on Housing in one of the most sweeping rent strikes in Harlem's history.

In the fall of 1963, the prominent Black writer and civil rights activist James Baldwin had asked a crowd gathered in Foley Square what effect a rent boycott by Harlem residents would have on the 'White economic power structure.'[39] Two months later residents put his rhetorical question into action. On December 1, with the support of the Community Council on Housing and energetic youth mobilized by HARYOU, 585 families in 50 tenement buildings in the neighbourhood of 117th and 118th Streets went on a collective strike. Until landlords corrected countless housing violations that threatened the health and safety of residents—garbage-strewn hallways, inadequate heat, falling plaster, walls littered with rat holes, broken toilets and windows, leaky plumbing and roofs, and rats the size of small dogs—tenants refused to pay rent. Within a matter of weeks, the strike had grown to 167 buildings and over 2,000 residents. An estimated $60,000 in rent did not flow out of Harlem into the New York City bank accounts of White landlords in January of 1964.[40] When Jesse Gray, the leader of the rent strike, orchestrated the mailing of 200 rubber rats, each with a letter signed by a Harlem resident urging emergency repairs in slum housing, to New York Governor Rockefeller, he was mobilizing nature, albeit synthetic, to make visible the structural inequalities at play in the urban ecology of the city and to organize Harlem residents around issues of health and housing as a means to gain political and economic control of their own community.[41]

In East Harlem, too, housing and health were at the centre of a battle waged by young Puerto Rican activists for the 'self-determination for all Latinos' and the 'community control' of their 'institutions and land.' Inspired by the Black Power movement, the Young Lords, with chapters in Chicago and New York City, formed a powerful political organization in the late 1960s that agitated for social justice and community empowerment in the urban barrios of America. Fighting against 'attacks' on their 'land by urban removal, highway destruction, universities and corporations' and the 'violence of hungry children, illiterate adults, diseased old people,' what was called 'the violence of poverty and profits,' the Lords launched a 'garbage offensive' in July of 1969. Their goal was to bring visibility to the miasma of want and disease that emanated from the streets of East Harlem. Armed not with guns but with brooms, Puerto Rican youth took to the streets to clean their neighbourhood and barricade the main thoroughfares of El Barrio—Madison, Lexington, and Third Avenues—with garbage that the city's sanitation department had failed to collect. The mayor's office got the message. But the garbage carried away by the city's trucks did not remove conditions of despair.[42]

By the fall of 1969, the Lords had grown their political base and extended their community reach through campaigns for free clothing drives, a day-care centre, a breakfast programme for school-aged children, and a free health clinic. But the Lords lacked an affordable space in which to house such programs. After a minister, a Cuban exile fearing another socialist revolution in his midst, refused to allow use of his Methodist church as a community centre during weekdays when the building was unoccupied, Lords activists and their supporters took control of the church on December 28 after Sunday services. The First Spanish Methodist Church, located in the heart of the Barrio, became *La Iglesia de la Gente*—the People's Church—servicing the needs of over 3,000 community residents for eleven days before helmeted police officers surrounded the Lords' sanctuary and forcibly removed and arrested more than 100 people.[43]

Undeterred by the arrests and eviction, the Lords continued their efforts in community activism. Tuberculosis and lead poisoning became a focus of political action for the Lords. These 'diseases of oppression' plagued the people of East Harlem and were seen as symptomatic of the dilapidated housing and overcrowded conditions in which New York City's Puerto Rican population lived. On Saturdays, the political and health revolutionaries devoted their time to giving tuberculin tests in the Barrio. In one instance, they stole a city TB truck and screened more than 1,000 community residents for tuberculosis in a single day. They also tested children for lead poisoning, using the results to prod health authorities to take action regarding the environmental risks posed to children growing up in the old tenements of East Harlem's slum.[44]

In the politicization of health and housing, youth groups such as HARYOU and the Lords made visible the environmental and health disparities faced by people of colour living in urban ghettos. Asthma was one such disparity. The struggle to breathe was just one symptom of a widespread pathology of urban decay grounded in economic, social, and racial inequalities. But asthma, newly visible in the urban ghetto in the 1960s, had yet to gain the political traction that more visible, serious diseases such as tuberculosis had in mobilizing community activists seeking an end to poverty and social injustice. During the 1980s, rates of asthma in the inner city again climbed and once again drew media and medical attention to the disease. In this new political climate, asthma became the signature disease around which activist groups rallied to make visible the disparate environments in which Americans live, work, and play.

CONCLUSION

In the 1970s, the news media, physicians, and public health experts, which had first drawn public attention to asthma as an emerging inner city disease, became relatively silent about the epidemic. By then, the spikes in asthma emergency room admissions seen in inner city hospitals during the 1960s had become less prominent. John Salvaggio, the physician at the Louisiana State

University School of Medicine and Charity Hospital who had spent more than a decade trying to discover the cause of New Orleans's fifth season, tracing it unsuccessfully to burning dumps, grain elevators, and pollen loads, looked back on the period less through the eyes of a biomedical researcher, and more through the lens of ecology and political economy. Poverty, substandard housing, and poor quality medical care combined to create a group of people ecologically vulnerable to the onslaught of allergens in their environment. The noticeable decline in asthma emergency room admissions in the early 1970s was due not to the disappearance of any one environmental allergen. Rather, many factors—the replacement of housing stock in the neighbourhood of Charity Hospital, the creation of Medicaid, which enabled indigent asthmatics to seek out private medical care, the establishment of an outpatient allergy and asthma clinic at Charity Hospital, and the availability of a new generation of asthma drugs—combined to create a breathing space in the inner city more like that experienced by White, middle-class Americans for whom asthma was a less serious disease.[45]

But the conditions that fostered a more equitable environment in the urban ghetto were short-lived. During the 1970s, the programmes put in place by the War on Poverty were gradually dismantled. Between 1974 and 1986, children's poverty increased at an alarming rate, particularly in the central cities, where 44 percent of Black children lived below the poverty line. The Reagan administration's war on welfare in the early 1980s slashed new housing starts for low-income residents, dismantled Community Development Block Grants that provided support for housing rehabilitation, and cut federal subsidies to maintain and operate public housing.[46]

The effects had become particularly acute in public housing projects erected by the federal government after the Second World War. While groups like HARYOU pushed for active participation by neighbourhood residents in the planning, repair, and rehabilitation of housing, federal housing policy had evolved in a different direction to the goals of community empowerment set forth by the War on Poverty. Under the Housing Act of 1949, Congress established a federal program for the construction of public housing targeted at the urban poor. Over the next two decades, however, bulldozers demolished more low-income housing in the name of urban renewal than was built. The old five- and six-story tenement buildings came tumbling down as local authorities, under the right of eminent domain, cleared tracts of dilapidated housing in urban slums. But little was done to relocate displaced tenants into affordable housing.[47] In Harlem, 2,000 new public or publicly assisted housing units were added each year between 1949 and 1970. At the same time, demolition for urban renewal projects or abandonment by private owners took 3,000 units per year off the rental market. By 1970, 20 percent of Harlem's total housing inventory consisted of public or publicly assisted high-rise buildings. In East Harlem, home to the greatest number of public-housing projects in New York City, one out of three residents in 1965 lived in government housing.[48]

The vast complex of stark towers that came to dominate the skyline of poor urban communities in Chicago, Detroit, New York City, and other American metropolises initially provided residents with central heating, sanitary housing, and less crowded living quarters. But they also transformed once vibrant neighbourhoods into concrete islands in the sky. The effect was to sever community bonds forged through daily interactions with friends and neighbours: gossiping on the front steps, shopping at the corner grocery store, watching children play on the streets. Most public housing, due to strict federal limits on building costs, was also poorly designed and shoddily built. As federal subsidies for maintenance and operation costs declined, housing authorities found themselves financially unable to address the deteriorating physical conditions that threatened the safety and health of residents. In these vertical cities—building complexes that might house upwards of 10,000 people—spires of concrete concentrated and magnified the physical, psychological, and social problems they were designed to alleviate. Malfunctioning elevators that might stop on only a few floors, faulty heating and ventilation systems, leaky plumbing, infestations of rats and cockroaches, and high rates of crime and drug addiction were just a few of the problems that began to surface in the late 1970s and through the 1980s.[49] Another was asthma.

By the late 1980s, after nearly two decades of relative quiet, public health officials, physicians, the popular press, and community activists again turned the national spotlight on an emerging public health crisis in America's inner cities. An initial wake-up call came when the Centers for Disease Control reported in the late 1980s that the number of individuals with asthma had increased 29 percent between 1980 and 1987. In 1998, the statistics were even more alarming: The prevalence of asthma between 1980 and 1996 had increased 75 percent.[50] Although changes in diagnosis might account for some of the observed increase, most medical and public health professionals saw the trend as a real effect and not as an artifact of changing classification categories. Mortality and morbidity patterns revealed widespread geographic variation. Prevalence and severity of asthma appeared especially acute among inner-city African-American and Hispanic populations. Between 1982 and 1986, for example, hospitalization rates for asthma in East Harlem were 16 times higher than those in Greenwich Village–Soho.[51] Minority children seemed especially vulnerable. Compared to Whites, African-American children were almost twice as likely to suffer from asthma and 2 to 5 times more likely to die of the disease.[52] In central Harlem, a 2005 study found one in four children has asthma. The national average was one in sixteen.[53] Suddenly the nation found itself confronting a 'new' urban asthma epidemic, while sadly oblivious to history and the lessons of the first epidemic outbreaks of urban asthma in the 1960s.

Medical opinion has once again divided over whether poverty or race accounts for the observed disparities in asthma.[54] Medical and public health researchers debate whether accessibility to health care, adverse affects of asthma medications, environmental exposures, or different genetic susceptibilities can explain the current trend. At the same time, these professionals acknowledge that no single factor is likely to offer an adequate explanation of the urban asthma epidemic, even as medical research largely views urban asthma through the lens of individual behaviour and pathology. Large, federally funded research projects like the National Cooperative Inner-City Asthma Study examine high levels of exposure to cockroach allergen, tobacco smoke, and other indoor materials in hopes of understanding and controlling inner-city asthma. Other studies, such as the decade-long Collaborative Study on the Genetics of Asthma, funded by the National Heart, Lung, and Blood Institute, search for underlying genetic difference both within and across African-American, Hispanic, and Caucasian populations. Such studies aim to unmask the genetic factors involved in asthma, including, for example, different genetic susceptibilities to cockroach allergens, in hopes of leading to new treatment therapies targeted at the molecular level. Despite different emphases on environment or heredity, these multi-million-dollar research efforts frame the problem of urban asthma largely around individuals and their ability to manage and control the disease and the spaces in which they live.[55] But is asthma one person's disease, or is it society's problem?

Community activists who live and work in inner-city asthma zones confront on a daily basis the burden the disease places on the lives of children. Such activists tend to see asthma in ways different from the views of the biomedical community. 'You can't just get rid of cockroaches and expect asthma to go away,' remarked one organizer of West Harlem Environmental Action (WE ACT). 'For that matter, you can't just put in better buses and expect asthma to go away. It's all got to be approached in a social justice framework.'[56] A puff of an inhaler might ease the symptoms of asthma, but it will not alleviate the underlying environmental and social conditions that exacerbate the disease.

Founded by Peggy Shepard and Vernice Miller-Travis in 1988, WE ACT is a nonprofit, community-based, environmental justice group built on the principles of self-determination and community empowerment to 'fight environmental racism and improve environmental health, protection and policy in communities of color.'[57] Shepard, a journalist by training, got her first taste of social activism working for New York State's Division of Housing and Community Renewal in the late 1970s. Over the next decade, she and others watched as people in poor communities of colour in Warren County, North Carolina, in Houston, and in other neighbourhoods drew upon protest strategies and legal actions learned during the civil rights era to speak out. These communities challenged in the courts the disproportionate share of hazardous waste facilities, garbage dumps, and polluting industries that ended up in 'poor, powerless, black and Latino communities, rather than in affluent, white suburbs.'[58] A new social movement, environmental justice, gathered political momentum in the 1980s. But its roots reached into the past, into the era of civil rights and the take-it-to-the-streets fight for health and social justice by groups like the Young Lords.

Asthma is a disease that is today at the centre of environmental justice groups in New York City like WE ACT and El Puente, a community learning and development organization based in the Greenpoint/Williamsburg neighbourhood in Brooklyn, where asthma rates are twice the national average. Asthma is, as Brown University sociologist Phil Brown wrote, a 'stepping point to a politicized view of the world.'[59] Through the research and educational efforts of groups like WE ACT and El Puente, people suffering from asthma in the inner city have begun to see themselves 'less as an individually sick person' and more as a collective of people living in a world where exposures, both indoor and out, are a consequence of an urban ecology—physical, economic, and social—shaped by a long history of racism and economic inequality in America.[60]

It is almost a half century since Flavio da Silva stepped off the plane in Denver, brought there to be cured because Americans took notice. It is also almost a half century since the first wave of urban asthma epidemics swept the United States. Since that fateful time that forever altered Flavio's life and hopes, three generations of children in America have grown up living in conditions of poverty, poor housing, and despair. How many epidemics of asthma does it take to notice the ecology of injustice that makes each breath a fight to survive?

NOTES

* This chapter was adapted from *Breathing Space: How Allergies Shape Our Lives and Landscapes,* pp. 130–166, published by Yale University Press.

1. Gordon Parks, 'Freedom's Fearful Foe: Poverty,' *Life* (June 16, 1961): 86–98.
2. 'Flavio's Rescue: Americans Bring Him From Rio Slum to Be Cured,' *Life* (July 21, 1961): 24.
3. Gordon Parks, *Flavio* (New York: W. W. Norton, 1978). 91–92.
4. Piri Thomas, *Down These Mean Streets* (New York: Vintage, 1974), xi.
5. W. Carr, L. Zeitel, and K. Weiss, 'Variations in Asthma Hospitalizations and Deaths in New York City,' *American Journal of Public Health* 82 (1992): 59–65; V. A. De Palo, P. H. Mayo, P. Friedman, et al., 'Demographic Influences on Asthma Hospitalization Rates in New York City,' *Chest* 106 (1994): 447–451; L. Stevenson and M. Kaminsky, 'Asthma Hospitalization and Mortality in New York City, 1987–1996,' in *Conference Proceedings, Working Together to Combat Urban Asthma* (New York: New York Academy of Medicine, 1998).
6. Scott Hamilton Dewey, *Don't Breathe the Air: Air Pollution and U.S. Environmental Politics, 1945–1970* (College Station: Texas A&M University Press, 2000). 'Smog is Really Smaze: Rain May Rout it Tonight,' *New York Times,* 21 November 1953, 1; 'Rain and Wind Lift City's 6-Day Siege of Smaze and Smog,' *New York Times,* 23 November 1953, 1.
7. Leonard Greenburg et. al., 'Air Pollution and Morbidity in New York City,' *Journal of the American Medical Association* 182 (1962): 161–164; Leonard Greenburg et al., 'Report of an Air Pollution Incident in New York City, November 1953,' *Public Health Reports* 77 (1962): 7–16

8. Leonard Greenburg, 'Air Pollution and Asthma,' *Journal of Asthma Research* 2 (1965): 195–198.
9. Leonard Greenburg, Carl Erhardt, Franklyn Field, and Joseph I. Reed, 'Air Pollution Incidents and Morbidity Studies,' *Archives of Environmental Health* 10 (1965): 351–356. Michael Earnest et al., 'Emergency Clinic Visits for Asthma,' *Public Health Reports* 81 (1966): 911–918.
10. Robert F. Lewis and Edward A. Cleave, *A Study of Relationships Between Meteorologic Variables and Asthma Admissions to Charity Emergency Center, New Orleans, Louisiana* (New Orleans: Tulane University, 1960); Robert Lewis, Murray M. Gilkeson, Jr., and Ray W. Robison, *Air Pollution and New Orleans Asthma* (New Orleans: Tulane University, 1962), 2 vols.; 'A City Chokes Up,' *Newsweek*, 14 November 1960, 104. On the Agriculture Street Landfill, known as Dante's Inferno, see Amanda Furness, 'Officials and Activists Join Forces to Clean Up Dump Sites,' *Louisiana Weekly*, 8 October 2001; Louisiana Office of Public Health, *Public Health Assessment. Agriculture Street Landfill. New Orleans, Orleans Parish, Louisiana. EPA Facility ID: LAD981056997*, 2 June 1999.
11. John D. Walsh and Vincent J. Derbes, 'The Fifth Season: New Orleans Asthma,' *NTA Bulletin* (December 1964): 8–9.
12. Kenneth B. Clark, *Dark Ghetto: Dilemmas of Social Power* (New York: Harper & Row, 1965), 22. Douglas S. Massey and Nancy A. Denton, *American Apartheid: Segregation and the Making of the Underclass* (Cambridge, MA: Harvard University Press, 1993); Steward E. Tolnay, 'The Great Migration and Changes in the Northern Black Family, 1940 to 1990,' *Social Forces* 75 (1997): 1213–1238.
13. These statistics are taken from HARYOU, *Youth in the Ghetto: A Study of the Consequences of Powerlessness and a Blueprint for Change* (New York: Orans Press, 1964). Quote appears on p. 316.
14. Richard Pomeroy, in collaboration with Robert LeJeune and Lawrence Podell, *Studies in the Use of Health Services by Families on Welfare: Utilization by Publicly-Assisted Families* (New York: Center for the Study of Urban Problems, 1969), 114.
15. Virginia E. Sánchez Korrol, *From Colonia to Community: The History of Puerto Ricans in New York City*, rev. ed. (Berkeley: University of California Press, 1994).
16. Thomas, *Down These Mean Streets*, 10.
17. Beatrice Bishop Berle, *80 Puerto Rican Families in New York City: Health and Disease Studied in Context* (New York: Columbia University Press, 1958). See also: Elena Padilla, *Up From Puerto Rico* (New York: Columbia University Press, 1958); Patricia Cayo Sexton, *Spanish Harlem: Anatomy of Poverty* (New York: Harper & Row, 1965).
18. 'Race Tension Shows Contrasting Pattern in North and South,' *New York Times*, 26 July 1964, E3; E. W. Kenworthy, 'Johnson Orders Full F.B.I. Inquiry in Harlem Riots,' 22 July 1964, 1; Paul L. Montgomery and Francis X. Clines, 'Thousands Riot in Harlem Area; Scores Are Hurt,' *New York Times*, 19 July 1964, 1.
19. John A. Osmundsen, 'Asthma Linked to Rights Drive,' *New York Times*, 26 July 1965, 25.
20. John A. Osmundsen, 'Asthma Linked to Emotions,' *New York Times*, 1 August 1965, E7.
21. See, for example, Michael Hirt, ed., *Psychological and Allergic Aspects of Asthma* (Springfield, IL: Charles C. Thomas, 1965). See also the chapter by Mark Jackson in this volume.
22. Abram Kardiner and Lionel Ovesey, *The Mark of Oppression: A Psychosocial Study of the American Negro* (New York: Norton, 1951), 310. On the history

of the damaged Black personality, see Daryl Michael Scott, *Contempt and Pity: Social Policy and the Image of the Damaged Black Psyche, 1880–1996* (Chapel Hill: University of North Carolina Press, 1997).
23. Osmundsen, 'Asthma Linked to Rights Drive,' 25.
24. Samuel C. Bukantz, 'Initial Medical Evaluation Conferences,' *Journal of Children's Asthma Research Institute* 1 (March 1961): 132. Samuel C. Bukantz, 'Final and Interim Medical Evaluation Conferences,' *Journal of the Children's Asthma Research Institute and Hospital* 1 (June 1961): 173–204.
25. On White privilege and imperception, see Michelle Murphy, 'Uncertain Exposures and the Privilege of Imperception: Activist Scientists and Race at the U.S. Environmental Protection Agency,' *Osiris* 19 (2004): 266–282.
26. See, for example, *West Side Story* (1961). For cultural histories of the cockroach, see Marion Copeland, *Cockroach* (London: Reaktion Books, 2003) and Richard Schweid, *The Cockroach Papers: A Compendium of History and Lore* (New York: Four Walls Eight Windows, 1999).
27. Harry S. Bernton and Halla Brown, 'Cockroach Allergy II: The Relation of Infestation to Sensitization,' *Southern Medical Journal* 60 (1967): 852–855.
28. Jane E. Brody, 'Allergy to Cockroaches Called One Possible Cause of Asthma,' *New York Times,* 2 September 1967, 15.
29. Michael K. Rust, John M. Owens, and Donald A. Reierson, eds., *Understanding and Controlling the German Cockroach* (New York: Oxford University Press, 1995); William J. Bell and K. G. Adiyodi, *The American Cockroach* (New York: Chapman and Hall, 1982).
30. Richard J. Brenner, Kathleen C. Barnes, Ricki M. Helm, and Larry W. Williams, 'Modernized Society & Allergies to Arthropods,' *American Entomologist* 37 (1991): 143–155; Angel M. Marchand, 'Allergy to Cockroaches,' *Bol. Asoc. Méd. P. Rico* (February 1966): 49–53.
31. R. C. Akers and W. H. Robinson, 'Spatial Pattern and Movement of German Cockroaches in Urban, Low-Income Apartments (Dictyoptera: Blattellidae),' *Proceedings of the Entomological Society of Washington* 83 (1981): 168–172; Erik S. Runstrom and Gary W. Bennett, 'Movement of German Cockroaches (Orthoptera: Blatellidae) as Influenced by Structural Features of Low-Income Apartments,' *Journal of Economic Entomology* 77 (1984): 407–11.
32. Gordon Parks, 'The Cycle of Despair,' *Life* (March 8, 1968), 50.
33. Warren Miller, *The Cool World* (New York: Fawcett Premier, 1959), 26.
34. Michael Katz, *The Undeserving Poor: From the War on Poverty ot the War on Welfare* (New York: Pantheon Books, 1989).
35. Richard A. Cloward, 'The War on Poverty: Are the Poor Left Out?' *The Nation,* 2 August 1965, 55.
36. Herbert Krosney, 'Mobilization for Youth: Feuding Over Poverty,' *The Nation,* 14 December 1964, 455–461.
37. Cloward, 'The War on Poverty,' 59.
38. HARYOU, Inc., *Youth in the Ghetto: A Study of the Consequences of Powerlessness and a Blueprint for Change* (New York, 1964), 355. On the history of HARYOU and community empowerment in Harlem, see *Children, Race, and Power: Kenneth and Mamie Clark's Northside Center* (New York: Routledge, 1999), 180–216.
39. 'Harlem Tenants Open Rent Strike,' *New York Times,* 28 September 1963, 44.
40. 'Tenants in 34 Tenements Join Growing Rent Strike in Harlem,' *New York Times,* 2 December 1963, 30; 'Slum Rent Strike Gains Momentum,' *New York Times,* 1 January 1964, 28.
41. '200 Rubber Rats Sent to Governor,' *New York Times,* 16 February 1964.
42. Jose Yglesias, 'Right on With the Young Lords,' *New York Times,* 7 June 1970, 86.

43. For an excellent account of the Young Lords in relation to environmental justice, see Matthew Gandy, *Concrete and Clay: Reworking Nature in New York City* (Cambridge, MA: MIT Press, 2002), 162–86.
44. 'Right on With the Young Lords;' Gandy, *Concrete and Clay.*
45. I. F. Goldstein and John Salvaggio, 'The Decline of New Orleans Asthma Epidemics,' *Reviews on Environmental Health* 4 (1984): 133–146.
46. Katz, *The Undeserving Poor,* 189–190.
47. R. Allen Hayes, *The Federal Government and Urban Housing: Ideology and Change in Public Policy* (Albany: State University of New York Press, 1995); James O. Wilson, (ed.), *Urban Renewal: The Record and the Controversy* (Cambridge, MA: MIT Press, 1966).
48. Harlem Task Force, *A Profile of the Harlem Area* (December 1973), SC-NYPL.
49. Alexander von Hoffman, 'High Ambitions: The Past and Future of American Low-Income Housing Policy,' *Housing Policy Debate* 7 (1996): 423–446.
50. 'Asthma—United States, 1980–1987,' *Morbidity and Mortality Weekly Report* 30 (1990): 493–497; D. Mannino et. al., 'Surveillance for Asthma Prevalence—United States, 1960–1995,' *Morbidity and Mortality Weekly Report* 47 (1998): 1–27. See, also, Kevin B. Weiss, Peter J. Gergen, and Ellen F. Crain, 'Inner-City Asthma: The Epidemiology of an Emerging US Public Health Concern,' *Chest* 101 (June 1992): 362S–367S; D. Mannino et. al., 'Surveillance for Asthma—United States, 1980–1999,' *Morbidity and Mortality Weekly Report* 51 (2002): 1–13.
51. W. Carr, L. Zeitel, and K. Weiss, 'Asthma Hospitalization and Mortality in New York City,' *American Journal of Public Health* 82 (1992): 59–65.
52. Brian P. Leaderer et. al., 'Dust Mite, Cockroach, Cat, and Dog Allergen Concentrations in Homes of Asthmatic Children in the Northeastern United States: Impacts of Socioeconomic Factors and Population Density,' *Environmental Health Perspectives* 110 (2002): 419–425.
53. Stephen W. Nicholas, 'Addressing the Childhood Asthma Crisis in Harlem: The Harlem Children's Zone Asthma Initiative,' *American Journal of Public Health* 95 (2005): 245–248.
54. Lawrence W. Wissow et. al., 'Poverty, Race, and Hospitalization for Childhood Asthma,' *American Journal of Public Health* 78 (1988): 777–782; D. M. Lang and M. Polansky, 'Patterns of Asthma Mortality in Philadelphia from 1969 to 1991,' *New England Journal of Medicine* 331 (1994): 1542–1546.
55. See, for example, David Rosenstreich et. al., 'The Role of Cockroach Allergy and Exposure to Cockroach Allergen in Causing Morbidity Among Inner-City Children with Asthma,' *New England Journal of Medicine* 336 (1997): 1356–1363; Jianfeng Zu et. al., 'Genomewide Screen and Identification of Gene–Gene Interactions for Asthma Susceptibility Loci in Three U.S. Populations: Collaborative Study on Genetics of Asthma,' *American Journal of Human Genetics* 68 (2001): 1437–1446. For an overview of the National Cooperative Inner-City Asthma Study, see http://www.niaid.nih.gov/factsheets/asthma.htm. For information on the Collaborative Study on the Genetics of Asthma, see http://www.csga.org.
56. Quoted in Phil Brown et al, 'The Health Politics of Asthma: Environmental Justice and Collective Illness Experience in the United States,' *Social Science and Medicine* 57 (2003): 461.
57. http://weact.org.
58. Peggy M. Shepard, 'Issues of Community Empowerment,' *Fordham Urban Law Journal* 21 (1994): 739. The literature on the history of environmental justice in America is rapidly growing. For a sampling, see Robert Bullard,

Dumping on Dixie: Race, Class, and Environmental Quality (Boulder, CO, 1990); Giovanna Di Chiro, 'Nature as Community: The Convergence of Environment and Social Justice,' in William Cronon (ed.), *Uncommon Ground: Rethinking the Human Place in Nature* (New York: W. W. Norton, 1996), 298–321; Michael Egan, 'Subaltern Environmentalism in the United States: A Historiographic Review,' *Environment and History* 8 (2002): 21–41; Gandy, *Concrete and Clay;* Robert Gottlieb, *Forcing the Spring: The Transformation of the Environmental Movement* (Washington, DC: Island Press, 1993); Ellen Maura McGurty, 'From NIMBY to Civil Rights: The Origins of the Environmental Justice Movement,' *Environmental History,* (1997), 39: 301–323; Laura Pulido, *Environmentalism and Economic Justice: Two Chicano Struggles in the Southwest* (Tucson: University of Arizona Press, 1996); Sylvia Hood Washington, *Packing Them In: An Archaeology of Environmental Racism in Chicago, 1865–1954* (New York: Lexington, 2004); Julie Sze, *Noxious New York: The Racial Politics of Urban Health and Environmental Justice* (Doctoral Dissertation, New York University, 2003).
59. Brown, 'The Health Politics of Asthma,' 461. On El Puente, see Jason Corburn, *Street Science: Community Knowledge and Environmental Health Justice* (Cambridge, MA: MIT Press, 2005).
60. Brown, 'The Health Politics of Asthma,' 461.

13 Social Science, Housing, and the Debate Over Transmitted Deprivation

John Welshman

INTRODUCTION

This volume is concerned with how historians and people in general have evaluated the role of families, parents, society, houses, and homes in the determination of health. A key concept in the recent literature on the relationship between living standards, poverty, and health has been that of 'deprivation.' Deprivation might be defined as suffering from hardship, or having been dispossessed, particularly of good medical, social, and educational facilities. However, it is also clear that deprivation can have many meanings. As early as 1976, Richard Berthoud suggested that it was an umbrella term to cover all the misfortunes that people could suffer in society, a phenomenon that was as much about the way society worked, or ought to work, as one existing in society itself. Berthoud suggested that deprivation seemed to imply a situation that was unacceptably below some minimum standard, even though more general inequality might be accepted as inevitable, if not desirable: 'If inequality can be seen as a hill, deprivation is a ravine into which people should not be allowed to fall.'[1] What was crucial for Berthoud was the distinction between the individual and the group, between internal and external weakness, or between structural factors and individual characteristics.

Subsequently Peter Townsend introduced the concept of 'relative deprivation,' writing in his monumental survey of poverty in the United Kingdom that 'individuals, families and groups in the population can be said to be in poverty when they lack the resources to obtain the types of diet, participate in the activities and have the living conditions and amenities which are customary, or are at least widely encouraged or approved, in the societies to which they belong. Their resources are so seriously below those commanded by the average individual or family that they are, in effect, excluded from ordinary living patterns, customs and activities.'[2] Earlier definitions of poverty, from Rowntree onwards, had tended to be based on some conception of 'absolute' deprivation or minimum needs. But the concept of relative deprivation also led to controversy, most notably between Townsend and Amartya Sen.[3]

Attempts have been made more recently to operationalise concepts of deprivation, through the compilation of indicators, usually combining indicators of conditions and people in some composite index. These have been used to identify 'underprivileged areas,' for instance the most deprived local authorities in London, or the most deprived areas in England, for example, in the North.[4] These have revealed difficulties in distinguishing between the measurement of deprivation in different areas, and the kind of people experiencing that deprivation. Later approaches built on the conceptual distinction between material and social forms of deprivation. Material deprivation was seen as the lack of goods, services, resources, amenities. and physical environment that were customary or widely approved in society. Thus, indicators of material deprivation might include unemployment, car ownership, home ownership, and overcrowding. Social deprivation, on the other hand, embraced non-participation in the roles, relationships, customs, functions, rights, and responsibilities implied by membership of a society and its sub-groups. The merits of the concept of deprivation were that it was non-monetary and multi-dimensional, whereas poverty was a one-dimensional monetary measure. Townsend himself was later to distinguish between objective deprivation, normative deprivation, and individual subjective or group deprivation, arguing that each could act as a basis for explaining social conditions, attitudes, and behaviour.[5]

In these respects, deprivation might be seen as an antecedent of the contemporary concept of social exclusion. At the same time, the systematic study of deprivation as a concept, other than relative deprivation, remained in its infancy in the 1980s. What is clear is that these debates were played out against the backdrop of debates about the cycle of deprivation, or transmitted deprivation, and it is these that are the real focus of this chapter. In June 1972, Sir Keith Joseph, then Secretary of State for Social Services, referred in a speech to a 'cycle of deprivation,' and a Joint Department of Health and Social Security (DHSS)–Social Science Research Council (SSRC) Working Party on Transmitted Deprivation was established. The large-scale Research Programme that was organised through the Working Party was to span eight years. It cost around £750,000 (1970s values), and by 1982 had generated some nineteen research studies, fourteen literature reviews, and four feasibility projects. Earlier research has provided a preliminary examination of this episode, exploring the background to the cycle speech, tracing the direction taken by the Research Programme, and illustrating the hostility of DHSS civil servants to the research and researchers.[6] However despite this work, both are only beginning to attract serious attention.

This chapter explores the cycle speech and Research Programme in respect to one theme—that of housing. It argues that the example of housing illustrates differing approaches taken by social scientists, and helps to explain them. Joseph had exhorted researchers to look at the interrelationship of behavioural and structural factors, including the role of the home; contemporary studies highlighted the influence of 'social reasons' for homelessness;

and a literature review noted that personal inadequacy and incompetence were independent of the wider housing situation, as were some aspects of educational attainment. However, apart from one study, researchers for the most part looked at housing rather than the home, and located this within a structural analysis, and this was especially true of the final report on the Research Programme as a whole. Therefore the hypothesis of the cycle of deprivation, and the Transmitted Deprivation Research Programme, are central to the broader themes of this volume. In both, the key issue was, in explaining disadvantage, how much emphasis should be placed on individual or familial factors on the one hand, and structural or social factors on the other.

SIR KEITH JOSEPH, THE CYCLE, AND DEPRIVATION

As the recent biography by Denham and Garnett makes clear, Keith Joseph (1918–94) is a fascinating political figure. Educated at Harrow School and Magdalen College, Oxford, his father had largely created the successful Bovis construction company. As MP for Leeds North East (1956–87), Joseph displayed a compassionate interest in questions of health care and social policy from the 1950s onwards. He first entered the Cabinet in 1962, under Harold Macmillan, as Minister of Housing and Local Government, but had been a junior minister from 1959. As Secretary of State for Social Services, 1970–74, Joseph played a central role in the background to the 1974 health service reorganisation. He was a key advocate of monetarism in the mid 1970s, as well as founding a think-tank, the Centre for Policy Studies. In the 1980s, he served in the Thatcher governments as Secretary of State for first Industry and then Education. Yet Joseph remained an enigmatic character whose honesty, belief in intellectual rigour, courtesy, agonising scrupulousness, and 'intensely nervous disposition' were apparent to all who met him.[7]

The cycle speech was given at a conference for local authorities organised by the Pre-School Playgroups Association, at Church House, Westminster, on 29 June 1972. It was in the second half of the speech that Joseph developed his main theme, asking why it was that, in spite of full employment, rising living standards, and the expansion of social services since the Second World War, deprivation and maladjustment 'so conspicuously' persisted. By deprivation, Joseph meant 'those circumstances which prevent people developing to nearer their potential—physically, emotionally and intellectually—than many do now.'[8] He acknowledged that deprivation took many forms and had complex causes, including those that were economic, personal, and to do with patterns of child rearing. But he continued, 'Perhaps there is at work here a process, apparent in many situations but imperfectly understood, by which problems reproduce themselves from generation to generation.'[9] There was not a single process. But it seemed that in a proportion of cases, the problems of one generation were repeated in the next. According to Joseph, social workers and teachers could often be sure that because of family background, a child was experiencing disadvantage and was likely to face the same difficulties as 'his' parents.

Part of Joseph's speech was a call for more research, and a recognition that the cycle was poorly understood. Joseph admitted that his theory was not underpinned by scientific research, but maintained that 'the cycle is not a process that we fully understand, but a number of objective studies do tend to bear out the subjective belief of many practitioners that cyclical processes are at work.'[10] Joseph acknowledged that poverty did play a role in its causation. For this reason, he said, the Government recognised the need to improve access to the benefits that already existed, to increase welfare spending, and to introduce new subsidies. Research was also needed into the dynamics of family poverty, the mechanisms and circumstances that led families into poverty, its duration and effects, and the forces that enabled some to leave whilst others remained locked in. Joseph therefore recognised that longitudinal studies were relevant to, and complementary to, the cycle. However in the meantime, his remedies were noticeably more limited. Apart from playgroups and services for the under-fives, they focused on family planning, support for parents, and attention to the needs of children.[11]

Joseph located the issue of deprivation within the context of rising living standards, and the role played by the home was implicit throughout the speech. For example, he suggested that 'many parents had no chance when they were children to learn what a happy home can be,' and he acknowledged that what he termed 'living conditions' could play a part—'bad housing and overcrowding and few opportunities for recreation.'[12] He acknowledged that the Government must continue to improve housing and abate poverty. Joseph argued that 'where parents with large families are immature and in danger themselves of marital breakdown, the more so when they are also poor and badly housed, the children are virtually sure to be deprived.'[13] But he also noted that the emotional and intellectual needs of children might not be met 'and this can be in homes that are not poor and in housing that is not bad,' noting that 'there are good parents in poor homes; and bad parents in prosperous homes. There are good parents of large families and bad parents of small families.'[14] Perhaps most importantly, he acknowledged the role played by material circumstances, including poor housing, but also argued that the emotional health of the home was important in the bringing up of children, so that his solutions focused on home helps and social workers tackling perceived problems.

The speech was reported in the main broadsheet newspapers, but met with a fairly muted immediate response.[15] Undeterred, in the months afterwards Joseph made numerous visits to inner-city areas looking for pilot projects for what was termed 'Preparation for Parenthood.' Some visits indicated the potential usefulness of area initiatives where a range of schemes—playgroups, adventure playgrounds, childminding, family planning, and the involvement of mothers—might enable families to escape the cycle. More broadly, in the autumn of 1972, the DHSS was involved in informal meetings with voluntary and professional organisations. Joseph's comments on these indicated some rethinking, since he stressed the debate about the cycle had not distracted the Government from its priorities in the areas of low income, unemployment, poor health, and poor housing. He conceded the term 'cycle' was 'a shorthand one and, as such, imprecise and open to much conceptual questioning.'[16] Better knowledge and greater sensitivity to the needs of her children could not on their own help a mother to fulfil her role if she was hindered by isolation, poor housing, and unsympathetic public agencies and staff.

THE INTELLECTUAL ORIGINS OF THE CYCLE SPEECH

In explaining the timing and content of the speech, Joseph's own background, his genuine concern with poverty, the concept of the problem family, and the policy context of the early 1970s all played a part. Denham and Garnett provide numerous examples of Joseph's charity work and concern with child poverty, vulnerable groups, and the homeless, which included the founding of the Mulberry Trust housing association and support for the Child Poverty Action Group.[17] Nevertheless, while there is no doubt Joseph's concern with poverty was genuine, his interest in low-income families was of a particular kind, and closely bound up with the concept of the problem family. In 1966, for example, Joseph had included, among categories of need, problem families whose poverty was not caused primarily by lack of income, but by difficulties in managing money and in using welfare services.[18] They were dominated by families of low income and low intelligence, with more than the average number of children. A cycle was created and repeated, whereby broken homes and bad parents were reproduced. Joseph saw poverty, bad housing, over-large classes in schools, and inadequate parenting as mutually reinforcing, but his solutions were more modest. More social workers and home helps should be recruited to provide care in the home, and while money was important, effective social services were also crucial.[19] With hindsight, this was a dry run for the cycle speech.

A similar discourse around 'unsatisfactory tenants' was a continuous thread in debates about housing management. A 1955 report from the Central Housing Advisory Committee, for example, had argued that 'the unsatisfactory tenants of today may very well produce the unsatisfactory tenants of tomorrow.'[20] The three main reasons given by local authorities for regarding tenants as unsatisfactory were rent arrears, neglect of the house or garden, and behaviour causing a nuisance to neighbours. The report argued that those owing rent comprised those on low incomes, those who would not pay rent regularly, and those who were 'so incompetent in managing their affairs generally that they are constantly in debt.'[21] It was this third group that posed the most difficult problem, since 'their houses are often ill-kept and dirty, their gardens uncultivated, their children uncontrolled and troublesome.'[22] The Committee considered various courses of action, including segregation in rehabilitation centres, and efforts by voluntary organisations such as Family Service Units.

The problem family concept, which exercised an important influence over public health doctors, social workers, and voluntary organisations in the 1940–70 period, was an essentially behavioural explanation of poverty and deprivation that emphasised household squalor.[23] Similarly homes and housing were persistent aspects of Joseph's thinking. With his private income enabling him to purchase a large house in Chelsea, Joseph had a happy domestic life with his wife and four children, and it was this awareness of his own privileged upbringing and circumstances that led to his compassion for others not so fortunate. In 1967, for example, Joseph had written of the 2–3 million privately rented homes that 'here are the overcrowded: the families living in single rooms carved perfunctorily out of unconverted, insanitary, multi-occupied rabbit warrens. Here are the seed-beds of delinquency and even crime.'[24] Moreover, in 1975 Joseph queried what had been achieved by compulsory purchase orders and slum clearance, noting that 'it is now realised that bulldozing did great social harm, destroying communities as well as property, and that many council estates were bound to become foci of social pathology.'[25] It was the Home-Start charity, which used volunteers to befriend families, and provide assistance to those struggling to bring up children, which Joseph later applauded from the Lords.

A further influence was a concern with inter-generational continuities. As Secretary of State for Social Services, in the early months of 1971 Joseph began to visit approved schools and remand centres, and these experiences confirmed his earlier suspicions that family background was a key factor in deprivation among families and adolescents. He became convinced that 'something in the parental background had virtually doomed these children,' and it was not poverty alone; many children survived poverty because the family bonds were strong.[26] Moreover Joseph was told by one Director of Social Services that 'we have 20,000 households in this city. Nearly all our problems—delinquency, truancy, deprivation, poverty and the rest—come from about 800 of them. And I think that most of the families have been known to us for five generations.'[27] This striking emphasis on inter-generational continuities has obvious echoes with earlier eugenic studies of 'bad' families, such as the Kallikaks.[28] Joseph's emphasis on heredity was to lead to his notorious Edgbaston speech, given in October 1974, where the clearly eugenic tone effectively ended his chances of assuming the leadership of the Conservative Party. In explaining the timing and form of the cycle speech, others have pointed to the broader policy context of the late 1960s.[29] However, the striking emphases on individual characteristics, inter-generational continuities, and social work solutions show how the cycle speech can be located in the context of a pathological emphasis on individuals and the family that had been a theme in debates about poverty over at least the previous 100 years.

THE RESEARCH PROGRAMME

The cycle speech led directly to the Transmitted Deprivation Research Programme, though there had been discussions between the DHSS and SSRC as early as March 1972. The Joint Working Party was formally convened in June and held its first meeting in July. The SSRC representatives comprised Professors Tony Atkinson, an economist then at Essex, Maurice Freedman from the Institute of Social Anthropology at Oxford, Roy Parker from the Department of Social Administration at Bristol, Michael Rutter, from the Institute of Psychiatry, University of London, and Peter Willmott, of the Institute of Community Studies. Its Chair was Professor Robin Matthews, then Chairman of SSRC. The SSRC members thus comprised specialists in anthropology, economics, psychiatry, social administration, and sociology. There were seven DHSS representatives on the Joint Working Party, including two each from the Local Authorities Social Services Division, the Social Work Services Division, and the Research Management Division. Key members included Joan Cooper and Geoffrey Otton. Like Otton, Cooper had been involved with the Children's Department at the Home Office, and has been specifically linked with a 'child care' view of delinquency.

The role played by the home in providing both the emotional context and material circumstances for the bringing-up of children provided a potentially interesting forum within which to debate the relative importance of behavioural and structural factors in creating deprivation. The Working Party from the start saw housing as a potentially important area for research. Its first report (1974), for instance, noted that follow-up studies of the children of families identified as living in very poor circumstances would be useful, especially if comparisons could be included with slum inhabitants who had been rehoused. There had been a few studies of the short-term effects of rehousing, but very little attempt to look at the longer-term effects on the next generation. The extent of bad housing and poor living conditions had been studied, but attention should be paid to these as part of multiple deprivation.[30] Similarly, in terms of intervention, it was noted that local authorities differed in their housing policies. Some segregated 'difficult families' in certain estates, while others distributed such families more widely. Some rehoused by two generation groups, while others aimed to place them on housing estates where families extended over three generations. It was suggested that investigations could be undertaken to determine the effects of these different policies, especially those for migrant families.[31]

Earlier research on housing had mainly been concerned with homelessness, which had been a long-term concern of the DHSS, started under Richard Crossman in the Labour government, but continued under Joseph. In

February 1969, for instance, Brian Abel-Smith had sought to dispel some of the prevalent myths.[32] Other reports had focused on homelessness in London, on policies and practice and on the role of Childrens' Departments, and asked what might be learnt from case records.[33] An influential report, by John Greve, had been critical of views that relied on concepts such as 'problem family,' arguing that ideas of the 'deserving' or the 'undeserving' should play no part as criteria in the allocation of services. Homeless families were predominantly young families in the early stages of bringing up their children, and the greatest need was for housing of a reasonable standard, at rents they could afford, and with security of tenure.[34] Moreover the report noted that 'home' was not synonymous with 'dwelling'; a dwelling or house was a physical structure, whereas a home was both a place and a set of personal relationships. This pointed to the need for a distinction between 'houselessness' and 'homelessness'; the latter was more complex being 'something multi-dimensional, involving the quality of life, and particularly of relationships between members of a family (or household), and not just the possession of a roof over one's head.'[35] Greve suggested the emphasis was shifting from 'house' to 'home,' with all that implied psychologically and emotionally.

Nevertheless other research had engaged more with familial issues and individual characteristics. Another study of homelessness, by Bryan Glastonbury, argued that its causes needed to be assessed on two levels—the immediate factor, and the underlying range of family problems in which its origins were to be found. While 'housing issues' were the main reasons for people entering temporary accommodation, what Glastonbury termed 'social reasons' were also important. Thus while Glastonbury gave attention to 'material circumstances,' including illness, and family size and structure, he was also interested in family relationships, including marital breakdown, domestic violence, and behavioural difficulties. Half the families in his survey had lost their homes because the family members could not get on with each other. He noted that many social workers attributed homelessness to behavioural difficulties, including gambling, sexual misbehaviour, poor domestic management, misuse of resources, domestic filth, and poor personal hygiene.[36] Sometimes a way of life could be handed down from generation to generation, and overall the causes of homelessness were complex and multi-causal.

By the time of its third report (1977), the Working Party had commissioned a paper on housing and transmitted deprivation from Clare Ungerson. She looked at values and housing, the values of those who allocated housing, and relationships between parents and children, making some suggestions about possible areas for research.[37] Moreover it had funded a Bristol-based research project into young adults from large lower status council estates, to determine which achieved upward social mobility in terms of housing, and which remained as local authority tenants. Part of the work was to see how far, for newly married couples suffering from multiple disadvantages, whose only hope of a home lay in the local authority sector, such an outcome was inevitable. But the researchers were also interested in the factors that contributed to the breaking out from this pattern by particular individuals. Exploratory interviews had been conducted with officials of local authority housing departments to discover the extent to which allocation policies and practices contributed to the transmission of inter-generational disadvantage in housing.[38] Overall, attempts were being made to correct the original focus on familial processes, and to look at the influence of broader structural factors.

THE HOME: LITERATURE REVIEWS AND ETHNOGRAPHIC FIELDWORK

This question of causation, raised by the cycle hypothesis, was to become much more significant in the Research Programme as a whole. In her referee's report on the Bristol application, for example, Ungerson had noted that 'what worries me is their apparent narrowing of *causation* to the allocation policies of local authorities.'[39] Moreover, an openness to differing explanations was apparent in the literature review that the Joint Working Party commissioned from Michael Rutter and Nicola Madge. Though this was not finally published until 1976, a large part was ready remarkably quickly, by June 1973. The Rutter and Madge literature review had an important bearing on the Research Programme as a whole, and its main thrust can be seen in the final published version. Rutter and Madge were to examine what evidence existed that might support the 'cycle of transmitted deprivation,' and to consider what it was that created alleged continuities between generations. But they admitted there were some serious problems with the brief they had been given, and changes had been necessary. Most importantly, they decided that they preferred the term 'disadvantage' to the original 'deprivation'; they substituted the plural 'cycles' for the singular 'cycle'; and they dropped the phrase 'transmitted.' It was from this point on that many researchers preferred to talk about cycles of disadvantage.

Rutter and Madge included an entire chapter on housing, outlining its general supply and adequacy in Britain, the situations in which disadvantage was most likely to be found, and the kind of people most likely to suffer. They noted that the study by Glastonbury had identified behavioural and relationship problems within families as the underlying causes of homelessness. The homeless 'frequently displayed elements of personal inadequacy and incompetence which were independent of the prevailing housing situation.'[40] However, they also noted that the earlier study by Greve had found that personal shortcomings were not the major factor in the majority of cases of homelessness, and 'socially inadequate' families formed only a small core. Greve had argued that the most important personal features influencing housing conditions were income level and family circumstances. Overall, Rutter and Madge conceded that very little was known about intergenerational continuities in housing, and while poor housing was associated with other forms of disadvantage including low educational attainment and delinquency, the associations were indirect and the mechanisms poorly understood.

Perhaps the most important point made by Rutter and Madge in connection with housing came in the conclusion to their literature review. They argued that it was sometimes assumed that nothing less than a complete change of the economic and social structure could influence cycles of disadvantage. But while they shared the outrage about the circumstances in which many families had to bring up children, and social inequalities between rich and poor, they argued that researchers were deluding themselves if they thought that nothing short of massive social change could influence cycles of disadvantage.[41] These were to be found at all levels of society, and associations with poor living conditions provided a poor guide to levels of disadvantage in other respects. Although overcrowded homes were twice as numerous in Scotland as in England, for example, Scottish children were much better readers, on average, than their English counterparts. Rutter and Madge concluded that 'if research into such cycles merely reconfirms that children disadvantaged in one respect are often also disadvantaged in other respects it will have failed. What are needed are investigations to determine why this is often *not* the case and how we can bring about discontinuities in cycles of disadvantage. This is the challenge for the future.'[42]

Among the projects funded by the Working Party was one that sought to examine the 'cycle of deprivation' through intensive case studies. The team led by Frank Coffield at Keele University realised that the very static, immobile, type of society found in the Potteries was ideal for an inter-generational study.[43] The project was interdisciplinary in scope, and aimed to combine the approaches of psychology, sociology, and anthropology to look at both individual and socio-economic factors. Housing was certainly central to the Keele study. Coffield and his team noted, for example, that each of their four families had previously lived in private rented rooms, and it was beyond the resources of all of them to buy their own home and have a valuable asset to pass on to their children. However, while each of their families was housed in local authority accommodation, only one of them was severely overcrowded, and in general housing was not a major problem. Coffield and his colleagues wrote that 'the problems which our families experienced were less easy to disentangle, as they were not so obviously the fault of the environment, of living amidst slum property, or of experiencing the rootlessness caused by rapid industrial change.'[44] The Barker family, for example, possessed insurance following a fire at their home, thereby disproving the familiar culture of poverty stereotype that poor people lived entirely for the present and failed to think about the future. Similarly, the Martin family looked after their garden, at least for a time, and the father was constantly repairing and improving household objects.[45]

The Coffield volume was the first of the original studies to appear in book form. But as with Rutter and Madge's literature review, its findings tended to challenge, rather than confirm, the cycle of deprivation theory. Coffield and his colleagues quoted Tawney that 'the duty of Governments is to create the environment which encourages the best, not the worst, in mankind.'[46] But overall, they argued from their fieldwork that the cycle of deprivation was too simple an idea to explain the complex lives of the families that they had spent so long studying in such minute detail. Employing a different metaphor, they concluded that 'the *web* of deprivation, rather than the *cycle* of deprivation, depicts more accurately the dense network of psychological, social, historical and economic factors which have either created or perpetuated problems for these families.'[47] Moreover, they wrote that to miss the compelling force of external circumstances on the performance of the roles of parent or child, and to imagine that the fragile household was not responsive to, and sometimes even torn apart by, the pressures of poverty, unemployment, and insecurity, was to attribute to poor people a freedom of choice and a control over their lives that did not stand up to scrutiny.[48] Coffield subsequently argued that 'distinctions between structural and individual factors more accurately reflect traditional academic divisions between sociology and psychology than real differences in the factors that impinged on the lives of the people we studied.'[49]

HOUSING: LONGITUDINAL STUDIES, ALLOCATION POLICIES, AND STRUCTURAL ANALYSES

Arguably the most interesting aspect of recent work on agency and social policy has been the suggestion that the response to the cycle speech provides insights into the outlook of a generation of social scientists. Richard Berthoud has argued that the research studies commissioned by the Transmitted Deprivation Research Programme were concerned with either economic factors or psychiatric factors, but not with the relationships between them.[50] Like Berthoud, Alan Deacon argues that academics did not respond to the challenge, regarding Joseph's research agenda as 'at best a red herring and at worst a distraction from the much more important issue of the generation and persistence of inequalities.'[51] Deacon has claimed that, by the 1970s, the alleged rejection of individualist or behavioural accounts of poverty by theorists such as Richard Titmuss had hardened into an approach that precluded any discussion of such factors. It was this 'quasi-Titmuss paradigm or school' that, in its hostility to explaining poverty by reference to the behaviour of the poor, created an intellectual void that was filled by neo-Conservative writers in the 1980s.

There is no doubt that many social scientists, certainly within the social policy community, were extremely hostile to the original Joseph hypothesis. Most famously, in March 1974, Peter Townsend condemned the cycle of deprivation as being 'a mixture of popular stereotypes and ill-developed, mostly contentious, scientific notions. It is a conceptual bed into which diverse travellers have scrambled for security and comfort.'[52] At the same conference, Barbara Castle, Joseph's successor as Secretary of State for Social Services, was careful to stress that study of a cycle of deprivation should be in parallel with a broader anti-poverty strategy, arguing there could not be any meaningful preparation for parenthood for families 'whose children are condemned to grow up in crowded homes, crowded schools, crowded streets, on meagre budgets under the shadow of endless nagging insecurity.'[53] Under Labour, there was a marked drop in Ministerial commitment to the Research Programme.

Deacon has argued that by the mid-1970s, social policy analysts were unwilling to enter debates about poverty, behaviour, and culture. This was shaped by the influence on the welfare debate of Marxist political economy, Anthony Crosland's view of socialism, the upsurge in unemployment from the mid-1970s, and the growth of inequality in Britain in the late 1970s and early 1980s.[54] Certainly by the mid-1970s the most radical critiques of the Community Development Projects had begun to appear.[55] In terms of housing, some argue by the late 1970s, explanations of 'problem estates' that emphasised the pathology of individual residents were replaced by studies that stressed the importance of design and management, and the changing demographic profile of council housing. Policies that were aimed at individuals or individual families were replaced by strategies aimed at economies and the employability of residents of particular areas. Although the debate in the 1950s had been about 'unsatisfactory tenants,' by the late 1970s the terminology had changed to that of 'difficult tenants.' This interpretation was influenced by theories on deviance, with the authors acknowledging that people could be victims of other tenants' notions of how people ought to behave—behaviour and tolerance were two sides of the same coin.[56]

Housing in some ways remained tangential to the Research Programme, which is in itself interesting, suggesting that the Joint Working Party struggled to attract applications from researchers working in this field, and providing partial support for the Deacon argument. Nevertheless, several studies into housing were commissioned, and housing was considered by researchers looking at other issues, such as health, psychiatric factors, and money. In his book-length literature review, Alan Murie argued that discussion of housing in relation to deprivation was not solely about cycles of disadvantage and transmitted deprivation, but was about cycles of advantage, accumulation of wealth and realisation of capital.[57] While Murie looked at low-income owner occupiers, he stressed two factors—the provision of housing aid and advice, and the system of housing finance and subsidy. Murie concluded that if housing inequality and its consequences were considered important, closer examination of the distributional aspects of policy and of the relationship between housing and other aspects of the social and economic structure were necessary.[58] Murie's work showed how discussion of housing had been dominated by writers such as David Donnison, Professor of Social Policy at the London School of Economics and, like Abel-Smith, a key adviser to the Labour Governments.

Other projects funded by the Research Programme employed an essentially structural analysis, and failed to respond to the challenge issued by Joseph or by Rutter and Madge in their literature review. Linda McDowell, for example, attempted to take an intergenerational approach to housing deprivation, using the National Survey of Health and Development (1946). Like Murie, McDowell noted that deprivation in general, and in the housing market in particular, was a reflection of the marked and persistent inequalities in the distribution of goods, resources and life chances in capitalist countries. The mechanisms of transmission, therefore, were extra-familial, located in the social and economic structure of society.[59] By 1961, housing conditions for all the survey members had improved markedly, because they moved out of the private rented sector into council housing and owner-occupation. Yet all the survey members who lived in the worst property in 1972 had experienced housing deprivation in 1948, and the privileged had largely maintained their position. McDowell concluded that housing mobility was a one-way process: while the majority of deprived and less-privileged survey members had moved up a category, it was very unusual for those initially in the most privileged category to move down.[60] Inequalities were reflected in a larger network of economic and social inequalities, in the education system and job market.

In the Bristol study of the allocation of council housing and its relation to social stratification, Bernard Ineichen noted that the failure of the market to provide adequate housing for the poorest households was an enduring feature of British society. Many of the poor were concentrated in the council sector. Ineichen explored the effects of allocation policies on the life chances of young people who grew up in the council sector, and attempted to relate them to the wider question of continuities in disadvantage. He noted, for example, that in the same way as dress, manner, and perceived life-style had been shown to influence the chances of applicants of obtaining a mortgage, the grading of prospective tenants had been a feature of the allocation process. Two surveys were undertaken, one of the allocation policies of six local authority housing departments in Avon, and the other of the housing aspirations of a group of young people who had grown up on a large local authority housing estate. In terms of allocation policies, intending tenants seldom had all the information they required, housing authorities had to allocate in terms of need, and the disorganised and sometimes chaotic personal relationships in the lives of some applicants for council housing was a further factor.[61] As Ungerson had noted at the outset, causation had been narrowed to the impact of allocation policies.

This structural emphasis was evident in Muriel Brown and Nicola Madge's final report on the Transmitted Deprivation programme (1982). They reported that many of the projects had favoured a structural rather than a personal or behavioural approach, noting that 'much of the research concerned with very broad definitions of deprivation has inevitably concluded that disadvantage is deeply rooted in the structure of our society.'[62] Age influenced the circumstances under which people lived, and there might be five housing stages experienced over the life cycle. Moreover, they drew on the Murie and McDowell projects to argue that, across the life cycle, socio-economic status had a more marked influence on housing conditions than did age or family circumstances, and that there was convincing evidence of intergenerational patterns of family continuity.[63] Housing circumstances contributed to the deprivation suffered by children and their families in terms of health, progress at school, and general well-being. However, Brown and Madge admitted that it was difficult to specify the causal nature of these relationships and to separate the effect of environmental stress from that of the social, economic, and personal problems that families living under the worst conditions were likely also to be facing.[64] Despite these caveats, Brown and Madge's analysis was primarily a structural one. They noted, for example, that 'housing both reflects the inequalities of income and wealth in society and, in an important sense, sustains and exacerbates them.'[65] Housing showed that deprivation was part of a network of structural disadvantages, and while housing conditions had improved enormously, the distribution of housing remained markedly unequal. They wrote that 'the will to tackle patterns of disadvantage in housing must be found if the persistent cycles of disadvantage in this field are to be reduced.'[66] A clear and uncontested implication of the evidence, they claimed, was that 'the better the housing stock becomes in terms of quantity and quality, the less absolute housing deprivation there will be.'[67] Therefore action was required not only to build and improve the housing stock, but also to 'tackle the question of the distribution of income and wealth in our society which is crucial to the question of access to housing.'[68]

Muriel Brown subsequently provided an insight into her own stance on deprivation and disadvantage. She wrote that it was originally thought that the clue to the persistence of poverty and deprivation in the midst of affluence might lie in its transmission across the generations as a result of cultural or psychological processes within the family. But much of the research that was set up moved the inquiry away from family failure to include a more socio-economic view of deprivation—'alongside work on problem families and psychological processes, work on such topics as employment prospects and housing opportunities was undertaken.'[69] The research found that intergenerational continuities, in areas such as poor housing, were far more likely to derive from the structural disadvantage of certain social groups than a coincidence of particular family lifestyles. Brown wrote that 'structural factors do not explain all the incidence of all deprivations but they do account for the largest part of material or socio-economic deprivations.'[70] Thus she concluded that 'social disadvantage is demonstrably a consequence of the structure of society. Certain groups are consistently exposed to deprivation in income, health, education, housing, employment and family life.'[71]

CONCLUSION

This chapter has been concerned with two main questions—tracing the origins of the cycle speech, and exploring the research on housing that was commissioned in the course of the subsequent Research Programme. The speech can be seen to have had both longer term antecedents and more immediate policy origins. However, in both the home was prominent. Joseph's own relatively privileged upbringing derived from the fact that his father had largely founded the Bovis construction company, and he himself was later a Director of the family firm. Joseph had a genuine interest in family background, homelessness, and poverty, illustrated by his founding of the Mulberry Housing Trust and support for the Child Poverty Action Group. He first entered the Cabinet in 1962, under Harold Macmillan, as Minister of Housing and Local Government, and he remained interested in housing issues. Through the 1950s and 1960s, Joseph was increasingly influenced by the concept of the problem family, which itself had fed into debates about 'unsatisfactory tenants.' From the Lords, Joseph later applauded the Home-Start charity, which used volunteers to befriend families and to provide assistance to those struggling to bring up children. The home and emotional or psychological health were therefore important components of his cycle of deprivation hypothesis.

The Transmitted Deprivation Programme itself provides insights into the approach of a generation of social scientists to the home and housing, and a means of testing the arguments of Berthoud and Deacon. There was evidence of research that tried to look at both behavioural and structural factors: by Bryan Glastonbury, Rutter and Madge, and the team led by Coffield. This reflected the disciplinary backgrounds of some researchers in psychology and psychiatry, as well as the influence of ethnographic and anthropological fieldwork in the United States, where culture was viewed as an adaptive response to environmental factors, and an awareness that explanations had become unnecessarily polarised. However, apart from the Coffield study, researchers for the most part looked at housing rather than the home. They located the role of housing within a structural analysis, and this was especially true of the final report on the Research Programme as a whole. Researchers working with longitudinal studies defined deprivation in terms of inequalities in goods, resources, and life chances in a capitalist society, and tended to stress the intergenerational continuities in housing experience of a minority of families. Housing was explored in terms of distributional aspects of policy, such as allocation systems for council housing, with researchers arguing that social stratification was a consequence of the failure of the housing market. These researchers tended to have backgrounds in social policy or social administration, they were influenced by the American literature on blaming the victim, and perhaps most importantly, their response to transmitted deprivation was itself a reaction against earlier casework approaches and problem family stereotypes.

It is interesting, if perhaps not particularly surprising, that some of those involved in these debates have continued to contribute to research into housing and what is now termed social exclusion. Some of this has again taken a predominantly structural approach, looking at the links between housing, housing tenure, relative deprivation, and poverty, and at the location of the poorest areas. It is claimed that social exclusion is concerned with more than issues of distribution, embracing concepts of social participation and citizenship.[72] Nevertheless, critiques of social exclusion have drawn attention to how discourses of 'poor neighbourhoods' and 'housing problems' have drawn on a moral underclass discourse, so that problems of housing are seen in terms of crime and anti-social behaviour.[73] It has been argued further that the Government's social exclusion initiatives concentrate on obvious symptoms of marginality, rather than on structural economic forces.[74] And this is reflected in punitive sanctions where tenants guilty of antisocial behaviour (again termed problem families) are to lose housing benefit if they refuse to take state help to address the underlying causes of their bad behaviour.[75] In these ways, there is much continuity in debates over the past thirty-five years. Overall, the cycle speech and studies commissioned for the Transmitted Deprivation Research Programme provide intriguing insights into the perceived relationships between health and the modern home through the lenses offered by social policy and contemporary history, and into contemporary assessments of the relative influences on behaviour of both personal characteristics and material circumstances.

NOTES

1. Richard Berthoud, *The Disadvantages of Inequality: A Study of Social Deprivation* (London: Macdonald and Jane's, 1976), 180.
2. Peter Townsend, *Poverty in the United Kingdom: A Survey of Household Resources and Standards of Living* (London: Penguin–Allen Lane, 1979), 31. See also W. G. Runciman, *Relative Deprivation and Social Justice: A Study of Attitudes to Social Inequality in Twentieth-Century England* (London: Routledge and Kegan Paul, 1966).
3. David Piachaud, 'Peter Townsend and the Holy Grail,' *New Society* 57 (1981): 419–21; Amartya Sen, 'Poor, relatively speaking,' *Oxford Economic Papers* 35 (1983): 153–69; Peter Townsend, 'A sociological approach to the measurement of poverty—A rejoinder to Professor Amartya Sen,' *Oxford Economic Papers* 37 (1985): 659–68; Amartya Sen, 'A sociological approach to the measurement of poverty: a reply to Professor Peter Townsend,' *Oxford Economic Papers* 37 (1985): 669–76.
4. Brian Jarman, 'Identification of underprivileged areas,' *British Medical Journal* 286 (1983): 1705–9.

5. Joanna Mack and Stewart Lansley, *Poor Britain* (London: George Allen & Unwin, 1985); Peter Townsend, Peter Phillimore and Alastair Beattie, *Health and Deprivation: Inequality and the North* (London: Routledge, 1989), 3–17, 30–40. See also Peter Townsend papers, Alfred Sloman Library, University of Essex, box 62, file 4: Peter Townsend, 'Deprivation' (n.d. but 1986).
6. John Welshman, 'Ideology, social science, and public policy: The debate over transmitted deprivation,' *Twentieth Century British History*, 16, 3 (2005): 306–41.
7. *The Times*, 12 December 1994, pp. 19, 21; Andrew Denham and Mark Garnett, *Keith Joseph* (Chesham: Acumen, 2001).
8. Keith Joseph, 'The cycle of family deprivation,' in Keith Joseph, *Caring for People* (London: Conservative Political Centre, 1972), 29–46, 32.
9. Ibid., 33.
10. Ibid., 34.
11. Ibid., 37, 39, 46.
12. Ibid., 32.
13. Ibid., 38.
14. Ibid., 41.
15. *The Times*, 30 June 1972, 17. See also Nicholas Timmins, *The Five Giants: A Biography of the Welfare State* (London: HarperCollins, 1995, new edn., 2001), 289–90.
16. DHSS, *The Family in Society: Preparation for Parenthood. An Account of Consultations with Professional, Voluntary and Other Organisations, October 1972 to February 1973* (London: HMSO, 1974), 5–8.
17. Terry Coleman, 'Captain of the second XI,' *Guardian*, 12 November 1973, 13; Denham and Garnett, *Keith Joseph*, 22, 55, 104, 232.
18. Keith Joseph, *Social Security: The New Priorities* (London: Conservative Political Centre, 1966), 7, 16.
19. Ibid., 33. See also Keith Joseph, 'Help for the really needy,' *Daily Telegraph*, 22 March 1966.
20. Ministry of Housing and Local Government, *Unsatisfactory Tenants: Sixth Report of the Housing Management Sub-Committee of the Central Housing Advisory Committee* (London: HMSO, 1955), 3.
21. Ibid., 4.
22. Ibid., 5.
23. See for example, John Macnicol, 'In pursuit of the underclass,' *Journal of Social Policy* 16 (1987): 293–318; John Macnicol, 'From "problem family" to "underclass," 1945–95,' in Rodney Lowe and Helen Fawcett (eds.), *Welfare Policy in Britain: The Road from 1945* (London: Macmillan/Institute of Contemporary British History, 1999), 69–93.
24. Keith Joseph, *Changing Housing* (London: Conservative Political Centre, 1967), 4.
25. Keith Joseph, *Freedom Under the Law* (London: Conservative Political Centre, 1975), 9.
26. Coleman, 'Captain of the second XI.'
27. John Cunningham, 'The family way,' *Guardian*, 4 June 1973, 9. This story has been much cited by later writers.
28. Henry Herbert Goddard, *The Kallikak Family: A Study in the Heredity of Feeblemindedness* (New York: Macmillan, 1912, Arno Press edn., 1973).
29. Macnicol, 'In pursuit of the underclass,' 296.
30. SSRC-DHSS, *Transmitted Deprivation: First Report of the DHSS-SSRC Working Party* (London: SSRC, 1974), para 18.4.
31. Ibid., para. 20.2.
32. National Archives, Kew, London (hereafter NA) BN 13/179: 'Note of a meeting held on 11th February 1969 to discuss homelessness,' 14/2/69.

33. Ibid.: J. Greve, 'Preliminary report of study of homelessness in Greater London,' 13/1/70.
34. John Greve, Dilys Page, and Stella Greve, *Homelessness in London* (Edinburgh and London: Scottish Academic Press, 1971), 255.
35. Ibid., 282.
36. Bryan Glastonbury, *Homeless Near a Thousand Homes: A Study of Families without Homes in South Wales and the West of England* (London: George Allen & Unwin, 1971), 74.
37. Clare Ungerson, 'Housing and transmitted deprivation—Some general thoughts on possible areas of research' (n.d. but 1976). Original SSRC copy now in the possession of the author.
38. SSRC-DHSS, *Transmitted Deprivation: Third Report of the DHSS-SSRC Working Party* (London: SSRC, 1977), paras 2.3.1, 2.3.2.
39. NA MH 152/83: Millerson and Ineichen, 'Housing factors in transmitted deprivation,' 9/75.
40. Michael Rutter and Nicola Madge, *Cycles of Disadvantage: A Review of Research* (London: Heinemann, 1976), 56.
41. Ibid., 327.
42. Ibid.
43. NA MH 152/85: Frank Coffield, Philip Robinson, and Jacquie Sarsby, 'A conceptual and empirical study of the transmitted deprivation thesis' (n.d. but 1974); interview between the author and Frank Coffield, Newcastle-Upon-Tyne, 8 April 2003.
44. Frank Coffield, Philip Robinson, and Jacquie Sarsby, *A Cycle of Deprivation? A Case Study of Four Families* (London: Heinemann, 1980), 22.
45. Ibid., 56, 66–7, 69, 161.
46. Ibid., 177.
47. Ibid., 163–64.
48. Ibid., 192.
49. Frank Coffield, '"Like father, like son": The family as a potential transmitter of deprivation,' in Nicola Madge (ed.), *Families at Risk* (London: Heinemann, 1983), 24. See also Berthoud, 'Transmitted deprivation,' 160, 166.
50. Richard Berthoud, 'Transmitted deprivation: the kite that failed,' *Policy Studies* 3 (1983): 161–2.
51. Alan Deacon, *Perspectives on Welfare: Ideas, Ideologies and Policy Debates* (Buckingham: Open University Press, 2002), 23–6. See also John Welshman, 'The unknown Titmuss,' *Journal of Social Policy* 33, 2 (2004): 225–47.
52. Peter Townsend, 'The cycle of deprivation: the history of a confused thesis,' in British Association of Social Workers, *The Cycle of Deprivation: Papers Presented to a National Study Conference, Manchester University, March, 1974* (Birmingham: BASW, 1974), 8.
53. Barbara Castle, 'The political challenge,' in BASW, *The Cycle of Deprivation,* 2.
54. Deacon, *Perspectives on Welfare,* 23–6.
55. See in particular Community Development Project, *Gilding the Ghetto: The State and the Poverty Experiments* (London: CDP, 1977).
56. Pauline Papps, 'Anti-social behaviour strategies—Individualistic or holistic?,' *Housing Studies* 13, 5 (1998): 641–3; Gerry Popplestone and Chris Paris, *Managing Difficult Tenants* (London: Centre for Environmental Studies, 1979).
57. Alan Murie, *Housing, Inequality and Deprivation* (London: Heinemann, 1983), 230.
58. Ibid., 236.
59. Linda McDowell, 'Housing deprivation: An intergenerational approach,' in Muriel Brown (ed.), *The Structure of Disadvantage* (London: Heinemann, 1983), 175.

60. Ibid., 188.
61. Bernard Ineichen, 'Council housing and disadvantage: The allocation of council housing and its relation to social stratification,' in Brown (ed.), *The Structure of Disadvantage*, 153–71.
62. Muriel Brown and Nicola Madge, *Despite the Welfare State: A Report on the SSRC-DHSS Programme of Research into Transmitted Deprivation* (London: Heinemann, 1982), 4–5.
63. Ibid., 83, 91–3.
64. Ibid., 242.
65. Ibid., 309.
66. Ibid., 310.
67. Ibid., 314.
68. Ibid., 311.
69. Muriel Brown, 'Deprivation and social disadvantage,' in Brown (ed.), *The Structure of Disadvantage*, 2.
70. Ibid., 6.
71. Ibid., 11.
72. Peter Lee and Alan Murie, *Poverty, Housing Tenure and Social Exclusion* (Bristol: Policy Press, 1997).
73. Peter Somerville, 'Explanations of social exclusion: where does housing fit in?,' *Housing Studies* 13, 6 (1998): 761–80; Paul Watt and Keith Jacobs, 'Discourses of social exclusion: an analysis of *Bringing Britain Together: A National Strategy for Neighbourhood Renewal*,' *Housing, Theory and Society* 17 (2000): 14–26.
74. David M. Smith, *On the Margins of Inclusion: Changing Labour Markets and Social Exclusion in London* (Bristol: Policy Press, 2005), vi–x, 39–62.
75. Patrick Wintour, 'Antisocial neighbours could face loss of housing benefit,' *Guardian*, 6 June 2006, 15.

14 The Home as Environment

Changing Understandings from the History of Childhood Lead Poisoning[1]

John Burnham

INTRODUCTION

In spite of the relentless processes of modernization and the efforts of modernists, the Victorian ideal of the home persisted to a substantial extent on both sides of the Atlantic through the twentieth century. The home was a safe moral sphere, dominated by a wife-mother. But this psychological haven was also a physical construction. Walls and screens kept the cruel, dangerous world shut outside. Housing therefore created a private place of material safety while the 'home within' provided a safe psychological environment. Particularly for children, the home sheltered youngsters from the physical elements and, at the same time, kept undesirable, worldly influences at bay.[2]

The fortress home was always under siege. At the turn of the nineteenth into the twentieth century, people saw how germs could come in and turn the home, previously a safe harbour, into a dangerous place. Inhabitants could, of course, cleanse and disinfect their houses and render them safe once again. As ideas of allergy developed, staying inside was one way to defend oneself against the irritating pollens, smokes, and fumes that caused so much misery to the allergic. During the twentieth century, however, as Mark Jackson has pointed out, experts came to believe that the house itself was a major source of allergens, particularly house dust and all of the components that went into that ubiquitous and complex substance that dominated the domestic environment. By mid-century, the house for many people had become anything but a refuge.[3] In the middle of the twentieth century, just as the idea of house dust was working from the inside to make the home a dangerous place, another change was taking place that also caused people to think of the home as a source of danger. The new factor was an alarming syndrome, known as childhood lead poisoning.

Even to conceptualize a disease syndrome involves having some idea about the cause of the syndrome. In the case of childhood lead poisoning, authorities agreed that originally the cause was a poison that existed in the home of the victim. At first, the supposed sources of lead, such as furniture and toys, were incidental to the home and easily controllable by care-givers. The new factor that emerged in mid-century was the discovery that the lead that was the source of dangerous lead poisoning in children was an integral part of the interior of their housing. Significantly, changing ideas of this disease syndrome provide striking opportunities for understanding how, in the past, the idea of home could change or, more particularly, how the house, conventionally a haven for children, first became itself a health hazard and then subsequently became reconstrued merely as part of the general environment that carried agents of impairment and illness.

Childhood lead poisoning, or childhood plumbism, refers to a syndrome that physicians began to differentiate from adult lead poisoning during the first three decades of the twentieth century. The literature initially was overwhelmingly dominated by investigations from the United States, where most of the cases were reported. In that literature, it was because the victims were very young children, usually toddlers who were exploring their immediate domestic environments, that understandings of childhood lead poisoning depended to a remarkable extent on ideas about the contents and boundaries of the home environment.

Experts' ideas about the syndrome went through three stages.[4] They believed first that the poison was introduced on specific objects such as the painted toys and furniture that would ordinarily be in a home. Around 1950, experts' attention turned to the walls, ceilings, and floors of the dwelling space. At that point, the care-givers who furnished the implicit psychosocial environment of the home also came into play. There were therefore two factors operating in the home, the physical environment and the psychosocial environment that caused children actively to ingest available lead. Beginning in the 1960s and 1970s, in a third stage, ideas about the general environment changed thinking not only about the syndrome of childhood lead poisoning but about the material boundaries of the home itself. Under these new circumstances, when the physical confines of the home dissolved in many ways, the psychosocial environment, the interaction of care-givers and children, also became much less relevant to children's health. Where once it had been possible to blame the child's care-givers for allowing the child to ingest a chemical, now it was possible to blame society as a whole for a dangerous, inescapable environment. The primary aim of this chapter is to explore these shifting constructions of childhood lead poisoning.

THE HOME AS ENVIRONMENT

In the 1920s and 1930s, physicians knew a rare paediatric malady, childhood lead poisoning, only in an acute form. In those cases, a small child would show alarming and often fatal symptoms of poisoning, typically encephalopathy (disease of the brain). Even when there was some recovery, serious neurological sequelae could persist. Lead poisoning was at best very difficult to diagnose, and, once diagnosed, treatment was not effective. Prevention therefore became a high priority for physicians and public health figures.

Physicians were able to trace the first reported cases directly to a child's chewing on a surface that had been covered with a leaded paint—typically a crib or cot in the child's immediate environment. Lead has a sweet taste and so was attractive. After a few years, another major obvious source appeared: a painted window sill, which was a favourite object of gnawing or sucking for children in the teething stage. Occasionally other items in the child's home, such as furniture or even a toy, might still be blamed. Public health authorities warned parents to keep children from dangerous painted objects just as they warned parents to keep children away from sharp objects or domestic poisons (such as lye) or anything else that might be found normally in otherwise safe housing.[5]

In the middle decades of the twentieth century, ideas about children's environments transformed the concept of childhood lead poisoning. Experts began to focus on the dwelling itself rather than items found within the living space. It was at that time that the first concrete notion of environment explicitly shaped medical discourse concerning children's plumbism. The change occurred because public health officials identified a new, more general material danger in the home: chips and flakes produced from deteriorating leaded paint on walls and ceilings in the interior of the housing.[6] Paint that peeled and flaked off the walls and ceilings was first reported by a Baltimore health worker in the United States at the end of the 1940s when she first had to go visiting in slum homes.[7]

Interpretation of these observations were influenced by epidemiology. As medical authorities became increasingly concerned about chronic rather than acute diseases, housing had become an urgent concern to public health officials in the 1930s. In the post-Second World War period, doctors came to view housing as a generalizable environment that affected health and that could be improved in order to prevent illness. The U.S. Public Health Service in 1956, for example, suggested that 'Health departments should start thinking in terms of preventing blight rather than handling complaints.'[8]

In medical reports explicitly focusing on lead poisoning in children, the connection between the housing environment and poisoning was often specific, as it had been even before mid-century. The author of one 1950s report noted: 'Almost without exception these children come from families in the poorest economic groups, whose homes or apartments are in poor repair, often with paint peeling off the walls.' Or, as another report put it: 'Contributing factors to this high incidence of lead intoxication seem to be related directly to the environment . . . these children live in houses where lead-containing paint, used many years ago, is now flaking and peeling from the surface.'[9] As this phrasing shows, not only did the authors of these reports use the housing-as-environment formulation, but they tied it directly to the idea of peeling and flaking paint in the interior of the dwelling. In the context of housing environment, then, one source of the interest in paint chips and flakes becomes clear: an environmental explanation of childhood lead poisoning was easily conceptualized in a tangible form.

This idea of environment in the home in turn shaped epidemiological thinking. In the 1950s, in Philadelphia, an Eastern U.S. city, when officials made lead poisoning a reportable disease, it was easy for public health staff members to draw maps showing the geographical concentration of cases, just as John Snow had traced cholera in London a century earlier.[10] In this way, the problem of childhood lead poisoning became linked to an idea of general physical environment: if the housing environment could be improved, the medical problems would resolve. As late as 1974, Donald Barltrop, a British pediatrician who worked on both sides of the Atlantic, concluded bitterly: 'Until effective standards for the domestic environment are devised, it is likely that children will continue to be employed as biological indicators of substandard housing.'[11]

Ironically, the 1950s emphasis on the victims' environment also contributed to another view of childhood lead poisoning, one that caused physicians and public health personnel dealing with children diagnosed with lead poisoning to put renewed emphasis on an old problem, pica—a compulsion to eat non-food materials. 'The universality of pica' in cases of childhood lead poisoning, noted two Chicago investigators in 1957, 'is a finding again to be underlined.' Significantly, introducing pica into the causal chain between children and lead gave 'environment' a number of different connotations in the 1950s.[12]

In addition to the physical aspects of the housing, clinicians had become well aware of the social environment of the child. As one pair of experienced pediatricians reported, 'there seems to be widespread ignorance or disregard of the hazards to the child' of eating particles of paint. 'Despite vigorous education campaigns . . . many parents continue to accept pica as a harmless manifestation of normal infantile development.' Furthermore, 'crowded conditions within the home, and in many instances the absence of supervision by adults who may be obliged to leave children to earn a living, allow the infant and preschool child opportunity to eat toxic material without restraint.'[13]

The epidemiology was clear: lead poisoning affected small children in slum housing. During this period, as experts discussed the problem, hardly any source other than ingested paint chips from interior surfaces was even hinted at. The solution was also clear: remove either the lead or the children from the houses. A 1969 writer commented: 'It's no use telling women not to let their children eat paint . . . it does about as much good as telling a child not to suck his thumb.' Moreover, she quoted a Chicago physician: 'You have to have a home safe enough to put a child down in while you do the washing and ironing. You can tie him down, but then he doesn't get to explore his environment . . . he's culturally deprived. If you live in a lead trap, you can't win.'[14]

These clinicians, then, identified the social environment of the children as a new part of the operating environment that led to plumbism in children.

And they concluded: 'Since this disease is essentially environmental, preventive measures are possible.'[15] That statement concerning human agency could apply equally well to the physical housing of the children as well as the behaviour of care-givers. But other clinicians went further. They, too, found that pica was an almost universal precondition for childhood plumbism, but they construed the cause even more specifically as the child's social and psychological environment. Such a view was not unusual at mid-century, for at that time physicians, and especially paediatricians, attributed much illness of all kinds to psychological factors. As other chapters in this volume demonstrate, this was the era of psychosomatic medicine.[16] The Lead Poisoning Clinic established at Children's Hospital in Washington in 1955, for example, had a psychologist and a social worker on the staff as well as physicians.[17]

Since only children with pica were showing up in the hospitals, it was natural to ask, why were the pica children different from other children? The explanation, according to two experts from Chicago, was that the victims had been orally aggressive to an extreme, to the point of persistently biting other children as well as painted surfaces: 'The aggressive biting by many of our patients suggests again an emotional basis for pica.' Another group, from the District of Columbia, took up the problem of 'the persistence of oral activities beyond the normal developmental period' in the poisoned children. Their cases suggested to them that 'a child may turn to excessive mouth activities if his normal dependent needs for satisfactions in early relationships are not met.' As was customary then, experts turned again to the psychosocial environment and, in line with other authorities such as psychologist John Bowlby writing about maladjustment and delinquency, asserted that 'the most important and consistent factor in pica . . . was the mother-child relationship.'[18]

The extraordinary way in which pica, beginning about 1955, came to occupy a central place in discussions of lead poisoning in children is therefore more understandable when it is recognized that the new social/psychological environmentalism, working in combination with epidemiology, reinforced the traditional interest that doctors took in individual cases. Physicians and other concerned professionals were asking what social and psychological factors caused a particular child to have pica.[19] But whatever the basis for the pica, once again there was hope that controlling pica in the family environment could mean controlling lead poisoning in children in any home.

For those working within this idea of environment, one obvious strategy, as I have suggested, was to continue an individual approach and, in a policy that echoed the use 'parentectomy' in asthmatic children, to remove children from dangerous home environments.[20] In 1953, J. Julian Chisolm, Jr., at Johns Hopkins took the extraordinary step of arranging for a local children's hospital to hold lead-poisoned children for extensive periods so that they could not go home and be poisoned again. The children were discharged only when the home had been cleared of lead or when other quarters were found for the family. The programme was still in place in Baltimore a quarter of a century later, when the average stay was 63 days, with a range of 20 to 104 days.[21] In focusing on removing children from their environments, it was possible for clinicians to avoid choosing between the youngsters' housing environment and psychosocial circumstances as the primary causative factor for childhood lead poisoning.

During the 1950s and 1960s, all articulate parties—specialist physicians, public health officials, and various representatives of the public—concurred and subscribed to the stereotyped portrait of childhood lead poisoning. They agreed that it was a disease of housing that was inadequately maintained. They also agreed that it was a disease of segments of the population who were ignorant of the risks they were running in the home environments in which they lived and reared children.[22] For public health personnel who worked within this framework of unfortunate people in an unfortunate environment, it was still necessary to explain why some children in bad physical surroundings became sick, and others did not, beyond the differences among the care-givers who provided the psychosocial environment. Mouthing behaviour in small children was normal behaviour. Why would lead find its way into the stomachs of some toddlers, and not others? It was clear that epidemiology did not always have the answers.

The geographic distribution of reported cases was particularly baffling. Most of the case reports of lead poisoning in toddlers came from the United States. A locally peculiar outbreak among older children in Australia had been contained decades earlier.[23] The extremely rare cases in Britain could almost always be traced to drinking water carried through old lead pipes. In the United States, the bulk of the cases had been reported from one city, Baltimore, where by coincidence interested and influential experts were working in the Johns Hopkins medical school located there. There were a few cases in other U.S. Eastern cities. Cincinnati also had some cases, but in mid-century, it was one of only three U.S. cities with adequate testing facilities. Some cases showed up irregularly in Chicago. But Pittsburgh, for example, and most of the far Western cities tended to be free of cases.[24]

The usual explanation for the unevenness in the incidence of childhood plumbism at that time was that physicians in many localities were not looking for lead poisoning in children, and so they did not see and report cases. New research suggests, however, that in fact different housing patterns in different cities could account for much of the variation in reports of cases of childhood lead poisoning—one of those material flows that, as Christopher Sellers points out, can confound cultural constructions of the environment.[25] Lead paint was expensive. Therefore settled slum areas, such as parts of New York City, where dwellings produced a baffling lack of childhood lead poisoning, simply never had that kind of paint applied to them.[26] This pattern of neighbourhood stability may also explain why slum areas in Europe did not report cases. In the late nineteenth and early twentieth centuries, most newer cities developed slums in peripheral areas, housing that also would never be painted with expensive oil paints containing lead. Only certain urban areas such as Baltimore had upscale housing that in the middle of the twentieth century had deteriorated into slum dwellings in which children were poisoned by lead paint. Indeed, it turns out that outside of Baltimore and a few other locations, most deteriorated housing had never been upscale at all, so that childhood lead poisoning was largely an accidental occurrence that would not fit normal epidemiological patterns.[27]

THE ENVIRONMENT TAKES ON NEW MEANINGS

During the post-war period, and particularly during the 1960s, broader cultural conditions were also changing, bringing new ways of viewing the world and novel social agendas. The 'environment,' which was initially implicated in lead poisoning in children who lived in deteriorated housing, also was evolving as a concept and was caught up in various social movements and indeed became a social movement in itself. The term *environmentalism,* as Christopher Sellers comments, did not function until the 1960s; when it did, it began to carry significances distinct from either the physical or the psychosocial home environment that was implicated in lead poisoning in children.[28] In particular, a shift in the meaning of the term environment, as well as changes in the environmental movement, included the development of what became an embryonic field of environmental health, affecting, to some extent, all medicine and public health.[29] It was under these changing circumstances that, from the late 1960s, the syndrome of childhood lead poisoning was reframed. From that point on, there were altered ways of seeing threshold dosage, sequelae, standards of normality, and, most dramatically, the means by which the lead entered children's bodies. From these novel perspectives, writers now emphasized not paint from the walls and woodwork of a home, but the air and dust that were everywhere.

By the beginning of the 1960s, large numbers of physicians, sensitive to changes in the culture around them, were attempting to think environmentally. Articles on 'environmental' factors in medicine, already present in the 1950s, proliferated during the 1960s. Special conferences on the subject attracted unprecedented requests for participation. As one public health physician commented in 1964:

> In the immediate years ahead, physicians can expect to find themselves forced into more and more concern with how environmental health knowledge can improve their arts of healing. How can a doctor adequately cope with the respiratory ills of a patient, for example, without knowledge about the air the man breathes in his community, the fumes to which he may be exposed in his workplace, and whether or not he smokes?[30]

Only at the end of the 1960s and continuing into the 1970s, however, did new phases in environmentalism intrude so that environmentalists themselves might have an interest in lead poisoning and, later, in childhood lead poisoning. At that point, changing ways of viewing plumbism in children began to become an important driver of the political environmental movement. In the new phase, the language continued to shift from 'pollution' (primarily air and water pollution, which were specific and localized, like the killing smog at Donora, Pennsylvania, or the 1952 London smog) to more general references to 'the environment.' The new phase was one centered on an adult thinking about him- or herself.[31]

From a later point of view, the outlook of environmental enthusiasts of the 1960s was still limited. Not least of their limitations was the fact that despite their growing activism, environmentalists were so slow to give attention to childhood lead poisoning. Indeed, much of the writing on environmentalism tended to move the attention of physicians and other health workers away from thinking of a specific disease agent (like lead)—that is, away from what was regarded as 'the fallacy of the "doctrine of specific etiology,"'—and towards broadly contextualized processes. In part, this thinking about the environment in terms of general ambience was a major trend among environmental thinkers. In part, too, the new epidemiology also tended to free environmentally oriented thinkers from specific processes in particular patients. As a figure in environmental medicine explained in 1968, when he spoke of epidemiology, he meant 'the totality of relationships between man and his environment to the extent that such relationships affect human health.'[32]

In addition to the optimistic activism of the 1960s, other fresh ways of thinking about the environment began to affect the reframing that overtook childhood lead poisoning. There was, to begin with, a series of additional concerns in that time period. When environmentalists more and more frequently spoke and wrote about unknown environmental factors that could affect health, they had in mind chiefly invisible radioactivity, fallout, and imperceptible chemicals. Donald Barltrop commented, for example, that 'although airborne lead as such may have limited importance, atmospheric fallout provides a continuing source of contamination for city soils and dusts.' Clearly, then, one of the factors that influenced this type of thinking was the Cold War. Atomic bombs and radiation were a topic of frequent remark, and public health officials, especially, had to think in terms of possible wartime disasters as well as the chemicals about which Rachel Carson famously wrote in *Silent Spring* in 1962.[33]

Moreover, around the same time, particularly by the 1970s, another major shift was occurring. Childhood lead poisoning ceased being exclusively a syndrome of obviously very sick youngsters. A new term was becoming commonplace in the medical, and especially the public health, literature on plumbism in children: asymptomatic or 'subclinical' lead poisoning.[34] By 1966, Harold Jacobziner of New York had formulated how the idea provided a new—and perhaps alternative but certainly, to him, modern and up-to-date—way of looking at the syndrome. For many years, lead poisoning had been recognized in children only when associated with lead encephalopathy—when clinical signs and symptoms of central nervous system irritation aroused the examining physician's suspicion of the possibility of lead poisoning. Little, if anything, was known by the average physician of the subclinical or asymptomatic phase. Epidemiology, Jacobziner wrote, had enabled medical workers to reconceptualize the natural processes of plumbism, and he now offered a striking analogy that other writers often quoted afterward: 'Lead poisoning in children may be compared to an iceberg, with the small visible portion being cases of lead encephalopathy and the major portion being the invisible and as yet asymptomatic patients.'[35]

People who were dealing with childhood plumbism were, like Jacobziner, making an inference. In the words of a Cleveland team as early as 1964: 'It is apparent that in any community where overt lead poisoning occurs, there must be a significant number of children whose cases can be classed as "subclinical."' A public health worker's 1968 formulation made explicit the fact that new medical technology created a new conceptualizations. There were two kinds of plumbism, symptomatic and asymptomatic: 'Childhood lead poisoning is almost entirely restricted to slum neighbourhoods, where lead poisoning affects about one of every fifteen children between the ages of one and five. Most display no symptoms . . . Asymptomatic lead poisoning is diagnosed from laboratory findings in the absence of other observed symptoms of lead poisoning.'[36]

By the end of the 1960s, the focus on sub-clinical or asymptomatic plumbism, plus concern about the bad consequences of even a very small burden of lead in a child, was greatly extending the possible medical interest in children who might possibly have been exposed to lead. As Chisolm concluded in 1968: 'Today every child with asymptomatic increased lead absorption should be hospitalized. A team approach to his problem should include the comprehensive efforts of the local health department, physician, medical social worker, and psychologist.'[37]

After another decade, by the late 1970s, much of the leadership among experts on childhood lead poisoning came, not from investigators who were in one way or another oriented to physiology, but from those who looked at circumstance—loosely interpreted as the environment—and epidemiology. Such people employed bench laboratory investigations of patients and their environments at only a relatively low level of priority. It was in this sense that childhood lead poisoning was a changed syndrome and was in new hands.

Most physicians rejected the idea that anyone outside the medical establishment could discuss the clinical issue of when a body had an excess load of lead or any other substance, that is, a load that could cause illness. But that did not prevent widespread, but vague, fears that the air was polluted with one more toxic substance that could subtly undermine health. And, of course, with the uncertainty of diagnosis, what was more subtle than lead? It can be no surprise, then, that by the 1970s, invisible radiation and the chemicals in smog had new company in the thoughts of those concerned about pathogens in their surroundings: The new factor was traces of lead carried in the air. Airborne lead had two aspects. One was direct inhalation, and the other was as fallout—lead particles in the atmosphere contaminated soil and water and dust just as radioactive fallout did. 'Fallout of lead from the air is believed to contribute significantly to the high lead content found in urban soil,' as a Connecticut team summarized the idea in 1975.[38]

From early in the twentieth century, in Europe and America, the idea of airborne poisons in industrialized areas was commonplace. Over time after 1950, motor car emissions grew in importance as a component of air pollution, especially after some of the obvious smoke and soot had been eliminated from the air by clean air legislation. People who saw danger in automobile exhausts were much more concerned, however, about known carcinogens in emissions than they were about lead poisoning. However, given the fact that within occupational safety and health, airborne lead emissions were a traditional concern, small-particle lead fumes took on more significance by the 1960s.[39]

Concern over air pollution had led to the passage of legislation in Western countries, even in the United States where a Clean Air Act had been passed in 1963, but lead was not a factor, not even the gasoline additive tetraethyl lead, which had proven so dangerous in occupational medicine. Indeed, lead became an issue in air pollution only because in California in the 1950s and 1960s, the campaign against motor car emissions was thwarted by the action of gasoline lead on catalytic converters. At exactly the same time, in addition to general concern about lead particles in the atmosphere, an additional idea about dangers in the air appeared: the possible effects of cigarette smoke in initiating a chronic but fatal disease, lung cancer, and perhaps other chronic diseases, all 'of insidious onset,' provided an alarming model for dangers that could be carried in the air. And incidentally, cigarette smoke at one time had carried some lead from pesticides applied to the leaves. It was no wonder that slowly a specific concern about lead residues in the air grew as environmentalists raised levels of concern about air pollution.[40]

By the late 1960s, a number of physicians were exploring the implications of airborne lead for medicine in general. 'Interest in the deleterious effects of lead has shifted recently from the industrial field to that of potential hazards to the community at large,' wrote Bryan T. Emmerson, the Australian best known among lead poisoning researchers for his work on lead neuropathy.[41] The community at large of course meant all people in an area, without regard to age or residence—independent of local geography or of the walls of any dwelling. Such was the clear implication of airborne lead.

However, there were several problems that environmental health activists faced before they could reformulate childhood lead poisoning into a general problem, entirely separate from individual cases. One of the questions raised by the notion of asymptomatic plumbism was: What was the 'normal' or 'natural' burden of lead in the human body, and to what extent might there be in the atmosphere, particularly from leaded gasoline exhausts, an amount of lead that, without anyone's realizing it, would constitute an environmental danger? Threshold values in general had become increasingly controversial in medicine. And very soon the environmental activists, too, fixed on the sometimes arbitrary nature of threshold doses and found reason to believe that sub-threshold exposures were undesirable as well.[42]

Those who were alarmed about lead in the environment faced the problem of showing exactly why lead was bad. Allegations that low levels of lead affected the cardiovascular system, the kidneys, and the nervous system negatively could not be confirmed consistently. Significantly, childhood lead poisoning was crucial to the final conceptualization. First, some investigators demonstrated through animal experiments that extremely young mammals were unusually susceptible to lead burdens. In particular, such very immature organisms could manifest lasting effects in their neurological development.[43] Second, great concern about mental retardation (developmental disability) and the hope of preventing or curing this affliction led to the possibility that sub-clinical, asymptomatic lead burdens were a major causal factor.[44] Third, screening programmes, especially those carried out with new technology in the United States, showed that small children who had substantial lead burdens often showed no obvious physical signs or symptoms.[45]

In 1971, an American occupational physician and social activist, Harriet L. Hardy, in a classic paper written with associates, finally put airborne lead together with asymptomatic plumbism. She worked within the framework provided by Clair Patterson's notion that the whole world had become poisoned with lead traces. In surveying where lead existed in the environment, including the streets of Boston, Hardy and her team returned repeatedly to the themes of lasting, cumulative effects from a lead burden, including neurological damage; of the importance of inhaled lead; and of the special risks to small children, especially of neurological impairment. This classic statement provided a template for environmentalists' concerns about lead for years afterward. Within one year, the authors of a U.S. National Research Council report on airborne lead concluded that urban youngsters had undesirably high exposures to lead in the air and to lead that had settled in dust and soils—again in the context of a possibly hazardous lead burden in asymptomatic children.[46]

In its new form, lead poisoning did not require pica and was not focused on dangerous areas and objects in the home. Rather, a wide range of more or less normal children mouthed dirt and dust found everywhere—even beyond breathing the air, which was not specific to any dwelling. Investigators in Rochester, New York, in 1974 were searching for 'a ubiquitous source of lead exposure,' exposure revealed by screening studies of both inner-city and suburban children. The investigators limited themselves to interior surfaces of houses and children's hands, constrained by the traditional view that the home was the site of poisoning. But they opened the possibility that the interior lead came from powdered paint or the air.[47]

A year later, a British team found substantial amounts of lead in the dust and dirt of Manchester, and they also found 'that a child can transfer from 5–50 mg of dirt from his hands (dirty from 30 min of activity in a normal urban playground) to a typical "sticky sweet"'. They went on to calculate the enormous amount of lead a child eating from two to twenty sweets could ingest in 24 hours.

> We conclude that children in urban surroundings, who may already be ingesting in food and drink an amount of lead approaching a tolerable limit, may considerably increase their daily lead intake by the accidental ingestion of dirt and dust in their surroundings in the course of their normal everyday activity.[48]

Already, then, not only the air and water from outside, but surrounding streets and playgrounds were rendering the boundaries of the home meaningless in terms of at least this one health hazard. Moreover, the problem was no longer confined to the slums. If children's body loads of lead were abnormal, it was because the youngsters lived in a polluted, unnatural world. Their home environment was effectively expanded almost indefinitely from the one that paediatricians and public health personnel had discussed in the 1950s. As two environmentalist activists put it, as new legislative and regulatory initiatives came into place, it did not matter that the new findings were imperfect: 'Effective preventive action must precede complete and final knowledge.'[49]

But the reorientation went further. From one point of view, the transformation of this paediatric syndrome into an environmental disorder was one of the first steps in a great reversal, the demedicalization of Western societies. Expertise concerning both cognitive and social changes around childhood lead poisoning moved away from physicians and away from medicine. The driving insights now came, typically, from non-medical professionals concerned about general environments, not about poisoned individual patients.[50] Although both elements, the medical and the non-medical, had been present before and continued after this fundamental reorientation, the emphasis shifted away from clinical diagnosis and care towards social action and technological fixes, most notably, and successfully, eliminating lead from motor fuels. By 1986, two New Jersey public health workers summarized the change: 'Lead poisoning [in children], long recognized as a medical problem, may more appropriately be considered a social problem since its prevention and eradication depend in such large measure on factors outside the medical profession.'[51]

CONCLUSION

Childhood lead poisoning of late twentieth-century environmental medicine was therefore different from the syndrome that medical thinkers had described in the middle of the century. Experts originally had been concerned about children with clinical symptoms who came from toxic home environments in which care-givers did not provide a protective psychosocial environment. Now experts were concerned with a different problem: children bearing hidden lead burdens from multiple environmental sources that put their neurological development at risk. This syndrome could be detected only with high-technology tests. The public health problem, lead in the general environment, likewise could be established only by laboratory-level investigation of commonly shared general environments, not individuals' homes.[52]

The configuration of the environment that carried lead to children therefore had changed away from home interiors or even areas of bad housing. By the 1970s, experts began to include the dirt and dust outside the home, dirt and dust in which children played as well as that in the air that they breathed. The home environment for toddlers did not stop at the interior walls. Dust and dirt distant from, as well as surrounding, a dwelling, plus the very air that everyone had to breathe, was, from both medical and demedicalized perspectives, a part of the home environment.

Some new evidence suggests that the breaking down of the assumed boundaries of toddlers' homes should not have been a total surprise to clinicians and public health figures, who had been following specific cases of acute plumbism. Evidence from the 1950s and 1960s suggests that the source of the lead in half or more of the cases was almost certainly not paint on the inside of the dwelling, but paint on the outside of the building. Moreover, similar statistics appear in contemporary reports from Baltimore and Boston: in at least half the cases, the lead source was exterior, not interior, paint—clearly a step into the environment outside the home.[53]

Moreover, the new viewpoint shifted the relation of the child to the environment. Where the child in a private, confined space once actively chewed or gnawed on sweet-tasting lead paint, now the child was a passive recipient of air or dust or dirt that pervaded every home in the area and did not differentiate one home from any other. From one point of view, this was just one aspect of a major shift in Westernized countries away from personal responsibility for the interface between technology and the individual or the parent–child unit.[54] Policymakers turned to engineering solutions, such as eliminating lead from motor car exhausts, that would protect everyone from harm, regardless of personal or socio-economic differences or whether the person was in a home environment or not.

Such considerations raise questions about the extent to which, in the history of medicine, blaming material conditions should obscure taking into account differences in class and culture. It may even be possible for some people still to use this history to justify urging care-givers who provide a psycho-social environment to watch active children carefully and to train those children to wash their hands, to avoid putting things into their mouths, and to observe other Western bourgeois standards. However, the modern home always existed in a context of ambivalence. In the middle of the twentieth century, many people (and not just Freudians) knew that little children had deeply mixed feelings about other people in their homes. And those people recognized the vulnerability of the small children (dramatically in the case of lead poisoning), and used the home as a protective haven against outside forces. Yet as other chapters in this book point out, the home itself was in an ambiguous position. On the one hand, homes should be constructed to incorporate the fresh air and light from the outside. On the other hand, toddlers could actively move and explore the inside, protected space of the home because outside dangers and discomforts were shut out.

Over the years, views changed. The child's body became the passive recipient of dangers that walls and interior parental watchfulness could not keep out.[55] Germs one could of course fight. But dust, dirt, and air carried to each body poisonous lead and other chemicals, regardless of physical or psychosocial boundaries. The home and family functioned at a much subordinated level when neither could protect the individual body from external forces.[56] The shifts in perception of childhood lead poisoning suggest that, regardless of the images of advertisers, the home itself cannot be exempted from what Gregg Mitman, Michelle Murphy, and Christopher Sellers have characterized recently as 'the multitudinous exposures permeating our modern world.'[57] In particular, the home has been continuously and intimately connected with children's health, but the ways in which people have conceptualized that connection has also changed their ideas about the contours of the home.

ACKNOWLEDGMENTS

A number of colleagues have offered helpful suggestions, and I have had particularly helpful readings from Marsha Hamilton, Mark Jackson, and John Sauer. This chapter was completed while the author was Scholar in Residence in the Medical Heritage Center at Ohio State University.

NOTES

1. Disclosure statement: in 1991–1995, I consulted with defense counsel in some cases dealing with lead poisoning. Almost all of the work reported on here, however, covers a later period and was researched at a later time and supported entirely by university and personal funding.
2. Tony Chapman and Jenny Hockey (eds.), *Ideal Homes? Social Change and Domestic Life* (London: Routledge, 1999), including Mike Hepworth, 'Privacy, Security and Respectability: The Ideal Victorian Home,' 17–29, especially 18;

Ellen M. Plante, *Women at Home in Victorian America: A Social History* (New York: Facts on File, 1997), especially 79.

3. Mark Jackson, *Allergy: The History of a Modern Malady* (London: Reaktion Books, 2006), 166–73.
4. Most of the publications came out of the United States, but by the end of the twentieth century, investigators and clinicians from other areas were sharing dominance with North Americans. One notable example was the Port Pirie studies from Australia; see, for example, David Wilson et al., 'Children's Blood Lead Levels in the Lead Smelting Town of Port Pirie, South Australia,' *Archives of Environmental Health* 41 (1986): 245–50.
5. The best general treatment is Peter C. English, *Old Paint: A Medical History of Childhood Lead-Paint Poisoning in the United States to 1980* (New Brunswick, NJ: Rutgers University Press, 2001). Another major account, with a different approach, is Christian Warren, *Brush with Death: A Social History of Lead Poisoning* (Baltimore, MD: Johns Hopkins University Press, 2000). The present chapter does not deal with epidemics of lead fumes generated by burning battery casings, which had no effect on conceptualization of the syndrome being discussed here.
6. English, *Old Paint.*
7. Margaret Galbreath, 'Lead Poisoning in Young Children: The Role of the Public Health Nurse,' *Public Health Nursing* 44 (1952): 551–52.
8. 'That New Look in Housing Shows Healthy Attitude,' *Public Health Reports* 70 (1955): 157. U.S. Public Health Service, *Annual Report,* 1956, 145. The appalling sanitary and structural conditions that fostered ill health are suggested in Sylvia Hood Washington, *Packing Them In: An Archaeology of Environmental Racism in Chicago, 1865–1954* (Lanham, MD: Lexington Books, 2005).
9. Arnold L. Tanis, 'Lead Poisoning in Children, Including Nine Cases Treated with Edathamil Calcium-Disodium,' *American Journal of Diseases of Children* 89 (1955): 325. J. Edmund Bradley and Samuel P. Bessman, 'Poverty, Pica, and Poisoning,' *Public Health Reports* 73 (1958): 467. Most of the public health literature on deteriorated housing in the mid-twentieth century focused on tenements and other dwellings that were originally cheap, not the converted and deteriorated housing that was originally expensive but that was the probable source of leaded paint. When people writing about plumbism discussed housing after World War II, they referred to formerly expensive dwellings.
10. Tanis, 'Lead Poisoning in Children,' 325. Theodore H. Ingall, Emil A. Tiboni, and Milton Werrin, in 'Lead Poisoning in Philadelphia, 1955–1960,' *Archives of Environmental Health* 3 (1961): 577, however, were driven by their data to observe that 'the over-all pattern is such as to raise suspicion that factors other than the distribution of lead in old paints may be involved in selected areas.' See later discussion.
11. Donald Barltrop, 'Children and Lead,' *American Journal of Diseases of Children* 127 (1974): 166.
12. C. David Jenkins and Robert B. Mellins, 'Lead Poisoning in Children,' *Archives of Neurology and Psychiatry* 77 (1957): 71. See, for example, the way in which J. Julian Chisolm, Jr., reporting in *A.M.A. American Journal of Diseases of Children* 90 (1955): 515–16, used the term 'environmental' to cover his particular focuses.
13. Bradley and Bessman, 'Poverty, Pica, and Poisoning,' 467.
14. Margaret English, 'Lead-Poisoned Kids,' *Look* (21 October 1969), 114.
15. Bradley and Bessman, 'Poverty, Pica, and Poisoning,' 468.
16. See, in particular, the chapters by John Stewart, Sarah Hayes, and Mark Jackson.

17. The amount of conspicuously psychological material in paediatric journals by the mid-1950s was considerable. George J. Cohen and Walter E. Ahrens, 'Chronic Lead Poisoning: A Review of Seven Years' Experience at the Children's Hospital, District of Columbia,' *Journal of Pediatrics* 54 (1959): 283.
18. Mellins and Jenkins, 'Epidemiological and Psychological Study;' and Frances K. Millican, Reginald S. Lourie, and Emma M. Layman, 'Emotional Factors in the Etiology and Treatment of Lead Poisoning,' *A.M.A. Journal of Diseases of Children* 91 (1956): 144–49.
19. Marcia Cooper, *Pica: A Survey of the Historical Literature as well as Reports from the Fields of Veterinary Medicine and Anthropology, the Present Study of Pica in Young Children, and a Discussion of Its Pediatric and Psychological Implications* (Springfield, IL: Charles C. Thomas, 1957). This book contains a summary of the literature on pica and is a symptom of the interest in pica at that time. The author was driven to believe that malnutrition caused pica in slum children and therefore that solving malnutrition would prevent plumbism in children.
20. As late as 1969, the American Academy of Pediatrics (quoted in English, *Old Paint,* 161) was insisting, 'The first precept is: *no child ever returns to a leaded house.*' On 'parentectomy' for asthmatic children, see the chapters by Mark Jackson and Gregg Mitman in this volume.
21. Paul Burgan, 'Role of the Pediatric Intermediate Care Facility in the Treatment of Children with Lead Poisoning,' in *Lead Absorption in Children: Management, Clinical, and Environmental Aspects,* eds. J. Julian Chisolm, Jr., and David M. O'Hara (Baltimore, MD: Urban & Schwarzenberg, 1982), 166–67. J. Julian Chisolm, Jr., and David M. O'Hara, 'Editors' Historical Note,' in ibid., 167–169.
22. Another contemporary document, again showing how complete the consensus was, was *Control of Lead Poisoning in Children* (pre-publication draft, U. S. Department of Health, Education and Welfare, Public Health Service, Bureau of Community Environmental Management, December 1970).
23. Allen Christophers, *Paediatric Lead Poisoning in Queensland: How and Why it Was so Different from Paediatric Lead Poisoning Elsewhere* (Melbourne: Department of Epidemiology and Preventive Medicine, Monash University, 1999); John C. Burnham, 'Biomedical Communication and the Reaction to the Queensland Childhood Lead Poisoning Cases Elsewhere in the World,' *Medical History* 43 (1999): 155–72.
24. John C. Burnham, 'Unraveling the Mystery of Why There Was No Childhood Lead Poisoning,' *Journal of the History of Medicine and Allied Sciences* 60 (2005): 445–77, where it is explained why childhood lead poisoning could have been called 'the Johns Hopkins disease.'
25. Ibid. Christopher Sellers, 'The Artificial Nature of Fluoridated Water: Between Nations, Knowledge, and Material Flows,' *Osiris,* 2nd ser. 19 (2004): 182–200.
26. Lead paint was most commonly used in the late nineteenth and early twentieth centuries.
27. Burnham, 'Unraveling the Mystery.'
28. See especially Christopher Sellers, 'Body, Place and the State: The Makings of an "Environmentalist" Imaginary in the Post-World War II U.S.,' *Radical History Review* 74 (1999): 31–64. An additional complication was added by formal accident theory, in which the host (person injured) and agent (actual material that inflicted the injury) were held to operate in 'the environment,' a very elastic term that included immediate circumstances and sometimes remote ones. Lead poisoning was technically an accident, but the customary analytic terms were almost never applied to it in practice.

29. The fundamental work on this transformation is Christopher C. Sellers, *Hazards of the Job: From Industrial Disease to Environmental Health Science* (Chapel Hill: University of North Carolina Press, 1997), especially chap. 6, generalized into Sellers, 'Body, Place and the State.' A general, and more political, account, particularly emphasizing social reform efforts, is Barbara Berney, 'Round and Round It Goes: The Epidemiology of Childhood Lead Poisoning, 1950–1990,' *Milbank Quarterly* 71 (1993): 3–39, especially 10–24.
30. See, for example, Esmond R. Long, 'Environment in Relation to Health and Disease,' *Archives of Environmental Health* 3 (1961): 545–58; Harold Jacobziner, 'Introduction,' *American Journal of Public Health* 54 (1964): Supplement iii; and Burt L. Davis, 'Welcome Address,' in *International Conference on Environmental Health* (Beograd: Izdaje, 1973), 7–9, who summarized some recent activity. Robert J. Anderson, 'The Physician and Environmental Health,' *Archives of Environmental Health* 9 (1964): 558.
31. Samuel P. Hays, *Beauty, Health, and Permanence: Environmental Politics in the United States, 1955–1985* (Cambridge: Cambridge University Press, 1987), especially 52–56. Sellers, *Hazards of the Job,* offers a parallel narrative. Barry G. King, A. F. Schaplowsky, and Edward B. McCabe, in 'Occupational Health and Child Lead Poisoning: Mutual Interests and Special Problems,' *American Journal of Public Health* 62 (1972): 1056–59, summarized the areas of overlap and distinctiveness in the two narrowly specialist areas of occupational lead poisoning and childhood lead poisoning—in the rapidly changing medical scene at the end of the 1960s and the beginning of the 1970s.
32. James W. Henderson, Jr., and Bailus Walker, Jr., 'Goals and Policies for Our Physical Environment,' *Archives of Environmental Health* 16 (1968): 451. Richard A. Prindle, 'Environmental Health: Clinical and Epidemiological Considerations,' *Archives of Environmental Health* 16 (1968): 70. A. Bradford-Hill, in 'The Environment and Disease. Association or Causation?' *Proceedings of the Royal Society of Medicine* 58 (1965): 295–300, writing especially in the shadow of the controversy over the relationship between lung cancer and smoking, wanted to plead for common sense, invoking clinical judgment to gauge environmental impact, rather than totally depending upon strict statistical tests of significance.
33. See, for example, the special supplement, 'Conference on the Pediatric Significance of Peacetime Radioactive Fallout,' *Pediatrics* 41 (1968): 165–378. Or 'The Radioactive "Fall-Out" Problem,' *Pediatrics* 25 (1960): 929: 'Fall-out products have been found in many parts of the world—In the air, in vegetation, soil, water and food, and in human tissues.' Luther L. Terry, 'The Public Health Service and the Environment,' *Archives of Environmental Health* 7 (1963): 92–5. Barltrop, 'Children and Lead,' 165. Rachel Carson, *Silent Spring* (Boston: Houghton Mifflin, 1962).
34. In the literature on other chemicals in the environment, a long precedent existed for examining chronic but asymptomatic poisoning, the most obvious perhaps carbon monoxide; see, for example, Milton A. Bell, 'Subacute Carbon Monoxide Poisoning,' *Archives of Environmental Health* 3 (1961): 108–110. Medical writers as early as the mid-1930s were dealing with asymptomatic lead poisoning routinely in occupational health. In adults, the idea was involved in both individual susceptibility and the never-ending problem of insurance compensation. 'The ever prevailing question in regard to 'sub-chronic' plumbism arises as in the case of all metals,' wrote C. N. Myers, Florence Gustafson, and Binford Throne, in 'The Distribution and Diagnostic Significance of Lead in the Human Body,' *New York State Journal of Medicine:* 35 (1935): 588, 584: 'various syndromes . . . may be associated with the "sub-chronic" type of lead poisoning.' 'It usually requires from 2 to 4 months

or longer of nibbling paint before any acute symptoms arise. The duration of this early period, called by McKhann 'latent lead poisoning,' depends not only on the amount of lead ingested but to some extent on the amount of calcium and vitamin D in the diet,' wrote John R. Ross and Alan Brown, in 'III—Poisonings Common in Children,' *Canadian Public Health Journal* 26 (1935): 240. Similar formulations can be found in the literature for many years. H. A. Waldron and D. Stöfen, *Sub-Clinical Lead Poisoning* (New York: Academic Press, 1974).

35. Jacobziner, 'Lead Poisoning in Childhood,' 277.
36. Robert C. Griggs et al., 'Environmental Factors in Lead Poisoning,' *Journal of the American Medical Association* 187 (1964): 703; on 707, they speculated that asymptomatic exposure 'may or may not result in sequelae which are not recognized or adequately appreciated at the present time.' 'Lead Paint Poisoning Still With Us,' *Maryland State Medical Journal* 12 (1963): 296. David Elwyn, 'Childhood Lead Poisoning,' *Scientist and Citizen,* April 1968: 53, 54.
37. J. Julian Chisolm, 'Lead Poisoning in Childhood—Comprehensive Management and Prevention,' *Journal of Pediatrics* 73 (1968): 942.
38. Martha L. Lepow, 'Investigations into Sources of Lead in the Environment of Urban Children,' *Environmental Research* 10 (1975): 416.
39. Some idea of the evolution of general concern is found in Stuart Bruchey and Gene Brown (eds.), *Energy and Environment,* (The Great Contemporary Issue Series, Set 2, Volume 9, New York: Arno Press, 1979), chap. 2. See also: Homer L. Skinner, Jr., 'The Lead Problem: An Outline of Current Knowledge and Opinion,' *Journal of Occupational Medicine* 3 (1961): 429–435; Ralph I. Larsen, 'Motor Vehicle Emissions and Their Effects,' *Public Health Reports* 77 (1962): 963–69.
40. A summary of the literature is in Ruth Schwartz Cowan, *A Social History of American Technology* (New York: Oxford University Press, 1997), 240–42. Another account is in Warren, *The Silent Epidemic,* chap. 10.
41. Bryan T. Emmerson, 'Atmospheric Contamination with Lead,' *Annals of Internal Medicine* 68 (1968): 488.
42. English, *Old Paint,* chaps. 13–14.
43. A. Pentschew and F. Garro, 'Lead Encephalo-Myelopathy of the Suckling Rat and Its Implications on the Porphyrinopathic Nervous Diseases,' *Acta Neuropathologica* 6 (1966); 266–78.
44. Peter L. Tyor and Leland V. Bell, *Caring for the Retarded in America* (Westport: Greenwood Press, 1984), chap. 6. Grace E. Woods and Ruth M. Walters, 'Lead Poisoning in Mentally Subnormal Children,' *Lancet* 2 (12 September 1964): 592.
45. Warren, *Brush with Death,* passim, especially chap. 12.
46. Harriet L. Hardy et al., 'Lead as an Environmental Poison,' *Clinical Pharmacology and Therapuetics* 12 (1971): 982–1002. *Lead—Airborne Lead in Perspective: Biologic Effects of Atmospheric Pollutants* (Washington, DC: National Academy of Sciences, 1971), especially 208–11.
47. James W. Sayres et al., 'House and Hand Dust as a Potential Source of Childhood Lead Exposure', *American Journal of Diseases of Children* 127 (1974): 167–70.
48. J. P. Day, M. Hart, and M. S. Robinson, 'Lead in Urban Street Dust,' *Nature* 253 (1975): 343–45.
49. Herbert L. Needleman and Vernon H. Houk, 'More on Long-Term Sequelae of Exposure to Lead,' *Journal of Pediatrics* 94 (1979): 681.
50. The most conspicuous non-physician was Clair Patterson, about whom much has been written; see especially *Clean Hands: Clair Patterson's Crusade*

Against Environmental Lead Contamination (Cormack, NY: Nova Science Publishers, 1999).

51. D. Jean Schneider and Marvin A. Lavenhar, 'Lead Poisoning: More than a Medical Problem,' *American Journal of Public Health* 76 (1986): 242.
52. One review article was Kathryn R. Mahaffey, 'Relation Between Quantities of Lead Ingested and Health Effects of Lead in Humans,' *Pediatrics* 59 (1977): 448–56.
53. Burnham, 'Unraveling the Mystery'; J. Julian Chisolm, Jr., and Harold E. Harrison, 'The Exposure of Children to Lead,' *Pediatrics* 18 (1956): 947–48.
54. Michelle Murphy, 'The "Elsewhere Within Here" and Environmental Illness; or, How to Build Yourself a Body in a Safe Space,' *Configurations* 8 (2000): 87–120, describes some extreme thinking about the relationship between the body and a pathogenic environment.
55. How much individual genetics in each body might have been involved in sensitivity to this environment is a question not yet settled.
56. Such a point of view of course could reflect the isomorphic intrusion of mass culture as well as lead in dust, dirt, and air.
57. Gregg Mitman, Michelle Murphy, and Christopher Sellers, 'A Cloud Over History,' *Osiris,* 2nd ser. 19 (2004): 16. Their essay and this whole issue of *Osiris* suggest many ways in which historians and others can view the history of childhood lead poisoning.

15 Into the Mouths of Babes

Hyperactivity, Food Additives, and the Reception of the Feingold Diet

Matthew Smith

INTRODUCTION

If you had looked at the health section of a bookshop during the 1970s, and if you were the parent of a rambunctious child, the boldly titled *Why Your Child Is Hyperactive*, by Dr. Ben Feingold (1899–1982), might have caught your attention. That a book on hyperactivity should be a big seller is not, in itself, all that surprising.[1] During the 1970s in North America, hyperactivity was a growing concern, a disorder of epidemic proportions. Estimates suggested that between 5 and 20 percent of North American children were afflicted.[2] Rarely mentioned in psychiatric journals prior to the 1960s, hyperactivity inundated the pages of journals such as the *American Journal of Psychiatry, Pediatrics,* and *Archives of General Psychiatry* by the 1970s. Moreover, most psychiatrists had ceased to conceptualize hyperactivity as a developmental problem that children eventually outgrew and now implicated the disorder in adult depression, criminal behaviour, and even schizophrenia. Indeed, the public seemed ripe for a popular book about hyperactivity.

But *Why Your Child Is Hyperactive* was not a typical hyperactivity handbook. Instead of finding the root of hyperactivity in ego disruption (as psychoanalysts suggested), in socio-economic problems (as social psychiatrists posited), or in genetically wired neurological dysfunction (as the increasing numbers of physiologically oriented psychiatrists proposed), Feingold's theory was rooted in allergy and blamed the preponderance of food additives in the North American child's diet. The corollary to this claim was that hyperactivity could be prevented by a diet free of the offending substances, a diet subsequently dubbed the Feingold diet. Moreover, Feingold's book targeted parents instead of physicians, making them responsible for preventing hyperactivity in their children. And while this empowering notion might have inspired some parents to make positive choices regarding their child's health, it also indicated to parents that the domestic environment was increasingly unhealthy. By arguing that hyperactivity could be a reaction to the food additives found in processed foods, Feingold's theory echoed contemporary concerns that clinical ecologists raised about the deleterious side effects of Western industrialization and the increasing incidences of multiple chemical sensitivity and food allergy.[3] But just as clinical ecologists and allergists experienced difficulty gaining respect and proving the existence of these conditions, Feingold and his followers struggled to earn the trust of mainstream medicine, especially in North America.

This chapter examines the rise and fall of the Feingold diet in North America. It explores Feingold's theory, outlines the reaction of the medical community to his unconventional ideas, and, finally, explains why his diet failed either to gain widespread acceptance or to encourage further research into the link between nutrition and behaviour, despite the existence of supportive scientific evidence. Indeed, the scientific evidence generated by interest in the Feingold diet became subsumed and undermined by a myriad of social factors, which, in turn, doomed Feingold's diet to the fringes of medicine. These factors include: Feingold's methods, personality, and ability to market his theory to the medical community; methodological difficulties in testing his thesis; and conflicts with the interests of the medical establishment (especially the newly physiologically-oriented psychiatric community), as well as those of the food chemical industry and pharmaceutical companies. In addition, this chapter explores the manner in which the difficulties that families faced in employing the Feingold diet at home, along with the presence of less challenging treatment alternatives, prevented the diet from gaining the grass-roots support necessary to countermand its censure by the medical community. In this way the fate of the Feingold diet exemplifies how medical treatments, irrespective of their scientific validity, are impotent unless they conform to prevailing familial and social contexts.

A NEW EXPLANATION FOR HYPERACTIVITY

The history of the Feingold diet is largely a story about American psychiatry,[4] but its roots originate in Feingold's work as an allergist. In 1951 Feingold joined the Kaiser Medical Program in San Francisco and embarked upon a research programme that centred upon flea bite allergies.[5] Feingold soon concluded that the reaction to flea bites was caused by a low-molecular-weight chemical, or hapten, present in the insect's saliva and began investigating haptens found in food additives and dyes.[6] Although Feingold cited the influence that contemporary clinical investigators, including Fred Speer, Max Samter, and Stephen D. Lockey, had on his thinking,[7] it is also likely that the work of allergists such as Arthur Coca and, especially, clinical ecologist Theron Randolph helped to shape his views.[8]

Indeed, Randolph's belief that food and chemical sensitivities could cause mental illness might well have played a role in the seminal event that led Feingold to connect food additives and hyperactivity.[9] In 1965 Feingold treated a 40-year-old woman suffering from hives. Suspecting that food additives might be responsible, he suggested a diet eliminating these substances and within 72 hours her symptoms had disappeared. Ten days later, Feingold received a strange phone call from a psychiatrist who, unbeknownst to him, was treating the same woman for psychotic behaviour. These symptoms, too, had mysteriously vanished shortly after she had started the elimination diet.[10] Curious, Feingold alerted his staff to be attentive to similar effects, but essentially carried on with his work as before. Then, while recuperating from illness and contemplating retirement during the late 1960s, he started reading about hyperactivity. Feingold had not dealt with hyperactivity during his early paediatric career from the 1920s to 1940s; he wondered why it had become so prevalent. Recalling the work of Bernard Dattner, a Viennese colleague of his at the Pirquet Institute in Vienna who, in the late 1920s, had linked nutrition and neurology,[11] as well as his own work on the allergenic effect of haptens, Feingold concluded that haptens in food additives and some natural foods were causing a great deal of the hyperactivity seen in children. As he would argue in a subsequent article, 'the growth of H-LD [Hyperkinesis-Learning Disorder] coincides with the rapid increase in the use of synthetic colors and flavors in our food supply. A graph of the estimated incidence of H-LD over the past ten years parallels Standard and Poor's curves for the dollar value of soft drinks and synthetic flavors over the same period.'[12]

By 1972, Feingold was treating hyperactive children in San Francisco with an elimination diet and encouraging entire families to participate. The diet, which he found to be effective in up to 50 percent of his patients,[13] eliminated food additives and fruits and vegetables containing natural salicylates. Culprits such as sugary breakfast cereals, prepared luncheon meat, and powdered pudding were banned along with high-salicylate fruits and vegetables such as apples, oranges, grapes, and tomatoes.[14]

Word about the diet spread quickly. In October 1972, Feingold was interviewed on San Francisco television and from then on parents learned about his diet from magazines, news reports, government hearings (such as his speech to Congress on 30 October 1973, at the behest of Senator Glen Beall of Maryland), television appearances on *Today* and the *Phil Donahue Show*, and, of course, his 1974 bestseller. Media coverage, such as a *New York Times* article provocatively entitled 'Why Are We Poisoning Our Children?,' tended to be supportive and hopeful that Feingold's diet might replace the pharmaceutical treatment of hyperactivity, which, at the time, focused heavily on the use of stimulants such as Ritalin, Cylert, and Dexedrine. Commenting on Feingold's publicity in 1977, paediatrician Esther Wender stated that 'the food-additive-free diet now occupies a definite spot on the American nutritional scene. Very few paediatricians remain who have not been asked by concerned parents about giving their child a special diet.'[15] By that time, parents who were convinced of the Feingold diet's efficacy had formed Feingold Associations across North America. Feingold went on to write *The Feingold Cookbook* in 1979, a book that demonstrated the diet's popularity by reaching number four on the *New York Times* non-fiction best seller list. Then, in March 1982, after less than a decade of spreading his message and urging the American Food and Drug Administration to legislate the labelling of food additives, Ben Feingold died at the age of 82 and, immediately, media interest faded away.

TESTING THE FEINGOLD DIET

The death of the charismatic Feingold certainly dampened interest in his diet, but there were other factors that relegated his ideas to medicine's margins. The scientific record, however, was not one of these factors. Despite the overwhelming medical perception during the past 30 years that the diet is ineffective, closer examination of the research literature unveils a far more ambiguous picture. Assessing the scientific research alone, it would be difficult for any physician to determine whether the Feingold diet worked or not.

The most intense period of research intended to test the Feingold diet occurred between 1974, when *Why Your Child Is Hyperactive* was published, and 1982, when Feingold died. The contradictory nature of the conclusions at which these researchers arrived is striking. Some investigators, such as Harley, a neuropsychologist, the psychiatrists Mattes and Gittelman, and Wender registered decidedly negative findings, stating, for example, that 'the overall results do not provide convincing support for the efficacy of the experimental (Feingold) diet,'[16] and that 'the more dramatic improvement . . . probably represents placebo effect.'[17] Indeed, many researchers, both supporters and detractors of the diet, suggested that the extra attention paid by parents to their children while on the diet was a key factor in improving behaviour.[18]

Other studies, such as those led by Cook and Woodhill, a child psychiatrist and nutritionist, Conners, a psychologist, and Brenner, a paediatrician, however, were positive. Australians Cook and Woodhill, for example, stated that 'findings appear to support Feingold, suggesting that the lives of many children have been adversely affected by the presence . . . of chemicals . . . which have been considered harmless.'[19] Conners was less definitive, but nonetheless added that '[the Feingold diet] reduces the perceived hyperactivity of some children suffering from hyperkinetic impulse disorder.'[20] On the other hand, Brenner found that many of the children he tested had 'an unequivocally excellent response as interpreted by schoolteachers, parents, and the paediatrician . . . [and that] medication could be discontinued permanently.'[21] Still others published mixed results.[22] Although methodological problems (mentioned later in this chapter) might account for some of these incongruities, it is clear that researchers developed very different perspectives of the Feingold diet.

Review articles compiled to analyze the dozens of experiments testing the Feingold hypothesis also contradicted each other wildly, reflecting how divisive Feingold's theory was within the medical community. Moreover, these articles often betrayed a lack of objectivity on the part of their authors; studies backing the diet's efficacy were condemned as methodologically unsound by some reviewers, yet hailed as conclusive by others. For example, in 1980 an unsupportive review by professor of paediatrics and neurology Gerald Golden concluded that 'well-controlled studies fail to document any improvement in the behaviour of children on the additive-free diet.'[23] However, Golden failed to describe what determined a 'well-controlled' study. By contrast, psychologist Bernard Rimland's opinion leaned heavily in the opposite direction, stating unequivocally that 'despite anti-Feingold bias . . . all studies, without exception . . . concede that some children react to additives and some children do respond to the diet.'[24] Nor did all reviewers agree that more research needed to be done. While a tentative review by Canadians Williams and Cram suggested that 'additional research should be done to test the [Feingold] hypothesis,'[25] Mattes, after stating that support for the diet was 'circumstantial' and accusing Feingold of clamouring for book sales, stated that conducting more research would be a waste of time and money.[26]

Nevertheless, Mattes's call for a halt to research into the Feingold diet differed from the tendency of most investigators to conclude that, notwithstanding their results, more research was warranted prior to making definitive statements about the diet. Australian researcher Rowe, for example, stated that 'the need for further research is of paramount importance.'[27] The 1982 National Institutes of Health's Consensus Development Conference on Defined Diets and Hyperactivity also 'called for more controlled research.'[28] Moreover, child psychologist Thorley stated that, even if Feingold's thesis was unsound, exploring the link between nutrition and behaviour was useful.[29] Psychologist C. Keith Conners concurred, stating that '*something* is going on which is worth pursuing. If there are *any* children whose behaviour is reliably worsened by food additives, then the problem is significant.'[30]

Feingold, himself, was not interested in further research. As Conners described in his book entitled *Food Additives and Hyperactive Children* (one of the few relatively balanced accounts of the Feingold diet): 'Dr. Feingold at 75 is a man in a hurry. He once told me while we were on a radio program together, "I don't have time for sacred cows of science, the double-blind placebo-controlled trials."'[31] Moreover, Feingold felt that 'it has been demonstrated that these children respond to dietary intervention. That is the immediate and urgent need to halt and reverse the persistent rise in scholastic failures, vandalism, delinquency, and crime.'[32] Feingold's somewhat understandable impatience notwithstanding, the consensus among most researchers was that more research was essential in order to make conclusive statements about the Feingold diet and the link between nutrition and behaviour.

Some further research was conducted, but not nearly as much as could have been expected, given the loud calls for deeper investigation into the Feingold diet. Despite the unanswered questions and calls for more attention, research waned considerably after Feingold's death in 1982. And, although many subsequent studies supported the link between nutrition and behaviour, they did not generate increased research or media coverage of the diet and its clinical efficacy.

THE CASE AGAINST FEINGOLD

What led to lagging interest in the Feingold diet? One answer is that the success of Feingold's theory was not in the interest of many parties, including the drug companies, the food chemical industry, and American psychiatrists. This is reflected in Williams and Cram's statement that 'there has been interest in testing [Feingold's hypothesis] if only to disprove it.'[33] For example, in *Why Your Child Is Hyperactive,* Feingold devoted two chapters to stating how his diet prevented the use of 'hazardous' and 'frightening' drugs like Ritalin, a million-dollar seller for its manufacturer, Ciba.[34] An anonymous editor for *The Lancet* agreed that drugs might become less necessary, suggesting that the diet 'would now seem to be the most promising form of treatment, at least in the United Kingdom, with stimulant drugs reserved for a small number of resistant cases.'[35] Jane Hersey, the current director of the Feingold Association of the United States (FAUS), has argued that drug manufacturers actively conspired against Feingold.[36] While there is no direct evidence to support this claim, drug companies would certainly not be interested in funding research into the Feingold diet, unless they were convinced that a negative outcome would result.[37] It could also be argued that psychiatric journals, which, by the 1970s and 1980s, sold reams of advertising to drug companies, and psychiatric researchers, who were increasingly funded by drug companies, would be reluctant to support the Feingold thesis.

Food additive manufacturers also had much to lose if Feingold's campaign for the labelling of foods containing additives was successful, an outcome recognised by many contemporary observers.[38] One of Feingold's goals was to mandate the labelling of all foods to indicate whether or not they contained artificial colours or flavours.[39] Such labelling was certainly not in the interest of the billion-dollar food chemical industry when, according to a *New York Times* reporter, '80% of the foods on supermarket shelves contain components he condemns.'[40] So, in a not particularly subtle initiative, the Nutrition Foundation, a consortium of food and drug manufacturers including Coca Cola and General Mills, funded a study into the Feingold research.[41] Their negative findings, despite the potential for bias, were often cited by Feingold's critics.[42]

The most influential group in the Feingold debate, however, was the psychiatrists themselves. Psychiatrists had led the research into hyperactivity during the disorder's emergence in the 1960s, and by the 1970s the explanations of biologically oriented psychiatrists had become predominant.[43] Furthermore, they assumed responsibility for heading further investigations into Feingold's thesis and deciding whether or not to prescribe his diet. Despite the cries for more research into the link between nutrition and behaviour, however, only a handful of studies emerged after Feingold's death. Why were psychiatrists not more inclined to do more research?

One issue hampering further research was methodological, or at least the perception that methodological difficulties made testing the Feingold thesis nearly impossible. In the words of one research group:

> a major reason for the dearth of controlled studies is the difficulty in performing them when food is involved: 1) unless the subjects are confined to a strictly controlled environment, cheating is all too easy; 2) children are difficult to persuade to stick to a prescribed diet. . . . 3) ideally the food being tested should be disguised so that the subjects are blind to what they are ingesting—and this is difficult to manage; and 4) the raters should be blind to what subjects are eating, and this, too, is difficult to arrange.[44]

Another observer stated that 'further investigations [into food additives and hyperactivity] have proved remarkably difficult' and that 'the [Feingold] hypothesis would be difficult to test even if the state of hyperactivity in children were a precise and readily recognisable entity. It is not.'[45] Yet another group suggested that 'complex methodological and data interpretation issues [need] to be resolved before Dr. Feingold's assertions can be scientifically supported or refuted.'[46] For example, Feingold asserted that 3,000 substances could cause hyperactive reactions in children, but not all children reacted to the same chemicals.[47] Since testing 3,000 substances individually was impossible, many researchers limited their inquiry to a single chemical, such as the food dye tartrazine yellow, thus testing only one of potentially thousands of culpable chemicals. Moreover, 'considerable confusion about suitable dosage levels'[48] meant that some children were tested using amounts of chemicals that were, according to other researchers, 'ridiculously small' and far below the average consumed by children.[49] When Swanson and Kinsbourne used a higher dosage, five times higher than the average cited by the Nutrition Foundation, 17 of the 20 of their hyperactive subjects performed poorly on learning tests when challenged.[50] Moreover, another research group admitted that 'the doses employed by us . . . are 50 times less than the maximum allowable daily intakes (ADI's) recommended by the Food and Drug Administration.'[51] Even an unsympathetic article stated that 'it is conceivable that previous studies (except that of Swanson and Kinsbourne) used inadequate doses of food colourings.'[52]

Recruiting reliable subjects for trials that ideally demanded large sample sizes was also difficult, expensive, and frustrating. Subjects were also difficult to retain. Pollock and Warner, for instance, stated that their 'drop out rate [was] disappointingly high.'[53] Parents who were convinced of the diet's effectiveness often prevented researchers from testing their children with food additives or withdrew their children shortly after the challenge period began.[54] Maintaining strict compliance to the Feingold diet during month-long trials was difficult to enforce and assess. Recognizing this problem, two studies tested children in hospital[55] and at a summer camp[56] in order to control their diets, but would testing childhood behaviour in an unnatural setting lead to valid results? Researchers also debated the validity of using parent and teacher rating scales and worried about the 'imprecise diagnostic criteria for hyperactivity.'[57] Order effect similarly caused problems in some studies, with the Feingold diet appearing to be more effective when it followed the control diet in the trial sequence.[58] In yet another case, the possibility of having teacher rating scales was quashed by a teacher strike.[59]

Although there were clear methodological problems facing researchers interested in investigating the Feingold diet, the willingness of researchers to overcome these problems is less clear. In other words, methodological problems might have provided a convenient excuse for researchers not to thoroughly test the diet. This, according to Canadian paediatric geneticist Steven Bamforth, is a problem that continues to weaken our overall understanding of hyperactivity. In his words, 'to say that something is too difficult to study is not an excuse.'[60] Some researchers, such as C. Keith Conners, did take steps to improve their initial double blind trials,[61] but overall, both positive and negative reviewers of the Feingold literature were comfortable making strong statements based on research that was admittedly flawed or inadequate. One limitation that could have been overcome relatively easily, albeit with some cost, was sample size. Many researchers, including Conners, based their confident statements about the Feingold diet on trials consisting of less than a dozen children. Given that so many researchers stressed the importance of investigating the Feingold diet, it is perplexing that methodological problems such as these acted as such an impediment.

But methodological difficulties were not the only discouraging factors. The Feingold thesis also put psychiatrists in a difficult position professionally. American psychiatry had long existed on the fringes of medicine in terms of respectability and influence.[62] The profession's experience with inhumane treatments such as lobotomy, quasi-medical psychoanalysis and heavy-handed institutionalization in the mid-twentieth century did little to bolster its reputation and led to a powerful anti-psychiatry movement led by outspoken critics such Thomas Szasz and Erving Goffman.[63] But, by the mid 1970s, the internal power struggles between psychoanalysts, social psychiatrists, and biologically based psychiatry had been won and a more scientifically respectable psychiatry rooted in neurology, genetics and pharmacotherapy had been re-embraced by both the public and the medical community.[64] Feingold, a paediatrician and allergist, threatened the new psychiatric paradigm by suggesting that nutrition was at the root of hyperactivity and that drugs were not the answer.

Perhaps more troublesome to some biological psychiatrists than Feingold's basic claim, which was nevertheless rooted in physiology, was the manner in which he came to it and described it. Feingold's theory emerged out of clinical and anecdotal evidence, a basis that was sufficient for him, and for many other allergists, but not for mainstream psychiatry.[65] Indeed one of the reasons allergists, especially those who practised immunotherapy as clinicians, had difficulty establishing their profession as a legitimate medical specialty was their trust in clinical versus laboratory based and statistically sound knowledge.[66] Moreover, Feingold's accounts of his clinical experiences harkened back to the familiar descriptive and narrative style employed by psychoanalysts, a style that, by the 1970s, had been replaced by the dry, laconic, and impersonal descriptions of double-blind, controlled trials. Although Feingold's writing style contributed to public interest and acceptance, it seemed unscientific, anachronistic, and unconvincing to other researchers. In the words of a reviewer in *The Lancet*, 'the dietary theory of hyperactivity has aroused strong emotions. Believers in the scientific method felt challenged by the speed of its public acceptance and the lack of objective evidence.'[67] Another observer stated that 'the conflict is a classic standoff between the plodding nature of rigorous scientific research and the public need for answers to costly, distressing problems.'[68]

Feingold's willingness to respond to this public need offended psychiatrists concerned with the legitimacy of psychiatric research. This concern was understandable, given psychiatry's history of flawed or morally unacceptable treatments. According to some, 'the widespread popularization of [Feingold's] hypothesis is regrettable,'[69] while to others it was their 'opinion that the publicity has far outstripped the research on which it should be based.'[70] Alarmed that 'despite the subjective nature of Feingold's evidence and generally negative commentary by professionals, the hypothesis received favourable media attention and a favourable and enthusiastic response from the general public,'[71] psychiatrists used strong language to criticize Feingold. Prominent child psychiatrist John Werry warned that 'the most chilling aspect of Feingold's work lies in the enthusiasm with which it has been embraced by the anti-medication, anti-psychiatry section of the American public and used as a cudgel to try to close down paediatric psychopharmacological research.' Werry added that Feingold was a 'medical Pied Piper [who has] not tested his hypothesis, but has written for the popular market.'[72] T. J. David added that inflicting a child with the Feingold diet was in the 'range of child abuse.'[73] Although some researchers found that children on the Feingold diet consumed above the recommended dietary allowance for important vitamins,[74] others warned that depriving children of salicylate-laden fruits and vegetables could lead to malnutrition.[75] This was despite the fact that Feingold urged that fruits and vegetables be carefully re-introduced following success on the diet, since it might be solely additives, and not fruit and vegetables, that were causing the hyperactivity of some children. Others feared the 'long-term psychological impact in assuring a child that his behaviour or school performance is controlled by what he eats, when in fact it is not,'[76] and bemoaned that 'the widely publicized clinical evidence and quasi-religious belief espoused by "Feingold

Associations" will make it difficult to depose the Feingold . . . diet as a treatment alternative for hyperactivity.'[77]

In retrospect, this last concern is ironic; mainstream medicine did succeed in quelling research into the diet. In a recent interview, for example, psychologist Bonnie Kaplan has admitted that she stopped researching the nutrition–behaviour link because it was hard to get her research recognized due to the fact that 'people's minds were closed' to the idea.[78] In 1988, Rowe recognised this lack of interest in the Feingold diet, observing that since '1980 controlled clinical trials examining the relationship between food colourings and behaviour have been conspicuous by their absence.'[79] Perhaps the most convincing evidence that minds have been closed to the Feingold thesis, however, comes from the fact that although several new studies have supported the link between nutrition and behaviour, [80] these have largely been ignored by physicians.[81]

The tendency of researchers to ignore key aspects of Feingold's theory also suggests that the medical establishment was unwilling to take Feingold seriously. For example, in his 1975 article in the *American Journal of Nursing,* Feingold stated that younger children are much quicker to respond to an elimination diet than adolescents.[82] Despite this qualification, a research team led by Harley chose to dismiss the fact that the sample of pre-school children in their study responded to the diet and, instead, based their negative conclusions about Feingold's theory on the responses of an older sample group. The team acknowledged this anomaly by stating that:

> the attentive reader of this report has undoubtedly sensed, if not specifically identified, our discomfort and uncertainty in the manner of presenting the results on the preschool sample. We have chosen to emphasize the results of the school-age sample because we believe our experimental design for this group meets our intended criteria with respect to sufficient number of subjects, employment of selection methods clearly appropriate for the age sample, and the availability of multiple sources of objective data regarding changes in hyperactive behaviours.[83]

Given this excuse for the positive results, the 'attentive reader' might also have asked why such flaws were allowed to exist in one sample and not another, especially considering Feingold's observation that younger children were particularly responsive to his diet.[84] Moreover, subsequent reviews of the Feingold research record also acknowledged the efficacy of the diet with younger children;[85] but, until 2004, no studies had focused solely on this age group.[86]

FAMILIES AND THE FEINGOLD DIET

Ultimately, it was parents who had to decide whether or not the diet was feasible. Despite the censure of mainstream medicine, over 200,000 families had tried the Feingold diet by the mid 1980s,[87] and FAUS, relying on word of mouth and the internet, still attracts adherents. But although thousands of families have found the diet to be beneficial, with many recounting their success stories in FAUS's newsletter, *Pure Facts,* and in FAUS director Jane Hersey's *Why Can't My Child Behave,*[88] the diet still exists on the fringes of hyperactivity treatment. Moreover, the reasons that families did not use the diet were dependent on the nature of the diet itself as well as medical opinion. In the Feingold diet, parents, and especially mothers, found 'a difficult and exacting regimen which put considerable strain on the whole family'[89] and made them responsible if their attempts failed.

The inherent difficulty in weaning children off artificial colours and flavours was described neatly in a 1987 trial conducted at a summer camp for learning disabled children: 'The children were not happy with the Feingold diet. The teachers had the feeling that there would have been a rebellion had it lasted longer than a week. They particularly disliked the colourlessness of the food, and missed the mustard and ketchup . . . The strict Feingold diet appears to be distasteful to the typical American child.'[90] Given the need for complete dietary compliance, and the fact that hyperactive children tended also to be defiant, distractible, and impulsive, a child's apathy or resistance was a significant obstacle. As another group of researchers contended, perhaps pessimistically, 'it was inevitable that children would eat foods with artificial colours and flavourings.'[91]

Criticisms such as these are refuted by Hersey; she argues that 'trying to deal with a difficult (or impossible) child is what puts the strain on the family. Changing some of your grocery brands is no big deal.'[92] Nevertheless, even Hersey admits in her book that 'experienced Feingolders can get complacent about label reading' and that it is often difficult to determine the additive content of common (and locally produced) foods like bread and dairy products.[93] More importantly, embracing the Feingold diet required parents to eschew conventional medical opinion and the opinions of other parents who believed the diet to be a fad or gimmick. While parents in the 1970s might have eagerly endorsed the idea that petrochemicals used in food dyes were hazardous to their children's health, they were less likely to believe that tomatoes, cucumbers, and oranges could cause hyperactivity. A certain stubbornness and eagerness to defy medical authority and conventional wisdom were required of Feingold parents and their children if they were to employ the diet successfully.

How, then, was compliance to be ensured? Given the gendered nature of family food preparation, the task of preventing hyperactivity and promoting mental and physical health in allergic children fell largely to mothers. As in other areas of domestic medical management, it was mothers who had to shop carefully, reading labels and purchasing only suitable foods, but many items, including most baked goods and candy, had to be homemade. Mothers also had to keep a diet diary, recording consumption and noting the resulting behaviour. Re-introducing potentially troublesome fruits and vegetables, as suggested by Feingold, required mothers to have considerable skills of observation and deduction. Controlling the diet outside the home forced mothers to investigate what their children consumed at school, at birthday parties, and at the convenience store; no fast food, coloured icing, or unapproved drinks were allowed. The diet also required that mothers be vigilant with respect to instructing relatives, school officials, and other parents as to what foods were unacceptable for their hyperactive child. These were lofty expectations for mothers already dealing with excessive family pressures, at a time, during the 1970s and 1980s, when increasing numbers of mothers in North America were in the workplace.[94]

And what if the diet did not work? Some suggested that 'the diet may help to reduce the parents' feelings of guilt or other negative emotions involving their hyperactive child because an "outside" causative agent has now been identified,'[95] but since mothers were responsible for feeding their family, they would inevitably shoulder the blame for failure. Echoing contemporary concerns about the role of parents (and particularly mothers) in maintaining the psychological health of their children (discussed elsewhere in this volume), opponents of Feingold were quick to condemn parents who tried the diet, emphasising the need to 'help children whose parents insist on keeping them on very restrictive diets' that caused 'nutritional deficiencies . . . social isolation, and possible emotional harm.'[96] Solace might come from Feingold's suggestion that food allergies were not the only cause, but with a diet this difficult to enforce, how could a mother know for sure that she had removed all additives from her child's diet? Most importantly, the standard genetic explanation for hyperactivity and corresponding stimulant therapy suggested by most physicians similarly acquitted parents of blame, but provided a much more facile treatment, at least on the surface. The Feingold diet required significant patience, time, attention to detail, perseverance, assertiveness, and the willingness to defy conventional medical opinion; that many families lacked these qualities might have been unfortunate, but not surprising.

CONCLUSION

Today, psychiatrists often describe the Feingold diet as if it were an adolescent phase, and as if past medical interest in it was a passing, inconclusive flirtation. In many ways they are correct; the Feingold diet, once popular enough to be heralded on national television, has failed since to become a respectable treatment for hyperactivity. Contemporary physicians and their predecessors are incorrect, however, in suggesting that careful scientific study discredited the diet. As this chapter has shown, scientific investigation into the validity of the Feingold hypothesis was incomplete, incomprehensive, inconclusive, and, in the end, inadequate for observers to have made careful judgements about the diet. Instead, other factors, such as the methods and death of the diet's charismatic promoter, and the threat it posed to drug companies, the food chemical industry, and psychiatrists, as well as the challenges it posed to families, prevented the hypothesis from being sufficiently tested, let alone proven and promoted by the medical establishment. Two decades after Feingold's death, it is still unclear whether or not there is a definitive link between food additives and hyperactivity. While this is troubling for those who struggle to treat and manage the disorder on a daily basis, it also raises disturbing questions about our knowledge of hyperactivity in general, not to mention other links between what we ingest and our mental health. Instead of dismissing the Feingold theory as a phase best forgotten, it would be better to take the steps to close conclusively this chapter of hyperactivity's history, for better or worse.

This chapter has contended that the reception of medical solutions is dependent on social conditions. Conditions change. In the case of the Feingold diet, many dynamics, including new information technologies, growing concern about drugs, and changes to our dietary habits, suggest that the diet might experience a rebirth. The Internet, for example, has re-introduced families and researchers to Ben Feingold and has been used by FAUS to market the link between diet and behaviour. Although attainment of Feingold's goal of food additive labelling remains unlikely, FAUS has been successful in producing comprehensive lists of foods that conform to his diet. Concern about peanut allergies has also led to increased labelling and awareness.[97] Furthermore, drug companies have recently come under intense suspicion as some of their best-selling products for pain relief, depression, and hyperactivity have been found to be dangerous. The best-selling hyperactivity drug Adderall, for example, was banned by Health Canada in February 2005 for its role in the sudden deaths of twenty children and adults (the Food and Drug Administration in the United States did not follow suit).[98] Food supply disasters such as the bovine spongiform encephalopathy (mad cow disease) crises in the United Kingdom and elsewhere, as well as the corresponding rise of the organic food movement and concerns about childhood obesity, point to renewed interest in what we consume. In the United Kingdom, for example, celebrity chef Jamie Oliver has spearheaded a campaign to improve the food served in school cafeterias, and in April 2005, the Blair government pledged £280 million to combat the problem. On his 'Feed Me Better' website, Oliver lists 'poor concentration,' 'hyperactivity and behavioural problems,' and mood swings' as effects of the 'processed junk foods' served in schools.[99] In a similar vein, a private member's bill in the Canadian Parliament, if passed, would take steps to ban trans-fats from the food supply.[100] Companies such as Voortman Cookies have anticipated such legislation and now offer trans-fat-free cookies. With developments such as these, it is possible that a revival of the Feingold diet could be in the offing, leading not only to renewed medical interest in this intriguing theory but also to renewed attention being paid to the role of families and the home in the maintenance of health and the prevention of illness.

NOTES

1. I use the term *hyperactivity* for what we now call attention-deficit/hyperactivity disorder (ADHD), partly because it was the most common term for the disorder during the 1970s, but also because it continues to be the term most patients, parents, and physicians recognize and understand.
2. I. Philips, 'Research directions in child psychiatry,' *American Journal of Psychiatry* 137 (1980): 1136.
3. Mark Jackson, *Allergy: The History of a Modern Malady* (London: Reaktion, 2006), 200–8.
4. Paediatricians, psychologists, neurologists, and allergists, delving into the traditional realm of psychiatry, also played a part in the history of the Feingold diet. In this story, professional jurisdictions and boundaries often blur. Nevertheless, the most influential profession involved in the debates about the Feingold diet, and hyperactivity generally, has been psychiatry, and therefore psychiatry has been used as a catch-all to describe a less discrete group of health professionals involved in researching and treating the disorder. Similarly, while Australian, British, and New Zealander physicians also debated the Feingold thesis, often with more favourable assessments, it was in North America that the diet generated the most initial excitement but, ultimately, the least acceptance. The focus here is chiefly on the North American context.
5. Ben. F. Feingold, *Why Your Child is Hyperactive* (New York: Random House, 1974), 3–4.
6. Ibid., 6.
7. Ibid., 8.
8. Jackson, *Allergy,* 200–2.
9. Jackson, *Allergy,* 201.
10. Feingold, *Why Your Child Is Hyperactive,* 1–3.
11. Ibid., 20.
12. Ben. F. Feingold, 'Hyperkinesis and learning disabilities linked to artificial food flavors and colors,' *American Journal of Nursing* 75 (1975): 798. It is unclear why Feingold chose to publish his first academic paper on this topic in the *American Journal of Nursing,* rather than a journal dedicated to psychiatry or allergy. It could be that he had trouble finding an academic publisher, but it might also have been that Feingold was seeking to find allies in the nursing profession, having found lukewarm support within mainstream medicine.
13. Feingold suggested that organic brain damage, crowded conditions in classrooms, socioeconomic problems, discrimination based on ethnicity, and other environmental influences caused hyperactivity in much of the remaining 50 percent. Feingold, 'Hyperkinesis,' 798.
14. Feingold, *Why Your Child Is Hyperactive,* 11–21.
15. Esther H. Wender, 'Food additives and hyperkinesis,' *American Journal of Diseases of Children* 131 (1977): 1204.
16. J. Preston Harley et al., 'Hyperkinesis and food additives: Testing the Feingold hypothesis,' *Pediatrics* 61 (1978): 826; Jeffrey A. Mattes and R. Gittelman, 'Effects of artificial food colorings in children with hyperactive symptoms,' *Archives of General Psychiatry* 38 (1981): 715.
17. Wender, 'Food additives,' 1206.

18. Anonymous, 'Additive-free diet doesn't correct behavioral problems,' *American Family Physician* 20 (1979): 146; J. Preston Harley, Charles G. Matthews, and Peter Eichman, 'Synthetic food colors and hyperactivity in children: a double-blind challenge experiment,' *Pediatrics* 62, (1978): 982; Carl Spring and Jonathan Sandoval, 'Food additives and hyperkinesis: A critical review of the evidence,' *Journal of Learning Disabilities* 9 (1976): 563; Arnold Brenner, 'A study of the efficacy of the Feingold diet on hyperkinetic children: some favorable personal observations,' *Clinical Pediatrics* 16 (1977): 655.
19. Peter S. Cook and Joan M. Woodhill, 'The Feingold dietary treatment of the hyperkinetic syndrome,' *Medical Journal of Australia* 2 (1976): 88.
20. C. Keith Conners et al., 'Food additives and hyperkinesis: a controlled double-blind experiment,' *Pediatrics* 58 (1976): 161.
21. Brenner, 'A study of the efficacy of the Feingold diet,' 653.
22. I. Pollock and J. O. Warner, 'Effects of artificial food colours on childhood behaviour,' *Archives of Disease in Childhood* 65 (1990): 77.
23. Gerald S. Golden, 'Nonstandard therapies in the developmental disabilities,' *American Journal of Diseases of Children* 134 (1980): 487.
24. B. Rimland, 'The Feingold diet: An assessment of the reviews by Mattes, Kavale and Forness and others,' Journal of Learning Disabilities 16 (1983): 332.
25. J. I. Williams and D. M. Cram, 'Diet in the management of hyperkinesis: A review of the tests of Feingold's hypothesis,' *Canadian Psychiatric Association Journal* 23 (1978): 246–47.
26. Jeffrey A. Mattes, 'The Feingold diet: a current reappraisal,' Journal of Learning Disabilities 16 (1983): 323.
27. K. S. Rowe, 'Synthetic food colourings and "hyperactivity": A double-blind crossover study,' *Australian Paediatric Journal* 24 (1988): 144.
28. L. Eugene Arnold, 'Alternative treatments for adults with attention-deficit hyperactivity disorder (ADHD),' Annals of the New York Academy of Sciences 931 (2001): 314.
29. Geoffrey Thorley, 'Pilot study to assess behavioural and cognitive effects of artificial food colours in a group of retarded children,' *Developmental Medicine and Child Neurology* 26 (1984): 56.
30. C. Keith Conners, *Food Additives and Hyperactive Children* (New York: Plenum Press, 1980), 40. Italics in the original.
31. Ibid., 12.
32. Feingold quoted in Harley, Matthews and Eichman, 'Synthetic food colors,' 982.
33. Williams and Cram, 'Diet in the management of hyperkinesis,' 243.
34. Ironically, Ritalin had been marketed to physicians in mainstream journals like the *Journal of the American Medical Association* as early as 1956 as a treatment for depression in senior citizens. By 1967, children became the new target.
35. Anonymous, 'Feingold's regimen for hyperkinesis,' *Lancet* 2 (1979): 618.
36. Telephone interview with Jane Hersey, 5 October, 2004.
37. It has also been claimed that in the 1950s drug companies conspired against Russian clinician Konstantin Buteyko's drug-free method of treating asthma because of the threat it posed to their profits and reputations. Jackson, *Allergy*, 138.
38. Anonymous, 'Feingold's regimen,' 617; John S. Werry, 'Food additives and hyperactivity,' *Medical Journal of Australia* 2 (1976): 281; J. Preston Harley and Charles G. Matthews, 'The hyperactive child and the Feingold controversy,' *American Pharmacy* 18 (1978): 44; C. W. Bierman and C. T. Furukawa, 'Food additives and hyperkinesis: Are there nuts among the berries?' *Pediatrics* 61 (1978): 932.
39. Feingold, 'Hyperkinesis,' 797.

40. R. Walters, 'Paperback talk,' *New York Times* (27 May 1979), BR6.
41. United States National Advisory Committee on Hyperkinesis and Food Additives, *Report to the Nutrition Foundation* (Washington, DC: The Nutrition Foundation, 1975).
42. Werry, 'Food additives and hyperactivity,' 281; Harley et al., 'Synthetic food colors,' 819; K. A. Kavale and S. R. Forness, 'Hyperactivity and diet treatment: A meta-analysis of the Feingold hypothesis,' *Journal of Learning Disabilities* 16 (1983): 324; J. I. Williams et al., 'Relative effects of drugs and diet on hyperactive behaviors: An experimental study,' *Pediatrics* 61 (1978): 811; Anonymous, 'Diet and hyperactivity: Any connection?' *Nutrition Reviews* 34 (1976): 154.
43. Matthew Smith, 'The Hyperactive State: The History of Attention-Deficit/Hyperactivity Disorder and American Psychiatry,' (MA thesis, University of Alberta, 2004).
44. M. D. Gross et al., 'The effects of diets rich in and free from additives on the behaviour of children with hyperkinetic and learning disorder,' *Journal of American Association of Child and Adolescent Psychiatry* 26 (1987): 53.
45. Anonymous, 'Feingold's regimen,' 617.
46. Harley, Matthews and Eichman, 'Synthetic food colors,' 975.
47. Rimland, 'The Feingold diet,' 331.
48. K. S. Rowe and K. J. Rowe, 'Synthetic food colouring and behaviour: a dose response effect in a double-blind, placebo-controlled, repeated measures study,' *Journal of Pediatrics* 125 (1994): 692.
49. Rimland, 'The Feingold diet,' 331.
50. J. W. Swanson and M. Kinsbourne, 'Food dyes impair performance of hyperactive children on a laboratory learning test,' *Science* 207 (1980): 1485–87.
51. B. Weiss et al., 'Behavioural response to artificial food colours,' *Science* 207 (1980): 1487–89.
52. Mattes and Gittelman, 'Effects of artificial food colorings,' 715.
53. Pollock and Warner, 'Effects of artificial food colours,' 76. Although this British study did not find the Feingold diet particularly helpful, it is interesting that the alternatives it suggests for treating hyperactivity, 'child guidance, clinical and educational psychologists, family therapy,' do not include pharmacotherapy.
54. B Bateman et al., 'The effects of a double blind, placebo controlled, artificial food colourings and benzoate preservative challenge on hyperactivity in a general population sample of preschool children,' *Archives of Disease in Childhood* 89 (2004): 507.
55. T. J. David, 'Reactions to dietary tartrazine,' *Archives of Disease in Childhood* 62 (1987): 119.
56. Gross et al., 'The effects of diets,' 53.
57. Rowe, 'Synthetic food colourings,' 143.
58. Bonnie J. Kaplan et al., 'Dietary replacement in preschool-aged hyperactive boys,' *Pediatrics* 83 (1989): 7; Mattes and Gittleman, 'Effects of artificial food colorings,' 714.
59. Mattes and Gittleman, 'Effects of artificial food colorings,' 714.
60. Telephone interview with Steven Bamforth, 5 March, 2005.
61. Conners, *Food Additivies,* 38–40.
62. Gerald N. Grob, *Mental Illness and American Society, 1870–1940* (Princeton: Princeton University Press, 1983); Charles E. Rosenberg, *Explaining Epidemics and Other Studies in the History of Medicine* (Cambridge: Cambridge University Press, 1992); Jack D. Pressman, *Last Resort: Psychosurgery and the Limits of Medicine* (Cambridge: Cambridge University Press, 1998).
63. Thomas Szasz, *The Myth of Mental Illness: Foundations of a Theory of Personal Conduct* (New York: HarperCollins, 1974); Erving Goffman, *Asylums:*

Essays on the Social Situation of Mental Patients and Other Inmates (Garden City, New York: Doubleday Anchor, 1961).

64. Smith, 'The hyperactive state,' 100.
65. The views of prominent British allergist and clinician John Freeman (1876–1962) are indicative of the tendency for mid-century allergists to favour clinical evidence; see Jackson, *Allergy,* 73–4.
66. Jackson, *Allergy,* 73–4, 193–5.
67. Anonymous, 'Feingold's regimen,' 617.
68. R. Wurtman quoted in J. E. Brody, 'Diet therapy for behavior is criticized as premature; diet–behavior link: The debate,' *New York Times,* 4 Dec 1984, C1.
69. M. D. Levine and C. B. Liden, 'Food for inefficient thought,' *Pediatrics* 58 (1976): 147.
70. Spring and Sandoval, 'Food additives,' 560.
71. Kavale and Forness, 'Hyperactivity and diet treatment,' 324.
72. Werry, 'Food additives and hyperactivity,' 281–82.
73. David, 'Reactions to dietary tartrazine,' 122.
74. Conners et al., 'Food additives and hyperkinesis,' 161, 164.
75. Wender, 'Food additives,' 1206; David, 'Reactions to dietary tartrazine,' 122.
76. A. Ribon and S. Joshi, 'Is there any relationship between food additives and hyperkinesis?' *Annals of Allergy* 48 (1982): 277.
77. Kavale and Forness, 'Hyperactivity and diet treatment.'
78. Phone interview with Bonnie J. Kaplan, 18 January, 2005.
79. Rowe, 'Synthetic food colourings,' 143.
80. According to Arnold, 'since then [the 1982 NIH Consensus Development Conference on Defined Diets and Hyperactivity], at least 8 controlled studies have shown either significant improvement compared to a placebo condition . . . or deterioration on a placebo-controlled challenge of offending substances after an open diet trial and open challenge to identify the substance.' Arnold, 314. Subsequent to Arnold's article, another study, that of Bateman et al., has found a positive link between food additives and hyperactivity. Bateman et al., 'The effects of a double blind,' 506–11.
81. R. Schnoll, D. Burshteyn, and J. Cea-Aravena, 'Nutrition in the treatment of attention-deficit hyperactivity disorder: a neglected but important aspect,' *Applied Psychophysiology and Biofeedback* 28 (2003): 63–75.
82. Feingold, 'Hyperkinesis,' 800.
83. Harley et al., 'Hyperkinesis and food additives,' 826.
84. Conners also recognized the hypocrisy of making conclusive statements based on one group and not another, stating that 'they [the authors] cannot have it both ways.' Conners, *Food Allergies,* 39.
85. Williams and Cram, 'Diet in the management of hyperkinesis,' 245–6; Thorley, 'Piolot study,' 56.
86. The most recent study to focus on pre-school children is that of Bateman and Warner's research group whose results, generated from a sample group of 277 children, were in favour of the link between nutrition and behaviour. Bateman et al., 'The effects of a double blind,' 506–11.
87. Mattes, 'The Feingold diet,' 319.
88. Jane Hersey, *Why My Child Can't Behave* (Williamsburg, VA: Pear Tree Press, 2006), 30–40.
89. C. M. Carter et al., 'Effects of a few food diet in attention deficit disorder,' *Archives of Disease in Childhood* 69 (1993): 564.
90. Gross et al., 'The effects of diets,' 54.
91. Williams et al., 'Relative effects of drugs and diet,' 816.
92. Email interview with Jane Hersey, 1 July, 2006.

93. Hersey, *Why My Child Can't Behave,* 68, 94, 102.
94. Spring and Sandoval contended, using dissonance theory, that this 'extra effort might be expected to result in mothers adopting an even more positive attitudes towards Feingold's hypothesis than they might have had with less effortful compliance.' Spring and Sandoval, 'Food additives,' 564. Although this might have been the case for a small number of mothers, it seems much more likely that the difficulties in maintaining the regimen would instead lead mothers to quit the diet and look for easier solutions.
95. Harley, Matthews, and Eichman, 'Synthetic food colors,' 982.
96. David, 'Reactions to dietary tartrazine,' 122.
97. Jackson, *Allergy,* 145–6.
98. 'Public health advisory for Adderall and Adderall XR,' www.fda.gov/cder/drug/advisory/adderall.htm (9 February 2005).
99. 'What is junk food?' www.feedmebetter.com/why/junkfood.html (2005).
100. 'Bill C-220: An act to amend the Foods and Drugs Act (*trans* fatty acids),' www.parl.gc.ca/38/1/parlbus/chambus/house/bills/private/C-220/C-220_1/C-220_cover-E.html (18 October 2004).

Contributors

John Burnham is Research Professor of History at Ohio State University and Scholar in Residence at the Medical Heritage Center there. His most recent book is *What Is Medical History?* (Polity, 2005). He is currently finishing a history of the idea of accident proneness.

Michael J. Clark is an Honorary Research Associate of the Wellcome Trust Centre for the History of Medicine at University College London, where he works on medico-legal practice in nineteenth-century Ireland and archival medical films as source materials for the history of medicine. He was formerly Head of the Wellcome Library's medical film and audio collections and has also published several articles on aspects of the history of psychiatry.

Jo Gill is Lecturer in twentieth-century literature at the University of Exeter. She is the author of *Anne Sexton's Confessional Poetics* (University Press of Florida, 2007), and the editor of *Modern Confessional Writing: New Critical Essays* (Routledge, 2006) and *The Cambridge Companion to Sylvia Plath* (Cambridge University Press, 2006).

Ali Haggett gained her BA and MA degrees at the University of Exeter. Funded by a Wellcome Trust studentship, she is completing her doctorate dissertation on neurosis in post-war housewives. Exploiting oral history as well as a range of documentary sources, her primary research interests are in the links between gender and medical history, and in representations of gender in medical and popular print sources.

Sarah Hayes is currently completing her doctoral thesis in the Centre for Medical History at the University of Exeter. This research is funded by the Wellcome Trust and explores the conceptualisation and application of the term 'maladjusted' as a medical label applied to certain children in the twentieth century.

Rhodri Hayward is Lecturer in the History of Medicine in the Department of History, Queen Mary, University of London. He is the author of *Resisting History: Religious Transcendence and the Invention of the Unconscious*

(Manchester, 2007), and has published on the history of emotions, neuropsychiatry, prophecy, dreams, demonology, electrophysiology, and cybernetics. He is now working on a new book project, provisionally entitled 'Self Cures: Psychology and Medicine in Modern Britain.'

Mark Jackson is Professor of the History of Medicine and Director of the Centre for Medical History at the University of Exeter. He is the author of *New-Born Child Murder* (Manchester, 1996), *The Borderland of Imbecility* (Manchester, 2000), and *Allergy: The History of a Modern Malady* (London, 2006). He is currently writing a book on the history of asthma and developing research on the history of stress.

Catherine Mills completed her PhD at the University of Exeter. Her doctoral studies focused upon nineteenth and early twentieth-century occupational health reform of the British mining industries. In 2006, she was awarded a three-year Wellcome Trust Research Fellowship to examine the relationship between respiratory diseases and the regulatory politics of clean air in post-war Britain.

Gregg Mitman is William Coleman Professor of History of Science and Professor of Medical History and Science and Technology Studies at the University of Wisconsin–Madison. His most recent book is *Breathing Space: How Allergies Shape Our Lives and Landscapes* (Yale University Press, 2007).

Stephen Mosley is Senior Lecturer in History at the School of Cultural Studies, Leeds Metropolitan University. He is the author of *The Chimney of the World: A History of Smoke Pollution in Victorian and Edwardian Manchester* (Cambridge: White Horse Press, 2001). His research interests are in urban culture and environmental history.

Matthew Smith is a PhD Student within the Centre for Medical History at the University of Exeter. His doctoral research explores the history of the Feingold diet and his studies are being funded by the Wellcome Trust and the Social Sciences and Humanities Research Council of Canada.

John Stewart is Professor of Health History at Glasgow Caledonian University. He is the author of several books, including *'The Battle for Health': A Political History of the Socialist Medical Association, 1930–1951* (Ashgate, 1999), and *Taking Stock: Scottish Social Welfare after Devolution* (The Policy Press, 2004). His current research interests include the history of child guidance in twentieth-century Britain, the Scottish Poor Law, and welfare states in post-war Europe.

Nancy Tomes is Professor of History at Stony Brook University. Her most recent monograph is *The Gospel of Germs: Men, Women and the Microbe* *in American Life* (1998). At present she is completing a book titled *A Patient Paradox: The Making of the Modern Health Consumer, 1930–1980.*

John Welshman is a historian based in the Institute for Health Research, Lancaster University, UK. His many publications include *Underclass: A History of the Excluded, 1880–2000* (London, 2006) and *From Transmitted Deprivation to Social Exclusion: Policy, Poverty, and Parenting* (Bristol, 2007).

Index

R